# PUBLIC HEALTH COMMUNICATION

## SCIENCE AND PRACTICE

ANTHONY J. ROBERTO

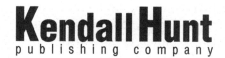

**Kendall Hunt** publishing company

Cover image © Shutterstock.com

# Kendall Hunt
publishing company

www.kendallhunt.com
*Send all inquiries to:*
4050 Westmark Drive
Dubuque, IA  52004-1840

Published in the United States of America

In loving memory of my grandparents,
Joseph Leonard Roberto and Rocca Lucia Grieco Roberto.

And for my wife, Karin Valentine.

# CONTENTS

# ACKNOWLEDMENTS

To begin, I gratefully acknowledge the many professors, professionals, graduate students, and undergraduate students that provided valuable feedback on this book. I am especially indebted to Judy Berkowitz (IQVIA) and Laura Martinez (Hugh Downs School of Human Communication, Arizona State University), who reviewed and provided feedback on most or all of the 13 chapters in this book. I am also grateful to the following individuals and students for reviewing and providing feedback on various chapters:

- Bradley Adame (Hugh Downs School of Human Communication, Arizona State University) and the graduate students in his Fall 2018 Applied Experimental Design class

- Kory Floyd (Department of Communication, University of Arizona) and the graduate students in his Fall 2018 Health Communication Theory seminar

- Alexis Koskan (College of Health Solutions, Arizona State University)

- Yanqin Liu (Banner MD Anderson Cancer Center)

- Paul Mongeau (Hugh Downs School of Human Communication, Arizona State University) and the graduate students in his Spring 2020 Persuasion and Social Influence seminar

- Summer Preston (University of Denver)

- YoungJu Shin (Hugh Downs School of Human Communication, Arizona State University) and the graduate students in her Fall 2018 Culture, Communication, and Health in Applied Contexts seminar

- Teresa Thompson (Department of Communication, University of Dayton; Editor-in-Chief, *Health Communication*)

- Sarah Tracy (Hugh Downs School of Human Communication, Arizona State University)

▶ The graduate students in my Spring 2019 Health Communication Campaigns seminar

▶ The undergraduate students in my Fall 2019 Health Communication and Social Marketing class

I also gratefully knowledge the following groups and individuals that directly or indirectly influenced this book in less obvious ways.

First, all the faculty, graduate students, and staff in the Department of Communication at Michigan State University during the time I received my PhD and beyond. A special thank you to Frank Boster, Jim Dearing, William Donohue, Sandi Smith, Steven Wilson (currently at the University of South Florida), Kim Witte, and the late Charles Atkin. I would be remiss if I did not also mention my friend and former office mate Gary Meyer (currently at Marquette University).

Second, the faculty, graduate students, and staff in the Hugh Downs School of Human Communication at Arizona State University. Everyone here has inspired me, but none more so than Jess Alberts, Benjamin Broome, Linda Lederman, Sarah Tracy, and the late Daniel Brouwer (one of the best teachers and kindest people I have ever met).

Third, this book was inspired by another book that I co-authored, *Health Communication in Everyday Life* (Lederman, Kreps, & Roberto, 2017). I am grateful for Linda Lederman (Hugh Downs School of Human Communication, Arizona State University) and Gary Kreps (Department of Communication, George Mason University) for encouraging me to expand my work on that project by writing this book.

Fourth, everyone at Kendall Hunt for supporting and giving me the time necessary to complete this book. Special thanks to Angela Willenbring and Paul Carty, my primary contacts throughout this project.

And, last but not least, thanks to my wife, grandparents, mom, sister, and the entire Miller family for your unconditional love and support.

# ABOUT THE AUTHOR

Anthony (Tony) Roberto received his MA in Advertising and his PhD in Communication from Michigan State University. He has held several academic and non-academic positions since completing his PhD in 1995 and is currently a professor in the Hugh Downs School of Human Communication at Arizona State University. Dr. Roberto's areas of interest and expertise include health communication, persuasion and social influence, and quantitative research methods. He has published extensively and received numerous awards for his research, teaching, and service in these and related areas. Tony lives in Arizona with his wife Karin, a miniature poodle named Brigitte, and a quarter horse named Peaches.

# SECTION 1

# Introduction to Public Health Communication Interventions

## CHAPTER 1

# Public Health, Health Communication, and Interventions

## CHAPTER OUTLINE

## INTRODUCTION

What if you held the key to a longer, healthier, and happier life? What would you *do* with it? Would you use it to open the door to health and wellness (or not)? I ask because one key to living a longer, healthier, and happier life is behavior; and healthy behavior can be difficult to sustain (Bouton, 2014). For example, behaviors such as physical inactivity, poor diet, excessive alcohol consumption, and tobacco use are the leading risk factors for premature death in the US (Centers for Disease Control and Prevention, 2018a). Thus, some keys to increasing your quality and quantity of life are to be physically active, eat well, not drink too much alcohol, and not smoke (see Table 1.1). Nevertheless, only 23% of American

| TABLE 1.1 | Guidelines for Four Leading Modifiable Health Behavior Risk Factors |
|---|---|
| Physical Activity | Adults should engage in at least 150 minutes (2 hours and 30 minutes) a week of moderate-intensity aerobic physical activity,[1] or at least 75 minutes (1 hour and 15 minutes) a week of vigorous-intensity aerobic physical activity,[2] or an equivalent combination of moderate- and vigorous-intensity aerobic activity (U.S. Department of Health and Human Services, 2008). |
| Dietary | A healthy eating pattern includes (1) a variety of vegetables from all of the subgroups—dark green, red, and orange, legumes (beans and peas), starchy, and other; (2) fruits, especially whole fruits; (3) grains, at least half of which are whole grains; (4) fat-free or low-fat dairy, including milk, yogurt, cheese, and/or fortified soy beverages; (5) a variety of protein foods, including seafood, lean meats and poultry, eggs, legumes (beans and peas), and nuts, seeds, and soy products; and (6) oils. A healthy eating pattern limits saturated fats and trans fats, added sugars, and sodium (U.S. Department of Health and Human Services and U.S. Department of Agriculture, 2015). |
| Alcohol Consumption | Excessive drinking includes binge drinking (four or more drinks on an occasion for women, five or more drinks on an occasion for men); consuming eight or more drinks a week for women or 15 or more drinks a week for men; or any alcohol use by pregnant women or those under the minimum legal drinking age of 21 (Centers for Disease Control and Prevention, 2014b). |
| Tobacco-Free Living | Tobacco-free living means avoiding use of all types of tobacco products—such as cigarettes, cigars, smokeless tobacco, pipes, etc.—and living free from secondhand smoke exposure (Surgeon General, 2014). |

[1] Examples of moderate intensity activity include walking briskly (at least 3 miles per hour), bicycling (less than 10 miles per hour), tennis (doubles), golfing (carrying clubs), weight training, general gardening, ballroom dancing, heavy cleaning, mowing the lawn, and so forth.

[2] Examples of vigorous-intensity activities include jogging, bicycling (over 10 miles per hour), tennis (singles), heavy gardening, aerobics classes, swimming laps, hiking uphill, many competitive sports (basketball, soccer, football, rugby, hockey, lacrosse), and so forth.

adults get the recommended amount of physical activity (Blackwell & Clarke, 2018), only 10% eat enough fruits and vegetables (Lee-Kwan et al., 2017), 30% drink excessively (Esser et al., 2014), and 16% smoke (Jamal et al., 2018).

Thus, nearly one million Americans die prematurely every year; and up to 40% of these deaths could have been prevented by making changes to behaviors that impact health (Centers for Disease Control and Prevention, 2014c; Yoon et al., 2014). Of course, physical activity, nutrition, and alcohol and tobacco use are just the four leading modifiable risk factors that impact to illnesses and death. Other modifiable risk factors include drug use, sun exposure, inadequate sleep, unsafe sexual practices, unsafe driving practices, and immunization and disease screening practices (Centers for Disease Control and Prevention, 2018a). And, as will be discussed in more detail later in this chapter, these modifiable health risk behaviors also impact our physical, mental, and social health and well-being (Dash et al., 2015; Knapen et al., 2015; Tayebisani et al., 2014).

That is where public health communication interventions come in. Public health communication interventions use messages to encourage healthy lifestyles that promote and protect the health of people and communities. But effective public health communication interventions do not happen by chance; they require careful planning and evaluation. The purpose of this book is to provide a systematic procedure to guide you through the process, a process that starts in this chapter where I will define (1) health and public health, (2) communication and health communication, and (3) interventions, strategies, campaigns, and programs. Before I do, however, I will provide some background information about the human papillomavirus (HPV) and the HPV vaccine, which will serve as the running example for this chapter.

HPV is the most common sexually transmitted infection (STI) in the US (Centers for Disease Control and Prevention, 2017b), and it is also the most common STI on college campuses (College Times, 2011). Most sexually active people will get HPV at some point in their lives. One key reason for this is that most cases of HPV do not have any symptoms, which increases the likelihood that an infected person will unknowingly transmit the virus to others. One of the most common manifestations of HPV infection in both men and women is genital warts. Persistent infection with certain strains of HPV is also a leading cause of several types of cancer, including cancer of the cervix, vagina, penis, anus, and throat (National Cancer Institute, 2015).

In 2006 the U.S. Food and Drug Administration approved an HPV vaccine recommended for females between the ages of 9 and 26, and in 2009 it approved an HPV vaccine recommended for males between the ages of 11 and 21 (Bixler, 2011). The HPV vaccine has been shown to be highly effective at preventing new infections of HPV in both females and males (National Cancer Institute, 2015). The best time to get the vaccine is before you are sexually active or before you are infected with HPV. Thus, the HPV vaccine is licensed for use in females and males aged 9 through 26 years, and the Advisory Committee on Immunization Practices recommends the multi-dose vaccine be administered to both girls and boys when they are 11 or 12 years old (Meites et al., 2016). To get the full benefits of the vaccine the recipient should get two (if ages 9 to 14) or three (if ages 15 to 26) doses over a 6- to 12-month period (Meites et al., 2016).

## HEALTH AND PUBLIC HEALTH

### HEALTH

The World Health Organization (1946; 2014) defines *health* as "a state of complete physical, mental, and social well-being" (p. 1). This definition highlights three important dimensions of health, which, in tandem, are often referred to as the "health triangle" (see Figure 1.1). That is, physical, mental, and social well-being are three essential factors that affect our ability to maintain a healthy quality of life and enjoy good health. Health is recognized as a fundamental right of every person as it enables individuals to realize aspirations, satisfy needs, and change or cope with the environment (World Health Organization, 1986).

*Physical well-being* refers to your body's ability to function properly. At its most basic level, this means that all your biological systems (e.g., circulatory, digestive, immune, nervous, reproductive, respiratory, etc.) are working well. Practically, this means you are

**FIGURE 1.1    Dimensions of Health (a.k.a., the Health Triangle)**

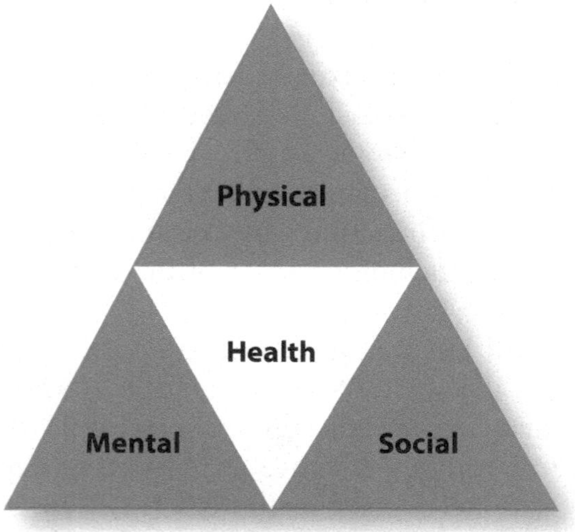

Adapted from The World Health Organization (1946; 2014).

physically fit enough to perform your daily activities without major restrictions (Rakhimov, 2018). *Mental well-being* refers to your cognitive and emotional state. Or, how well you feel about and deal with everyday life. For example, are you happy, how well do you cope with stress, are you able to adapt to different social situations, do you express your feelings in an appropriate manner, do you learn from and accept responsibility for your mistakes, and so forth (Kent, 2019)? *Social well-being* refers to your ability to establish and maintain satisfying interpersonal relationships. In other words, how do you relate to or connect with other people, such as friends, family, coworkers, and so forth? Communication is a key part of social health, as it affects how you interact or react to others (and how they interact or react to you).

Physical, mental, and social health and well-being are interrelated in a number of important ways. Not only do they mutually influence each other, but they are also influenced by a number of common behaviors. For example, numerous studies have found both exercise (Knapen et al., 2015; Tayebisani et al., 2014) and diet (Dash et al., 2015; Liu & Raine, 2017) to be positively related to physical, mental, and social health for a wide variety of individuals and contexts.

While the World Health Organization's definition of health has largely stood the test of time, a few concerns have been raised. For example, some have taken exception with the inclusion of the word "complete," noting that this "would leave most of us unhealthy most of the time" (Smith, 2008). This is especially relevant given that the number of people living with chronic diseases is increasing worldwide (Huber et al., 2011). Others argue that "health" and "well-being" are different concepts. Some common distinctions between the two include: (1) "health is physical, well-being is mental, emotional, spiritual," (2) "health is part of well-being," and (3) "one can be great, the other not" (Look, 2016). However, the notion that health has several interrelated dimensions, and the idea that physical, mental, and social well-being are all important components of health, remain important to this day.

### *Leading Causes of Death*

Table 1.2 lists the 10 leading causes of death in the US in 1900 and in 2016 (Centers for Disease Control and Prevention, 2018a; Jones et al., 2012). The three leading causes of death in the US in the early 1900s were influenza/pneumonia, tuberculosis, and gastrointestinal infections. All three of these are or result from *infectious diseases,* which are caused by organisms such as bacteria, viruses, or parasites. Infectious diseases can be spread from person to person (i.e., HPV and other STIs), through insect or animal bites (i.e., malaria or rabies), or by ingesting contaminated food or water (i.e., norovirus and salmonella).

| TABLE 1.2 Top 10 Leading Causes of Death and Percentage of All Deaths in the United States (1900 vs. 2017) | | | |
|---|---|---|---|
| **Leading Causes of Death in 1900** | **%** | **Leading Causes of Death in 2017** | **%** |
| 1. Pneumonia or Influenza * | 11.8 | 1. Diseases of Heart ** | 23.0 |
| 2. Tuberculosis * | 11.3 | 2. Cancer ** | 21.2 |
| 3. Diarrhea and Enteritis * | 8.3 | 3. Accidents | 6.0 |
| 4. Diseases of Heart ** | 8.0 | 4. Lung Disease ** | 5.7 |
| 5. Stroke ** | 6.2 | 5. Stroke ** | 5.2 |
| 6. Kidney Disease ** | 5.2 | 6. Alzheimer's Disease ** | 4.3 |
| 7. Accidents | 4.2 | 7. Diabetes Mellitus ** | 3.0 |
| 8. Cancer ** | 3.7 | 8. Influenza and Pneumonia * | 2.0 |
| 9. Senility ** | 2.9 | 9. Kidney Disease ** | 1.8 |
| 10. Diphtheria * | 2.3 | 10. Suicide | 1.7 |

Adapted from Jones et al. (2012) and Centers for Disease Control and Prevention (2017a).

* Infectious diseases are marked with an asterisk.

** Chronic diseases are marked with a double asterisk.

An *epidemiological transition,* or changes in disease patterns and causes of death, began around the mid-1900s. Today, people are more likely to die of *chronic diseases*, which develop and slowly worsen over time. Today, 7 of the top 10 leading causes of death in the U.S. are chronic diseases—heart disease, cancer, lung disease, stroke, Alzheimer's disease, diabetes, and kidney disease. In tandem, two thirds of all deaths in the US are attributed to these seven causes, with the top two accounting for 45% of all deaths (Centers for Disease Control and Prevention, 2018a). In addition, these and other chronic diseases also lower the quality of life for millions of individuals and cost hundreds of billions of dollars to treat each year.

### Non-Modifiable and Modifiable Health Risk Factors

A *risk factor* is anything that increases a person's chances of experiencing a disease or injury. Risk factors can be non-modifiable or modifiable. *Non-modifiable risk factors* are those that cannot be changed. Biological sex, age, race, ethnicity, and family history are all examples of non-modifiable risk factors. *Modifiable risk factors* are those that can be changed or treated. Many modifiable risk factors result from lifestyle or behavior choices that people make and are therefore subject to change. Examples of modifiable risk factors that can be changed include lack of physical activity, poor nutrition, excessive alcohol consumption, and tobacco use. Examples of modifiable risk factors that can be treated include hypertension or high blood pressure, abnormal glucose levels, and cholesterol profile.

There is overwhelming evidence that lifestyle and behavioral choices affect life expectancy, health, and well-being of people in the US and around the world (World Health Organization, 2002, 2009). For example, and as noted at the outset of this chapter, physical inactivity, poor nutrition, excessive alcohol consumption, and tobacco use are major causes of chronic disease worldwide. And, these unhealthy behaviors are associated with higher risks of heart disease, cancer, lung disease, stroke, Alzheimer's disease, diabetes, and kidney disease (Centers for Disease Control and Prevention, 2014a). Further, alcohol use is also a risk factor for unintentional injuries and suicide (Centers for Disease Control and Prevention, 2018b). Fortunately, evidence also indicates that the same behavioral risk factors that cause chronic disease can be modified, thereby positively influencing both quality and quantity of life. This is where public health, health communication, and interventions are important.

## PUBLIC HEALTH

*Public health* is the science and art of promoting and protecting the health of people and the communities where they live, learn, work, and play (American Public Health Association, 2018; Winslow, 1920). Public health includes anything that "we, as a society, do collectively to assure the conditions for people to be healthy" (Institute of Medicine, 1988, p. 1). Public health involves any activities designed to create healthy communities, to encourage healthy lifestyles, or to preserve or improve the well-being of a population via the prevention and control of diseases and injuries. Public health is a collaborative effort between global, national, state, and local governments, public and private organizations, communities, families, and individuals.

The public health and medical approaches represent distinct, yet complementary perspectives on health and health care (Fineberg, 2011). To illustrate, public health emphasizes disease and injury prevention for whole communities. Further, public health employs a wide variety of interventions (i.e., education, policy, screening, vaccination, built environments that support health, etc.) in a wide variety of settings (i.e., communities, schools, worksites, etc.) to improve health and reduce the risks of populations. Medicine, on the other hand, emphasizes diagnosing and treating illnesses and conditions after they occur, for one patient at a time, and typically in a clinical or health care setting. In short, the public health approach focuses primarily on preventing populations from getting sick or injured in the first place, while the medical approach focuses primarily on diagnosing, treating, and caring for individuals who are already sick or injured.

### Public Health in America

The Public Health Functions Project (1997) provides a vision and mission statement for public health in America (see Table 1.3). A *vision statement* looks forward and describes what a field hopes to achieve in the future. A *mission statement*, on the other hand, focuses on the present and describes what a field does and how it does it. In short, a vision focuses on what the future will look like if the field accomplishes its mission. The vision for public health in America is "healthy people in healthy communities," and its mission is to "promote physical and mental health and prevent disease, injury, and disability" (Public Health Functions Project, 1997, p. 21). Together, these vision and mission statements identify the guiding framework and describe the fundamental purpose of public health.

Table 1.3 also identifies the three core functions of public health and lists the 10 essential public health services (Institute of Medicine, 1988; Public Health Functions Project,

### TABLE 1.3    Public Health in America

**Vision**
- ► Healthy people in healthy communities

**Mission**
- ► Promote physical and mental health and prevent disease, injury, and disability

**Public Health**
- ► Prevents epidemics and the spread of disease
- ► Protects against environmental hazards
- ► Prevents injuries
- ► Promotes and encourages healthy behaviors
- ► Responds to disasters and assists communities in recovery
- ► Ensures the quality and accessibility of health services

**CORE FUNCTIONS OF PUBLIC HEALTH AND 10 ESSENTIAL PUBLIC HEALTH SERVICES**

**Assessment**
- ► Monitor health status to identify and solve community health problems
- ► Diagnose and investigate health problems and health hazards in the community

**Policy Development**
- ► Inform, educate, and empower people about health issues
- ► Mobilize community partnerships and action to identify and solve health problems
- ► Develop policies and plans that support individual and community health efforts

**Assurance**
- ► Enforce laws and regulations that protect health and ensure safety
- ► Link people to needed personal health services and assure the provision of health care when otherwise unavailable
- ► Assure competent public and personal health care workforce
- ► Evaluate effectiveness, accessibility, and quality of personal and population-based health services

**Serving All Functions**
- ► Research for new insights and innovative solutions to health problems

Sources: Institute of Medicine (1988); Public Health Functions Project (1997).

1997). I will not repeat the 10 essential public health services here, but I will define and provide some additional examples of the three core functions of public health as they serve as the foundation for the essential health services and are used to assess public health's progress toward its mission and vision. The three core functions of public health are assessment, policy development, and assurance.

The first core function of public health is assessment. *Assessment* involves collecting, analyzing, interpreting, and sharing information about a community's health needs and the resources available to meet those needs. For example, what are the health problems, how many people do they affect, who is at risk, what resources exist to address them, what other assets are needed to deal with the health threats, and so forth. The second core function of public health is policy development. *Policy development* entails consulting with stakeholders to develop plans to prioritize and support the health of the community. For example, based on the information obtained through assessment activities, you might work with a community to determine the best ways to inform, educate, and empower people regarding a health issue. This could include anything ranging from collaborating with schools, churches, or work sites to provide accessible health information, to creating or changing local, state, or federal plans or policies to address priority health needs. The third core function of public health is assurance. It makes little sense to help a community assess its health problems or develop policies and plans to address them if the community does not have the means or resources to do so. *Assurance* involves making sure a community's health needs are safely and effectively met by encouraging, requiring, or providing the services and resources necessary to address its priority health needs. This includes working with communities to make sure laws get enforced, that needed health services are made available, that interventions are implemented as intended, and that interventions effectively and efficiently inform and educate the intended audience.

### The Public Health Approach

The *public health approach* is a systematic process for solving public health problems. It is guided by the three core functions of public health reviewed in the previous section (assessment, policy development, and assurance). The public health approach provides a framework for defining and identifying a health problem, and for developing and implementing effective health promotion and disease prevention strategies to address the problem. It provides a comprehensive way to address a health problem by focusing on both individual and environmental factors when developing interventions. This four-step approach is rooted in the scientific method, with each step informing the next (Centers for Disease Control and Prevention, 2018d). The four steps are (1) defining the problem, (2) identifying risk and protective factors, (3) developing and testing prevention strategies, and (4) assuring widespread adoption. A visual representation of the public health approach is provided in Figure 1.2, and a brief discussion of each of these four steps is provided on the following page.

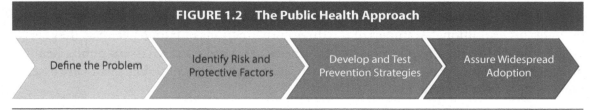

**FIGURE 1.2    The Public Health Approach**

Define the Problem  |  Identify Risk and Protective Factors  |  Develop and Test Prevention Strategies  |  Assure Widespread Adoption

Adapted from Centers for Disease Control and Prevention (2018d).

- ▸ **Step 1** involves identifying and defining the problem through systematic data collection. The goal here is to figure out what the health problem is, how big it is, who it affects, and so forth.

- ▸ **Step 2** consists of identifying risk and protective factors for the health problem. In other words, what causes the problem? What risk factors increase the likelihood that a person will experience the health problem? What protective factors decrease the likelihood that a person will experience the health problem?

- ▸ **Step 3** focuses on developing and testing prevention strategies to reduce risk factors or increase protective factors. For example, you might identify or adapt an existing intervention, or develop a new one. The goal here is to determine what works to prevent the health problem for a specific health threat or intended audience.

- ▸ **Step 4** entails assuring widespread adoption of effective and promising interventions. Here, the aims are to replicate successful interventions across a wider range of settings or populations, and to evaluate them in these new contexts.

I will review two different applications of the public health approach in Section 2 of this book, which focuses on intervention planning. For example, in Chapter 3 I will review social marketing and the Health Communication Program Cycle (National Cancer Institute, 2001), which adopt a consumer-based perspective to the public health approach. Also, for example, in Chapter 4 I will discuss the PRECEDE-PROCEED Model (Green & Kreuter, 2005), which embraces an ecological perspective to the public health approach.

### Three Levels of Prevention

Public health communication interventions include actions taken to avert a health problem altogether or to control the course of a health problem before it gets worse. Prevention can occur before (primary prevention), during (secondary prevention), and after (tertiary prevention) the onset of a health problem (Roberto, 2014). As "The Prevention Pyramid" presented in Figure 1.3 was designed to illustrate, the number of individuals impacted by

## FIGURE 1.3    The Prevention Pyramid

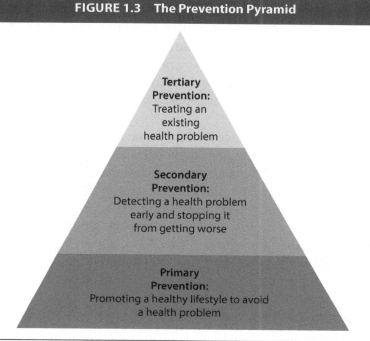

Adapted from Bromfield & Holzer (2008).

the prevention effort decreases as you move from primary prevention to tertiary prevention (Bromfield & Holzer, 2008). In other words, primary prevention has the potential to impact the largest number of individuals in the general population before they experience a health problem. This is followed by secondary prevention which impacts a smaller number of people who are most at risk or show early signs of the health problem. And finally, tertiary prevention, which focuses on individualized plans to treat people with the health problem. Below is a brief discussion of the three levels of prevention.

**Primary Prevention.** *Primary prevention* is designed to get people to take steps to avoid the health problem before it occurs. Examples include legislation (e.g., mandatory vaccinations for vaccine preventable diseases) and education (e.g., steps you might take to reduce your risk). To illustrate, here are just a few of the steps you might take to reduce your risk of contracting an STI: abstain from vaginal, oral, or anal sex; have fewer partners; use condoms correctly every time you have sex; and get the HPV and hepatitis B vaccines.

**Secondary Prevention.** *Secondary prevention* focuses on reducing the impact of a health problem that has already occurred through early detection and timely treatment. Screening tests are a good example of secondary prevention, especially since many STIs often have no or mild symptoms until their later stages. The goal here is to identify the disease in its early stages (usually before any symptoms occur) so it can be more easily treated or managed, and its most severe consequences avoided. For example, screening tests exist for many common STIs, including chlamydia, gonorrhea, HIV, genital herpes, and syphilis. Similarly, there are screening tests for numerous types of cancer, including the Papanicolaou (Pap) test used to screen for cervical cancer, one outcome caused by persistent infection with HPV.

**Tertiary Prevention.** Finally, the goal of *tertiary prevention* is to slow or stop the progression of the health problem after a person demonstrates symptoms. Ideally, the goal is to make the person healthy again. Alternatively, and at a minimum, the goal is to manage the health problem to prevent further deterioration or complications. For example, according to the Centers for Disease Control and Prevention (2017c), many STIs are curable and all are treatable. STIs caused by bacteria, such as chlamydia, gonorrhea, and syphilis, can be cured using penicillin or other antibiotics. Other STIs, like HIV, herpes, and some strains of HPV, cannot be cured, but they can be treated to minimize the impact of ongoing illness. For HPV, this might involve excision of cancerous lesions or other treatments to prevent further spread of the cancer.

In sum, the importance of public health should not be underestimated. As the Institute of Medicine (1988) notes, "many of the major improvements in the health of the American people have been accomplished through public health measures" (p. 1). For example, life expectancy of Americans increased from 45 years in the early 1900s to 75 in the early 2000s. Research indicates that 25 of those 30 additional years of life can be attributed to improvements in public health, including the control of infectious diseases, cleaner food, water, and air, improved motor-vehicle and workplace safety, and increases in knowledge about healthy and unhealthy behaviors (Schneider, 2014; Turnock, 2009).

## COMMUNICATION AND HEALTH COMMUNICATION

*Communication* is a social process by which people create meaning through the exchange of messages (Alberts et al., 2016). Many communication classes and textbooks focus on a single communication context, such as interpersonal, small group, organizational, mass, intercultural, or computer mediated communication. I define *health communication* as messages intended to influence health-related decisions. As this definition implies, health communication is a broad topic that intersects with all communication contexts. To illustrate, Thompson (2006) identified emerging themes based on articles published in the first 75 issues of *Health Communication*, a leading journal in the field. The most common topics were extremely varied, and included patient-physician interaction, health campaigns, risk communication, aging, language, media issues, social support, inter- or multicultural concerns, technology, families, health information, end-of-life concerns, and pediatrics. Also consider this quote from the *Healthy People Initiative*:

> Health communication can contribute to all aspects of disease prevention and health promotion and is relevant in a number of contexts, including (1) health professional-patient relations, (2) individuals' exposure to, search for, and use of health information, (3) individuals' adherence to clinical recommendations and regimens, (4) the construction of public health messages and campaigns, (5) the dissemination of individual and population health risk information; that is, risk communication, (6) images of health in the mass media and the culture at large, (7) the education of consumers about how to gain access to the public health and health care systems, and (8) the development of telehealth applications.

> *(U.S. Department of Health and Human Services, 2000, p. 11–3)*

Table 1.4 lists a few sample applications of health communication topics in each of the traditional communication contexts. You probably noticed that this list is neither

| TABLE 1.4 Sample Health Communication Topics by Communication Context | |
| --- | --- |
| **Context** | **Sample Topics** |
| Interpersonal | Patient-provider communication<br>Advocate/family-provider communication<br>Social support |
| Small Group | Support groups<br>Health care teams<br>Health decision-making |
| Organizational | Employee wellness<br>Stress and burnout in organizations<br>Health care policy |
| Mass | Health campaigns<br>Entertainment education<br>Health media literacy |
| Intercultural | Intercultural communication competence in the health care context<br>Cultural conceptions of health and illness<br>Intervention cultural adaptation |
| Computer-Mediated | Digital health literacy / Online health information<br>Computer tailored messages<br>Telemedicine |

exhaustive nor mutually exclusive. It is not exhaustive because it is incomplete and represents only a partial list of all possible topics that fall under the broad umbrella of health communication. Other examples include patient satisfaction, end-of-life communication, stigma and stigma reduction, health information seeking, health literacy, and so forth. It is not mutually exclusive because many of these areas overlap. For example, computer mediated communication overlaps with (1) patient-provider communication via patient portals and telemedicine, (2) small group communication via online support groups, (3) mass media and health campaigns via computer tailored messages, and (4) intercultural communication via health information technology that provides individuals in under-served communities with increased access to expert and better health care without having to travel far. These are also just a few of the many possible ways these areas overlap with health communication and each other.

Even if you narrow the topic down to public health communication interventions, the focus of this book, considerable overlap remains. The goal of such interventions is to directly or indirectly influence health behaviors of an intended audience, and they do so by designing, implementing, and evaluating messages distributed via interpersonal or small group communication (e.g., in-person individual or group interventions), small media (e.g., posters, pamphlets, videos), mass media (e.g., television, radio, magazines, newspapers, billboards), or social media (e.g., blogs, wikis, Facebook, Instagram, Twitter, video sharing websites) (U.S. Department of Health and Human Services, 2018).

In sum, health communication is a broad topic that "encompasses the study and use of communication strategies to inform and influence individual and community decisions that enhance health" (U.S. Department of Health and Human Services, 2000, p. 11-3). For example, health communicators study or use messages to improve (i.e., influence) patient-provider communication, health decision-making, employee wellness, or in the case of this book, to more effectively influence individuals' health-related beliefs, attitudes, and behaviors. Earlier in this section I defined health communication as (1) messages (2) intended to (3) influence (4) health-related decisions. Each of these four key words in this definition of health communication was selected for specific reasons, which are discussed in more detail below in the context of public health communication interventions.

## MESSAGES

Public health communication interventions designed to change behavior are communicative acts (Rimal & Lapinski, 2009). That means they involve the exchange of messages. *Messages* are the content of the communication, or the information and ideas the source wants to communicate or deliver to the receiver. In the realm of public health communication interventions, messages are designed by the planner (the source) to promote healthy changes in individuals or communities (the receiver/s). As will be discussed in more detail below, though the words "intervention," "strategy," "campaign," and "program," have slightly different meanings, they all involve the creation and exchange of messages.

Health messages can be communicated using many different channels. *Communication channels* refer to the medium through which a message is transmitted from the source to the receiver. Communication channels can be divided into two main categories: interpersonal communication and mass communication. *Interpersonal communication* traditionally involves face-to-face communication that takes place without any mediating technology (such as communication between individuals, in small groups, in organizations, etc.). *Mass communication*, on the other hand, refers to channels used to transmit information to larger audiences where the source and receiver are separated in time or space. Mass communication can be further broken down into a variety of categories including print media (such as books, newspapers, and magazines), broadcast media (such as radio, television, and films), and digital media via the internet and mobile devices (such as email, websites, and social networking sites). As noted previously, technology has blurred many of the lines between these traditional distinctions. For example, face-to-face interactions can now take place using Skype, FaceTime, or Zoom, and you can read your favorite newspaper or watch your favorite television shows and movies online. Regardless of the channel selected, the U.S. Department of Health and Human Services (2000) outlines 11 principles for effective health communication message development (see Table 1.5 on the following page).

## INTENDED

*Intended* means the message has a predetermined purpose. Or, as Du Pré (2010) notes, "people are actively involved in health communication. They are not passive recipients of information" (p. 7). In other words, health communicators deliberately study or use messages to improve health or communication. For example, and as will be discussed in detail in Chapter 2, public health communication interventions are designed with explicit goals (i.e., the overall health improvement that the intervention was designed to achieve), objectives (i.e., the cognitive and behavioral changes that must take place to achieve your goal), and strategies (i.e., the communication activities undertaken to accomplish your objectives) in mind. Further, intervention designers purposefully incorporate formative evaluation to gain insight and input from the intended audience during intervention development, process evaluation to make sure the intervention is being delivered as planned, and outcome and impact evaluation to make sure the intervention had the desired effects. Further, all aspects of the planning process are intentionally guided by previous theory and research.

| TABLE 1.5 Attributes of Effective Health Communication | |
|---|---|
| Attribute | Definition |
| Accuracy | The content is valid and without errors of fact, interpretation, or judgment. |
| Availability | The content (whether targeted message or other information) is delivered or placed where the audience can access it. |
| Balance | Where appropriate, the content presents the benefits and risks of potential actions or recognizes different and valid perspectives on the issue. |
| Consistency | The content remains internally consistent over time and also is consistent with information from other sources. |
| Cultural Competence | The design, implementation, and evaluation process that accounts for special issues for select population groups and also educational levels and disability. |
| Evidence Base | Relevant scientific evidence that has undergone comprehensive review and rigorous analysis to formulate practice guidelines, performance measure, review criteria, and technology assessments. |
| Reach | The content gets to or is available to the largest possible number of people in the target population. |
| Reliability | The source of the content is credible, and the content itself is kept up to date. |
| Repetition | The delivery of/access to the content is continued or repeated over time, both to reinforce the impact with a given audience and to reach new generations. |
| Timeliness | The content is provided or available when the audience is most receptive to, or in need of, the specific information. |
| Understandability | The reading or language level and format (including multimedia) are appropriate for the specific audience. |

Source: U.S. Department of Health and Human Services (2000).

I should note that some people may disagree with the inclusion of the word "intended" in this definition. For example, people can say or do things that informally or incidentally influence others without necessarily meaning to do so (Cline, 2003). And, interventions can have unintended consequences such as creating confusion (instead of reducing it) or reducing the likelihood that the intended audience engages in the recommended behavior (instead of increasing it) (Cho & Salmon, 2007). Nonetheless, the inclusion of the word "intended" is consistent with other commonly cited definitions of health communication

(National Cancer Institute, 2001; U.S. Department of Health and Human Services, 2000, p. 11-3). This is most likely because even health communicators who study incidental messages or unintended consequences intentionally do so to gain a better understanding of and improve communication. Thus, at the very least, intention is an essential component in the context of this book on public health communication interventions.

## INFLUENCE

*Influence* means the aim of the message is to modify a person's or community's response in some way. Usually that means getting people to believe, feel, or behave differently. As such, public health communication interventions inform, persuade, or motivate by increasing knowledge and awareness or reducing confusion and misconceptions. Such modifications or transformations fall into three main categories: response shaping, response changing, or response reinforcing (Miller, 1980).

### Response Shaping

*Response shaping* involves introducing a person to a new behavior that did not exist or that they did not know about before. Notably, the term "new" is relative here. It could be *new* because it did not exist before, or it could be *new* to a person because they were not aware of or had not seen or experienced it before. To illustrate, when the HPV vaccine was approved in 2006, most people were not aware of its existence or that getting vaccinated against HPV was even an option. Thus, a primary task of health professionals and pharmaceutical companies at that time became one of shaping people's initial beliefs, attitudes, and behaviors regarding the vaccine.

Given how common and contagious HPV is, knowing that it causes such serious diseases, and the fact that the HPV vaccine has been shown to be highly effective at preventing the most common types of HPV in both males and females, you might think it would be easy to create positive initial impressions of the vaccine and achieve high vaccination rates. However, this was not the case for some social and religious conservatives. Given the recommended age at which the vaccine should be administered (i.e., 11 or 12 years old), some were concerned that getting the vaccine would lead children to have sex earlier, have more sex, or have sex with more people. However, numerous studies have found that none of these things have come to pass (CBS News, 2012; Mayhew et al., 2014). Despite this, only about 60% of girls and 40% of boys have been vaccinated against HPV. And, while the vaccination rates are increasing slightly each year, they remain well below those for other vaccine-preventable diseases (Reagan-Steiner et al., 2015).

To provide another related example, when pharmaceutical companies get approval for a new drug, they often go to great lengths to shape how both consumers and prescribers view it. This could be as simple as coming up with the right brand name for the drug. For example, when it came time to market its new HPV vaccine, Merck marketed it under its brand name "GARDASIL®" (which implies protection and is much easier to remember) rather than the vaccine's generic or official name, "Human Papillomavirus Quadrivalent (Types 6, 11, 16, and 18) Vaccine, Recombinant." Or, it could be as complex as a large multi media marketing campaign. For example, in 2012, pharmaceutical companies spent over $3 billion on direct-to-consumer advertising, and five times that (or $15 billion) in face-to-face marketing activities designed to persuade the prescribers (Pew, 2013). Much of this was spent to market new drugs, or drugs that were at least new to the intended audience.

Another great example of response shaping that you may have seen is The Meth Project's "Not Even Once" campaign (see Figure 1.4A). Given that meth is highly addictive and can quickly lead to all sorts of severe consequences, the campaign is trying to influence people's beliefs, attitudes, and behavior *before* they ever try this dangerous drug.

### Response Changing

The HPV vaccine has been approved for over 10 years now, and many parents and young adults are aware that the vaccine exists. People are generally aware that the vaccine is approved for females and males of certain ages, that it is recommended for boys and girls when they are 11 or 12 years old, and that it reduces the risk of genital warts and several

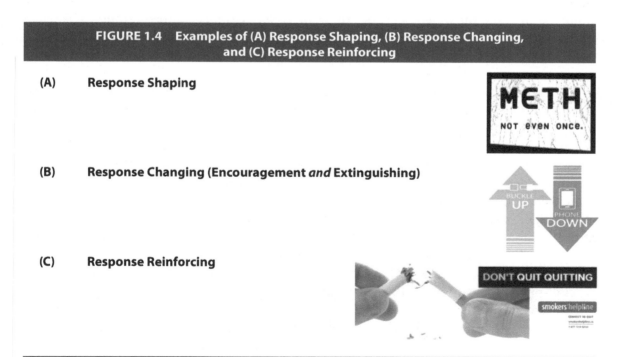

**FIGURE 1.4    Examples of (A) Response Shaping, (B) Response Changing, and (C) Response Reinforcing**

**(A)    Response Shaping**

**(B)    Response Changing (Encouragement *and* Extinguishing)**

**(C)    Response Reinforcing**

(A) © Partnership for Drug-Free Kids. *Reprinted by permission*; (B) © Ruwan Muhandirm/Shutterstock.com; (C) © StepanPopov/Shutterstock.com.

types of cancer. Based on this information, each person will decide whether to get their child (or themselves) vaccinated. For those who have decided to get the vaccine, response shaping efforts have done their job (though it may still be important to focus on response reinforcing, which is discussed below). For those who have decided *not* to get the vaccine, the issue now shifts from shaping their behavior to changing it. This brings us to the second way health communication messages may try to influence us.

*Response changing* occurs when you want a person to behave differently. In the context of public health communication interventions this typically means one of two things (Gass & Seiter, 2007). First, sometimes you want someone who is engaging in an unhealthy behavior to stop doing so; this is called *response extinguishing*. Examples include helping a family member who is smoking to quit, encouraging a classmate who is binge drinking to stop, or urging a friend who is engaging in risky sexual behaviors to refrain from doing so. Second, sometimes you want someone who is not engaging in a healthy behavior to start doing so; this is called *response encouragement*. For example, Merck's "Did You Know" campaign targeted parents who have not or might not vaccinate their children against HPV to encourage them to reconsider and do so.

Another great example of response changing is the Missouri Coalition for Roadway Safety's and the Missouri Department of Transportation's "Buckle Up, Phone Down" campaign (see Figure 1.4B). Notice how they are cleverly engaging in both response encouragement (i.e., "Buckle Up") and response extinguishing (i.e., "Phone Down") in this one simple message.

Finally, it is important to note that while response extinguishing and response encouragement are often discussed as two separate processes, they are often opposite sides of the same coin. For example, you may decide to urge a friend who is engaging in risky sexual behavior to stop doing so (extinguishing) by giving them condoms and telling them to start using them (encouragement). The important point to keep in mind is that public health communication interventions include both preventing unhealthy behaviors and promoting healthy ones.

### Response Reinforcing

Once a person decides to get the HPV vaccine, and even after they get the first dose of the vaccine, that is not the end of the matter. Like many other vaccines such as the Hepatitis B vaccine, the varicella (a.k.a., chickenpox) vaccine, and the measles, mumps, and rubella (MMR) vaccine, a person needs to get multiple doses of the HPV vaccine to be fully protected (Centers for Disease Control and Prevention, 2018c). As you might imagine, many things can happen between the first, second, and third doses. For example, a person might not like getting injections and simply decide not to get the second and third doses of the vaccine. Or, they may lose their insurance or otherwise not have enough money to pay for the additional doses. Or, a person might simply forget to return after 1 or 6 months to get the final two doses. Therefore, once a person decides to get the HPV vaccine, the task shifts to reinforcing the decision to make sure they follow through with the full schedule of doses.

*Response reinforcing* is designed to get a person to stay committed or become more committed to a choice they have already made. This is related to treatment compliance or adherence, which refers to how well or consistently a person follows advice from a medical or public health professional. Thus, response reinforcing includes any steps you can take to make sure a behavior stays changed (i.e., that it does not happen again in the case of response extinguishing, or that it continues in the case of response encouragement). In other words, once a person receives the first dose of the HPV vaccine, it is important to help that individual maintain or even strengthen their resolve to get the second or third doses. This might include something as simple as sending a reminder as the due date for a follow-up dose approaches, so the person does not forget about the commitment they have already made. Other ways to reinforce a behavior include offering genuine praise and support for the decision, reminding a person of the serious consequences of HPV, or making sure they have the time and money (or insurance) to get the additional doses as prescribed.

Another great example of response reinforcing is the Central East Tobacco Control Area Network's "don't quit quitting" smoking prevention program (see Figure 1.4C). This program is designed to help smokers who have decided to stop smoking remain consistent with this commitment. Similarly, while one key goal of Alcoholics Anonymous is to help alcoholics achieve sobriety (response changing), another important goal is to help those in recovery to stay sober (response reinforcing). Finally, while getting people to eat well and start exercising is important, it is equally important to reinforce the behavior, so it is maintained in the future.

In sum, influencing behavior "is seldom, if ever, a one-message proposition; instead, people are constantly in the process of being persuaded" (Miller, 1980, p. 19). And, while the focus has so far been on shaping, changing, and reinforcing behavior, it is important to keep in mind that this process is applicable to a variety of other important concepts as well. To illustrate (and as will be discussed in more detail in Chapters 6 through 10), behavior is often a product of many underlying factors including beliefs, norms, attitudes, and intentions. So, when you first teach a person about a new health issue, you introduce new facts and knowledge to shape their beliefs about the topic. Or, when a person incorrectly perceives a norm, it becomes important to change the perceived norm. And, if a person already feels positively toward a recommended behavior, it becomes important to reinforce this already existing positive attitude.

## HEALTH-RELATED DECISIONS

*Decision* refers to the act of choosing between two or more possibilities. This means that the recipient of the public health communication intervention has options available to them; they get to decide to behave in healthy or unhealthy ways. In other words, the objective of public health communication interventions is to influence personal health choices, or modifiable health risk factors. Even if part of the intervention involves a new policy or law (such as wearing a seatbelt or not texting and driving), everyone gets to decide whether to follow the law. Those who do not follow the law usually hope they do not get caught or are stuck having to pay a fine if they do.

Similarly, and as you will see when I introduce the behavioral ecological model in Chapter 4, many factors that influence behavior may be (or at least appear to be) outside a person's control. For example, smoking is addictive, or there may be few safe, convenient, or affordable places to exercise. However, even though adopting a healthy behavior may be difficult, a person usually still has options available to them, as does the intervention developer. For example, a person might choose to smoke a little less, or to exercise a little more. Or, an intervention developer might provide professional or financial assistance, attempt to alter the environment, or start by changing beliefs, attitudes, norms, and intentions—and eventually behavior.

## INTERVENTIONS, STRATEGIES, CAMPAIGNS, AND PROGRAMS

*Intervention* (n.d.) means "to come between" or to "interrupt." In other words, public health communication interventions are designed to come between or interrupt the link between unhealthy behaviors and health outcomes. For the purposes of this book, I define public health communication *interventions* as any activity or combination of activities designed to improve health by influencing behavior (or the precursors of behavior, such as beliefs, attitudes, and intention). For example, tobacco use, alcohol consumption, physical activity, diet, and sexual practices are all behaviors that exert a strong influence on health. Nonetheless, some people smoke cigarettes, drink too much alcohol, do not get enough exercise, eat poorly, or engage in risky sexual activity. Thus, public health communicators intervene by (1) preventing people from engaging in an unhealthy behavior in the first place—response shaping, (2) getting people who are engaging in an unhealthy behavior to start behaving in a healthier one—response changing, or (3) encouraging people who are engaging in a healthy behavior to continue doing so—response reinforcing. Intervention is a general term that may refer to a specific strategy, a large campaign, or a comprehensive program. And, while there is some overlap between these terms, there are also some differences, which I will review next.

A *strategy* is a specific communication activity or message designed to accomplish one or more objectives (i.e., the cognitive and behavioral changes you want to produce). Put somewhat differently, objectives focus on what you want to do, and strategies focus on how to do it. The term "strategy" is probably most closely related to what people typically mean when they use the words "message" or "intervention." Some common public health communication strategies were mentioned earlier, and include interpersonal or small group communication, small media, mass media, and social media.

Rogers and Storey (1987) define *campaigns* as follows: "(1) a campaign intends to generate specific outcomes or effects (2) in a relatively large number of individuals, (3) usually within a specified period of time and (4) through an organized set of communication activities" (p. 821). Businesses use campaigns to help sell their products and services, interest groups use campaigns to encourage or prevent changes in public policy, politicians use campaigns to help get themselves elected, and health communicators use campaigns to help people live longer and healthier lives. In short, campaigns are a specific type of strategy designed to reach many people over a short period of time and with a predetermined end date.

Green and Kreuter (2005) define a *program* as, "a set of planned and organized activities carried out over time to accomplish specific health-related goals" (p. 1). Programs generally include a coordinated set of strategies, interventions, and campaigns aimed at reaching an overarching goal (i.e., the overall health improvement the program wishes to achieve—such as improved quality and quantity of life). Programs are more comprehensive, focus on longer-term goals, and are less likely to have a specific end date. Ideally, a program will continue as long as it is making progress toward achieving its goal.

In sum, while there are some differences between the terms "intervention," "strategy," "campaign," and "program," there is also some overlap between these four terms. For example, intervention and strategy are often used synonymously, a campaign is a specific type of strategy, and a program is usually comprised of several interrelated strategies, interventions, and campaigns. Further, they all aim to interrupt the link between an unhealthy behavior and health outcomes, and to promote health and prevent disease by focusing on their underlying causes. In this book I use the word "intervention" broadly to mean any activity or combination of activities designed to improve health by influencing beliefs, attitude, and behavior.

## OVERVIEW AND SCOPE OF THIS BOOK

### OVERVIEW

The overarching goal of this book is to provide you with the tools needed to design and evaluate public health communication interventions. To help achieve this goal, this book includes four sections. Section One, which is made up of the introductory chapter you are reading now, introduces several overarching principles that serve as the foundation for the rest of the book: health and public health, communication and health communicating, and interventions, strategies, campaigns, and programs.

Section Two includes three chapters focusing on the intervention planning process. Chapter 2 provides an introduction and overview of the planning process by defining several recurring terms, such as various types of evaluation, as well as goals, objectives, and strategies. Chapters 3 and 4 introduce two different, but overlapping, approaches to intervention planning: social marketing and the Health Communication Program Cycle (National Cancer Institute, 2001) and the ecological approach and PRECEDE-PROCEED Model (Green & Kreuter, 2005).

Section Three focuses on theory. This section begins with a general overview of theory, meta-analyses, and conceptual and operational definitions. This is followed by five chapters on well-established theoretical perspectives that are commonly used to guide public health communication interventions (i.e., the health belief model, social cognitive theory, the extended parallel process model, the reasoned action approach, the transtheoretical model). In addition to describing each theory, I also provide conceptual and operational definitions for all key variables and summarize select meta-analysis results.

Section Four includes three chapters focusing on research methods that are commonly used to evaluate public health communication interventions: focus groups, survey research, and experimental design.

## SCOPE

It should also be noted that while this book includes a fair amount of information about public health and health communication in general, several important decisions had to be made to keep the presented material both focused and manageable. Here, I review three particularly important decisions that impact the scope of this book.

First, public health is a very broad subject that encompasses a wide variety of disciplines and topics (see Table 1.3). The same can be said for health communication (see Table 1.4). However, this book focuses on just one important aspect of these fields: the planning and evaluation of public health communication interventions designed to influence modifiable health risk behaviors. So, it is important to keep in mind what public health communication interventions can and cannot do (see National Cancer Institute, 2001). For example, public health communication interventions can influence knowledge, beliefs, attitudes, and intentions. They can also prompt action and lead to sustained behavior change when combined with other strategies. However, public health communication interventions alone cannot compensate for inadequate health care or access to health care services, produce sustained change in complex health behaviors without the support of a larger program, or be equally effective at addressing all topics and intended audiences.

Second, while public health communication practitioners have dozens of theories and models to choose from during the planning process, only a few have been used regularly and over a long period of time (Glanz et al., 2008, 2015). In this book I devote a full chapter to the four theories and models that are most commonly used to guide the planning and evaluation process—the health belief model, the theories of reasoned action and planned behavior, the transtheoretical model, and social cognitive theory. I also included a full chapter on the extended parallel process model as it shares many things in common with these other approaches, and makes some very specific recommendations about designing effective health risk messages. This is important given that the usefulness of fear appeals remain a disputed topic even after more than 60 years of research. However, I do address a few other common approaches as part of other chapters. For example, I discuss social marketing as part of Chapter 2 and the ecological model as part of Chapter 3.

Third, and as will be stressed in Chapter 4 which reviews the ecological approach to health promotion, a wide variety of individual, relationship, community, and societal factors influence behavior. While all four levels are important, this book focuses largely on influencing individual and relationship level variables such as beliefs, attitudes, norms, intentions, and behaviors. That said, both the Health Communication Program Cycle (Chapter 3) and especially the PRECEDE-PROCEED Model (Chapter 4) do address community and societal level influences during their respective planning and strategy development stages or phases. Further, all the theories included in this book do factor into community and societal influences via variables such as benefits and barriers or self-efficacy (see Chapters 6 through 10). In short, while this book emphasizes the individual and relationship levels, it acknowledges the importance of targeting multiple levels at various points in several different chapters.

## CONCLUSION

This introductory chapter provided an overview of public health communication interventions. It began by defining health and public health, highlighting three important dimensions of health—physical, mental, and social well-being, and identifying three types of prevention—primary, secondary, and tertiary. Next, it defined health communication as messages intended to influence health-related choices, described what was meant by each key word in this definition, and distinguished between three different types of influence—response shaping, response changing, and response reinforcing. Finally, it reviewed the scope and limitations of this book, so you will know exactly what it is and is not designed to do. As you read the rest of this book, you will learn more about these and other related topics which will put you well on your way to becoming an expert in designing and evaluating public health communication interventions.

# REFERENCES

Alberts, J. K., Nakayama, T. K., & Martin, J. N. (2016). *Human communication in society* (4th ed.). Prentice Hall.

American Public Health Association. (2018). *What is public health?* https://www.apha.org/what-is-public-health

Bixler, J. (2011, October 26). *CDC committee recommends boys receive HPV vaccine.* http://www.cnn.com/2011/10/25/health/hpv-vaccine/

Blackwell, D. L., & Clarke, T. C. (2018). State variation in meeting the 2008 federal guidelines for both aerobic and muscle-strengthening activities through leisure-time physical activity among adults aged 18–64: United States, 2010–2015. *National Health Statistics Report, 112,* 1–22. https://www.cdc.gov/nchs/data/nhsr/nhsr112.pdf

Bouton, M. E. (2014). Why behavior change is difficult to sustain. *Preventive Medicine, 68,* 29–36. http://dx.doi.org/10.1016/ j.ypmed.2014.06.010

Bromfield, L., & Holzer, P. (2008). *A national approach for child protection: Project report.* Australian Institute of Family Studies.

CBS News. (2012, October 15). *HPV vaccine won't make girls promiscuous, study finds.* http://www.cbsnews.com/news/hpv-vaccine-wont-make-girls-promiscuous-study-finds/

Centers for Disease Control and Prevention. (2014a). *CDC national health report highlights.* https://www.cdc.gov/healthreport/previous/2014/publications/Compendium.pdf

Centers for Disease Control and Prevention. (2014b). *Most people who drink excessively are not alcohol dependent.* https://www.cdc.gov/media/releases/2014/p1120-exessive-driniking.html

Centers for Disease Control and Prevention. (2014c). *Up to 40 percent of annual deaths from each of the five leading causes are preventable: Premature deaths from each cause due to modifiable risks.* https://www.cdc.gov/media/releases/2014/p0501-preventable-deaths.html

Centers for Disease Control and Prevention (2017a). Deaths and mortality. https://www.cdc.gov/nchs/fastats/deaths.htm

Centers for Disease Control and Prevention. (2017b). *Genital HPV infection—fact sheet.* https://www.cdc.gov/std/hpv/stdfact-hpv.htm

Centers for Disease Control and Prevention. (2017c). *Sexually transmitted diseases (STDs).* https://www.cdc.gov/std/general/default.htm

Centers for Disease Control and Prevention. (2018a). *2018 behavioral risk factor surveillance system (BRFSS) questionnaire.* https://www.cdc.gov/brfss/questionnaires/pdfques/2018_BRFSS_English_Questionnaire.pdf

Centers for Disease Control and Prevention. (2018b). *Fact sheet—alcohol use and your health.* https://www.cdc.gov/alcohol/fact-sheets/alcohol-use.htm

Centers for Disease Control and Prevention. (2018c). *Recommended immunization schedule for children and adolescents aged 18 years or younger.* https://www.cdc.gov/vaccines/schedules/downloads/child/0-18yrs-child-combined-schedule.pdf

Centers for Disease Control and Prevention. (2018d). *The public health approach to violence prevention.* https://www.cdc.gov/violenceprevention/publichealthissue/publichealthapproach.html

Cho, H., & Salmon, C. T. (2007). Unintended effects of health communication campaigns. *Journal of Communication, 57*(2), 293–317. https://doi.org/10.1111/j.1460-2466.2007.00344.x

Cline, R. J. W. (2003). Everyday interpersonal communication and health. In T. L. Thompson, A. Dorsey, Katherine I. Miller, & Roxanne Parrott (Eds.), *Handbook of health communication* (pp. 285–313). Lawrence Erlbaum Associates.

College Times. (2011, February 25). *STDs in college: 3 most common STDs among college students include HPV, chlamydia, and genital herpes.* https://collegetimes.co/stds-in-college/

Dash, S., Clarke, G., Berk, M., & Jacka, F. N. (2015). The gut microbiome and diet in psychiatry: Focus on depression. *Current Opinion in Psychiatry, 28*(1), 1–6. https://doi.org/10.1097/YCO.0000000000000117

Du Pré, A. (2010). *Communicating about health: Current issues and perspectives* (3rd ed.). Oxford University Press.

Esser, M. B., Hedden, S. L., Kanny, D., Brewer, R. D., Gfroerer, J. C., & Naimi, T. S. (2014). Prevalence of alcohol dependence among US adult drinkers, 2009–2011. *Preventing Chronic Disease, 11*, E206. https://doi.org/10.5888/pcd11.140329

Fineberg, H. V. (2011). Public health and medicine. Where the twain shall meet. *American Journal of Preventive Medicine, 41*, S149–S151. https://doi.org/10.1016/j.amepre.2011.07.013

Gass, R. H., & Seiter, J. S. (2007). *Persuasion: Social influence and compliance gaining* (3rd ed.). Pearson.

Glanz, K., Rimer, B. K., & Viswanath, K. (2008). Theory, research, and practice in health behavior and health education. In K. Glanz, B. K. Rimer, & K. Viswanath (Eds.), *Health behavior and health education: Theory, research, and practice* (4th ed., pp. 23–41). Jossey-Bass.

Glanz, K., Rimer, B. K., & Viswanath, K. (2015). Theory, research, and practice in health behavior. In K. Glanz, B. K. Rimer, & K. Viswanath (Eds.), *Health behavior: Theory, research, and practice* (5th ed., pp. 23–41). Jossey-Bass.

Green, L. W., & Kreuter, M. W. (2005). *Health promotion planning: An educational and ecological approach* (4th ed.). McGraw-Hill.

Huber, M., Knottnerus, J. A., Green, L., van der Horst, H., Jadad, A. R., Kromhout, D., Leonard, B., Lorig, K., Loureiro, M. I., van der Meer, J. W. M., Schnabel, P., Smith, R., van Weel, & Smid, H. (2011). How should we define health? *British Medical Journal, 343*, d4163. https://doi.org/10.1136/bmj.d4163

Institute of Medicine. (1988). *The future of public health.* The National Academies Press.

Intervention. (n.d.). Vocabulary.com. https://www.vocabulary.com/dictionary/intervention

Jamal, A., Phillips, E., Gentzke, A. S., Homa, D. M., Babb, S. D., King, B. A., & Neff, L. J. (2018). Current cigarette smoking among adults—United States, 2016. *Morbidity and Mortality Weekly Report, 67*(2), 53–59. http://dx.doi.org/10.15585/mmwr.mm6702a1

Jones, D. S., Podolsky, S. H., & Greene, J. A. (2012). The burden of disease and the changing task of medicine. *The New England Journal of Medicine, 366*, 2333–2338. https://doi.org/10.1056/NEJMp1113569

Kent, L. T. (2019). *Health triangle facts.* https://www.livestrong.com/article/42697-health-triangle/

Knapen, J., Vancampfort, D., Morien, Y., & Marchal, Y. (2015). Exercise therapy improves both mental and physical health in patients with major depression. *Disability and Rehabilitation, 37*, 1490–1495. https://doi.org/10.3109/09638288.2014.972579

Lee-Kwan, S. H., Moore, L. V., Blanck, H. M., Haris, D. M., & Galuska, D. (2017). Disparities in state-specific adult fruit and vegetable consumption—United States, 2015. *Morbidity and Mortality Weekly Report, 66*(45), 1241–1247. http://dx.doi.org/10.15585/mmwr.mm6645a1

Liu, J., & Raine, A. (2017). Nutritional status and social behavior in preschool children: The mediating effects of neurocognitive functioning. *Maternal and Child Nutrition, 13*(2), 1–15. https://doi.org/10.1111/mcn.12321

Look, M. (2016). Why defining health and well-being is important—and why it isn't. https://hart.blog/why-defining-health-and-well-being-is-important-and-why-it-isnt-eb52eb69079c

Mayhew, A., Kowalczyk Mullins, T. L., Ding, L., Rosenthal, S. L., Zimet, G., Marrow, J., & Kahn, J. A. (2014). Risk perceptions and subsequent sexual behaviors after HPV vaccination in adolescents. *Pediatrics, 133*(3), 404–411. https://doi.org/10.1542/peds.2013-2822

Meites, E., Kempe, A., & Markowitz, L. E. (2017). Use of a 2-dose schedule for human papillomavirus vaccination—Updated recommendations of the Advisory Committee on Immunization Practices. *American Journal of Transplantation, 17*(3), 834–837. https://doi.org/10.1111/ajt.14206

Miller, G. R. (1980). On being persuaded: Some basic distinctions. In M. E. Roloff & G. R. Miller (Eds.), *Persuasion: New directions in theory and research* (pp. 11–28). SAGE.

National Cancer Institute. (2001). *Making health communication programs work.* US Department of Health & Human Services.

National Cancer Institute. (2015). *HPV and cancer.* http://www.cancer.gov/about-cancer/causes-prevention/risk/infectious-agents/hpv-fact-sheet#q2

Pew. (2013). *Persuading the prescribers: Pharmaceutical industry marketing and its influence on physicians and patients.* http://www.pewtrusts.org/en/research-and-analysis/fact-sheets/2013/11/11/persuading-the-prescribers-pharmaceutical-industry-marketing-and-its-influence-on-physicians-and-patients

Public Health Functions Project. (1997). *The public health workforce: An agenda for the 21st century.* Public Health Services.

Rakhimov, A. (2018). *Physical health definition and simple body oxygen DIY test.* https://www.normalbreathing.com/e/physical-health.php

Reagan-Steiner, S., Yankey, D., Jeyarajah, J., Elam-Evans, L. D., Singleton, J. A., Curtis, C. R., MacNeil, J., Markowitz, L. E., & Stokley, S. (2015). National, regional, state, and selected local area vaccination coverage among adolescents aged 13–17 years—United States, 2014. *Morbidity and Mortality Weekly Report, 64*(29), 784–792. https://doi.org/10.15585/mmwr.mm6429a3

Rimal, R. N., & Lapinski, M. K. (2009). Why health communication is important in public health. *Bulletin of the World Health Organization, 87,* 247. https://doi.org/10.2471/BLT.08.056713

Roberto, A. J. (2014). Disease prevention. In T. L. Thompson (Ed.), *Encyclopedia of health communication* (pp. 353–358). SAGE.

Rogers, E. M., & Storey, J. D. (1987). Communication campaigns. In C. R. Berger & S. H. Chafee (Eds.), *Handbook of communication science* (pp. 817–846). SAGE.

Schneider, M. J. (2014). *Introduction to public health* (4th ed.). Jones & Bartlett.

Smith, R. (2008). *The end of disease and the beginning of health.* http://blogs.bmj.com/bmj/2008/07/08/richard-smith-the-end-of-disease-and-the-beginning-of-health/

Surgeon General. (2014). *National prevention strategy: Tobacco-free living*. https://www.surgeongeneral.gov/priorities/prevention/strategy/tobacco-free.pdf

Tayebisani, S. M., Azidi, Y., Maleki, H., Saadatifar, A., Zeinoddin, F., & Ghemi, B. (2014). The relationship between physical activity and mental health in active and inactive employees. *European Journal of Experimental Biology, 4*(3), 366–368. https://www.imedpub.com/articles/the-relationship-between-physical-activity-and-mental-health-in-active-and-inactive-employees.pdf

Thompson, T. L. (2006). Seventy-five (count 'em—75!) issues of *Health Communication*: An analysis of emerging themes. *Health Communication, 20*(2), 117–122. https://doi.org/10.1207/s15327027hc2002_2

Turnock, B. J. (2009). *Public health: What it is and how it works* (4th ed.). Jones & Bartlett.

U.S. Department of Health and Human Services. (2000). *Healthy People 2010* (2nd ed.). U.S. Government Printing Office.

U.S. Department of Health and Human Services. (2008). *2008 physical activity guidelines for Americans*. https://health.gov/paguidelines/pdf/paguide.pdf

U.S. Department of Health and Human Services. (2018). *Evidence-based resource summary*. https://www.healthypeople.gov/2020/tools-resources/evidence-based-resource/health-communication-and-social-marketing-campaigns

U.S. Department of Health and Human Services and U.S. Department of Agriculture. (2015). *2015–2020 dietary guidelines for Americans* (8th ed.). https://health.gov/sites/default/files/2019-09/2015-2020_Dietary_Guidelines. pdf

Winslow, C.-E. A. (1920). The untilled fields of public health. *Science, 51*(1306), 23–30. https://doi.org/10.1126/science.51.1306.23

World Health Organization. (1946). *Constitution of the World Health Organization*. Author. https://www.who.int/governance/eb/who_constitution_en.pdf

World Health Organization. (1986). *Ottawa charter for health promotion*. Author. https://www.euro.who.int/__data/assets/pdf_file/0004/129532/Ottawa_Charter.pdf

World Health Organization. (2002). *The World Health report 2002: Reducing risks, promoting healthy life*. Author. https://www.who.int/whr/2002/en/

World Health Organization. (2009). *Global health risks: Mortality and burden of disease attributable to selected major risks*. Author. https://www.who.int/healthinfo/global_burden_disease/GlobalHealthRisks_report_full.pdf

World Health Organization. (2014). *Basic documents* (48th ed.). Author. https://apps.who.int/gb/bd/PDF/bd48/basic-documents-48th-edition-en.pdf

Yoon, P. W., Bastian, B., Anderson, R. N., Collins, J. L., & Jaffe, H. W. (2014). Potentially preventable deaths from the five leading causes of death—United States, 2008–2010. *Morbidity and Mortality Weekly Report, 63*(17), 369–374. https://www.cdc.gov/mmwr/pdf/wk/mm6317.pdf

# SECTION 2

# Intervention
# Planning

## CHAPTER 2

# Introduction to Intervention Planning and Evaluation

## CHAPTER OUTLINE

## INTRODUCTION

Planning, implementing, and evaluating a successful public health communication intervention is no easy task; and it does not happen by chance. It requires careful preparation based on a wide variety of information. Thus, intervention planning is an ongoing process that involves assessing needs; setting objectives and goals; and developing, implementing, and evaluating message strategies to reach these objectives and goals. Intervention planning is a multistep approach that provides a practical and systematic method for collecting and analyzing a wide variety of information about a problem and using this information to guide decision-making and improve intervention performance. A good intervention planning tool will break down the planning process into several manageable stages or phases. As Crosby and Noar (2011) note, intervention planning "is a necessary first step in any health promotion endeavor. It is not a luxury or an extra step" (p. S9). Or, as an old proverb states, "Failing to plan is planning to fail."

With this in mind, this chapter will introduce several key aspects of the planning process. More specifically, this chapter will begin with a brief introduction to logic models. Next, it reviews how to develop appropriate goals, objectives, and strategies. After that, it will review the role various types of evaluation play throughout the planning and implementation process. This chapter will conclude by identifying several planning models and providing brief introductions to the Health Communication Program Cycle and the PRECEDE-PROCEED Model, which will be discussed in detail in Chapters 3 and Chapter 4, respectively. The running example throughout this chapter will be a public health communication intervention designed to increase physical activity among college students that is guided by the health belief model. Thus, before continuing, I will provide some background information regarding the relationship between physical activity and college student health and provide a brief overview of the health belief model.

As you may recall from Chapter 1, physical inactivity is a modifiable risk factor that is associated with many chronic diseases, such as heart disease, stroke, numerous types of cancer, and diabetes. Thus, the U.S. Department of Health and Human Services (2008) recommends that each week adults engage in (1) at least 150 minutes of moderate-intensity aerobic physical activity, (2) at least 75 minutes of vigorous-intensity aerobic physical activity, or (3) an equivalent combination of moderate- and vigorous-intensity aerobic activity. Examples of moderate-intensity activity include walking briskly (at least 3 miles per hour), bicycling (less than 10 miles per hour), tennis (doubles), golfing (carrying clubs), weight training, general gardening, ballroom dancing, heavy cleaning, mowing the lawn, and so forth. Examples of vigorous-intensity activities include jogging, bicycling (over 10 miles per hour), tennis (singles), heavy gardening, aerobics classes, swimming laps, hiking uphill, many competitive sports (basketball, soccer, football, rugby, hockey, lacrosse), and so forth.

Numerous longitudinal studies indicate that college students tend to gain about 5 pounds during their freshman year, and 10 pounds over 4 years in college (Gropper et al., 2012; Holm-Denoma et al., 2008; Pope et al., 2017; Racette et al., 2005). Further, the number of students classified as overweight or obese nearly doubles to around 36% over 4 years in college (Gropper et al., 2012; Pope et al., 2017). This is not surprising given that less than half of college students get the recommended amount of physical activity each week, and that physical activity tends to decrease with age or year in college (American College Health Association, 2009; Buckworth & Nigg, 2004; Huang et al., 2003; Racette et al., 2005). In short, college represents a critical developmental window for establishing healthy physical activity and weight management practices that continue into adulthood. Thus, college students are an important intended audience for public health communication interventions focused on physical activity and weight control.

A detailed discussion of the health belief model is presented in Chapter 6. However, I will briefly review it here given it is intricately related to the goals, objectives, and strategies that will be discussed throughout this chapter. Put succinctly, the health belief model posits that the following five variables impact behavior:

1. Perceived severity refers to one's beliefs about the significance or magnitude of a health threat.

2. Perceived susceptibility concerns one's beliefs about the likelihood of experiencing a health threat.

3. Perceived benefits include any pros or advantages that help or encourage a person to engage in the recommended behavior.

4. Perceived barriers include any cons or disadvantages that hinder or discourage a person from engaging in the recommended behavior.

5. Perceived self-efficacy concerns a person's belief about their ability to perform the recommended behavior under various challenging circumstances.

According to the health belief model, perceived severity, susceptibility, benefits, and self-efficacy should be positively related to the performance of a behavior, while perceived barriers should be negatively related to the performance of a behavior. Please keep this information about physical activity and the health belief model in mind as you read the remainder of this chapter.

## LOGIC MODELS

A *logic model* provides a graphical representation of how and why an intervention plan is supposed to work (Berkowitz et al., 2014). That is, it illustrates the thinking behind the intervention plan, and shows how each intervention component is related to the outcomes and impacts you hope to achieve. To illustrate, a basic logic model is presented in Figure 2.1 (W. P. Kellogg Foundation, 2001). This section provides a general overview of five key components of a logic model, and subsequent sections of this chapter and book will explain each component in detail.

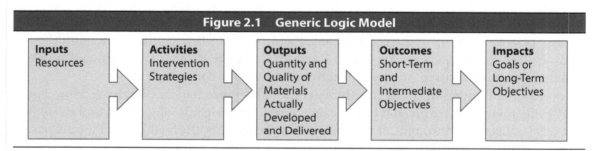

**Figure 2.1    Generic Logic Model**

| **Inputs** | **Activities** | **Outputs** | **Outcomes** | **Impacts** |
|---|---|---|---|---|
| Resources | Intervention Strategies | Quantity and Quality of Materials Actually Developed and Delivered | Short-Term and Intermediate Objectives | Goals or Long-Term Objectives |

Adapted from W. K. Kellogg Foundation (2001).

The inputs, activities, and outputs components of the basic logic model collectively represent the planning or process elements of an intervention. The first component, *inputs*, refers to the resources available for the intervention. This includes the staff, time, money, and infrastructure needed to design, implement, and evaluate an intervention. The second component of a logic model is *activities*, or what you do with the resources. This includes the specific intervention strategies you develop and how they are disseminated. The third component of a logic model is outputs. *Outputs* are the tangible products that were produced or achieved. For example, was the intervention implemented as planned, who did it reach, how many times did it reach them, and how did the intended audience perceive the intervention?

The outcomes and impacts components of the basic logic model focus on the intended results or effects of the intervention. To illustrate, the fourth component of a logic model is *outcomes*, which focuses on the objective-based changes that come about because of the intervention. For example, short-term objectives typically focus on beliefs, attitudes, and intentions, whereas intermediate objectives typically focus on the behaviors impacted by these new beliefs, attitudes, or intentions. The fifth component of a logic model is *impacts*, which are based on the intervention's goal or long-term objective. For example, how did health, social, economic, or environmental conditions change as a result of the intervention; or, more likely, as a result of a series of related interventions?

In sum, a good logic model will help you plan and evaluate your intervention. It will demonstrate why your intervention is a good solution to a health problem by explicating the relationships between its inputs, activities, outputs, outcomes, and impacts. Further, it will help you determine what evaluation questions to ask during the various stages or phases of the planning process. Those interested in seeing an excellent example of actual logic models in action are referred to Huhman et al. (2004), who present the logic model for the VERB campaign, which was designed to influence physical activity among 9- to 13-year-old children.

## GOALS, OBJECTIVES, AND STRATEGIES

In the previous section I mentioned the terms goals, objectives, and strategies in passing. In this section, I will discuss them in detail. Take a look at Figure 2.2 on the following pages, which provides some hypothetical examples for each component in a logic model. To illustrate, impacts are represented by the intervention's goals, outcomes are represented by the intervention's short-term and intermediate objectives, activities and outputs are represented by the intervention's strategies, and inputs include formative research collected through surveys, individual interviews, and focus groups. Also notice how the process involves "backwards planning" in that you must begin at the end. To illustrate, you begin with your goal or long-term objective (see the far-right-hand column of Figure 2.2) and then work backwards to develop a plan to achieve this goal. Thus, every objective should lead to this goal, and every strategy should be explicitly linked to one or more objectives. I will refer back to specific parts of Figure 2.2 that exemplify some important points throughout this section.

### GOALS

*Goals* (sometimes called *long-term objectives*; Centers for Disease Control and Prevention, 2009) refer to the overall health improvement, or impact, that you want your public health communication intervention to make. Goals represent long-term objectives that "are more distant in time, less attributable to the program, and harder to measure" (Centers for Disease Control and Prevention, 2009, p. 11). For example, the overarching goal or long-term objective of our hypothetical physical activity promotion intervention (the far-right column of Figure 2.2) is to improve college students' health, fitness, and quality of life through daily physical activity (U.S. Department of Health and Human Services, 2016). Goals such as this may be difficult for a single public health communication intervention to accomplish all by itself. But when combined with the efforts of other interventions and over time, such large-scale goals are achievable.

| FIGURE 2.2 | Example Strategies, Objectives, and Goals | |
|---|---|---|
| **6.** ➡ **(Formative Evaluation)** | **5. STRATEGIES/ ACTIVITIES** ➡ **(Process Evaluation)** | **4. SHORT-TERM OBJECTIVES** ➡ **(Outcome Evaluation)** |
| Campus-wide survey assessing students' perceptions (i.e., susceptibility, severity, benefits, barriers, and self-efficacy) and behavior regarding aerobic and muscle-strengthening physical activity. | Require all incoming students to attend a mandatory presentation at the student recreation center that identifies, explains, and provides examples of the recommended amount of physical activity, the health benefits of engaging in such activities, and proven ways to improve chances for success. | Increase by 40% the number of college students who believe that physical *inactivity* leads to serious health problems by the end of the fall semester. |
| | Place point-of-decision (or, cues-to-action) posters by all elevators to encourage students to use the stairs and remind students of the health or weight loss benefits of taking the stairs. | Increase by 40% the number of college students who believe that they are susceptible to health problems associated with physical *inactivity* by the end of the fall semester. |
| Individual interviews with college students to get an in-depth understanding of (1) the perceived benefits of physical activity—and how to enhance these benefits, and (2) the perceived barriers of physical activity—and how to diminish these barriers. | Distribute a "Personal Fitness Contract" and/or an "Exercise Buddy Agreement" to every student via the web and email and provide a list of reasons such contracts and agreements are effective. | Increase perceived benefits of physical activity among college students by 40% by the end of the fall semester. |
| | Send messages through social media and the campus-wide announcement system to encourage students to use active transportation and remind them of the health or weight loss benefits of using active transportation. | Reduce perceived barriers of physical activity among college students by 40% by the end of the fall semester. |
| Focus groups with college students to identify and get feedback on potential strategies for influencing beliefs and behavior regarding physical activity. | Create a campus walking group and campus walking events to promote physical activity and health awareness. | Increase by 40% the number of college students who believe they can engage in the recommended amount of physical activity by the end of the fall semester (i.e., self-efficacy). |

| FIGURE 2.2    Continued | | |
| --- | --- | --- |
| **3. INTERMEDIATE SUB-OBJECTIVES** (Outcome Evaluation) ➡ | **2. INTERMEDIATE OBJECTIVES** (Outcome Evaluation) ➡ | **1. GOAL or LONG-TERM OBJECTIVES** (Impact Evaluation) ➡ |
| Increase by 20% the number of college students who set and monitor fitness goals by the beginning of the spring semester. | | |
| Increase by 20% the number of college students who use active transportation by the beginning of the spring semester. | Increase by 10% the number of college students that get at least 150 minutes of moderate physical activity or 75 minutes of vigorous physical activity (or a combination of the two) each week by the end of the spring semester. | Improve college students' health, fitness, and quality of life through daily physical activity. |
| Increase by 20% the number of college students who enlist social support via "personal fitness contracts" or "exercise buddy agreements" by the beginning of the spring semester. | | |
| Increase by 20% the number of college students who join a campus walking group or attend a campus walking event by the beginning of the spring semester. | | |

## OBJECTIVES

*Objectives* are the specific cognitive and behavioral changes you want your public health communication intervention to produce. These are changes that, if achieved, should lead to your overarching goal. Most interventions will have some mix of short-term, intermediate, and long-term objectives. Long-term objectives (or goals) were discussed in the preceding paragraph, and a discussion of intermediate and short-term objectives follows.

*Intermediate objectives* are the interim changes in behaviors that provide a sense of progress toward reaching the long-term objectives (Centers for Disease Control and Prevention, n.d.). As illustrated in Figure 2.2, we have four intermediate sub-objectives, and one intermediate primary objective. Our four intermediate sub-objectives are to increase by 20% the number of college students who (1) set and monitor fitness goals, (2) use active transportation, (3) enlist social support, and (4) join a campus walking group or attend a campus walking event. Our primary intermediate objective is to increase by 10% the number of college students that get at least 150 minutes of moderate physical activity or 75 minutes of vigorous physical activity (or a combination of the two) each week.

Finally, *short-term objectives* represent the most immediate changes you expect the intervention to have on the intended audience. Short-term objectives usually target variables that are easier to change, such as knowledge, beliefs, and attitudes. For example, the short-term objectives in Figure 2.2 focus on increasing perceived severity, susceptibility, benefits, and self-efficacy (and decrease perceived barriers) by 40%.

### Creating SMART Objectives

When creating short-term, intermediate, or long-term objectives, it is important that they be SMART. SMART is an acronym that stands for **S**pecific, **M**easurable, **A**chievable, **R**elevant, and **T**ime-bound (Centers for Disease Control and Prevention, 2015). First, objectives should be *specific*; they should clearly identify what you want to achieve, such as the variables and intended audience you wanted to change. In our example, our short-term objectives focus on five specific variables—severity, susceptibility, benefits, barriers, self-efficacy; our intermediate objectives focus on four specific behaviors; and all of our objectives focus on one specific intended audience—college students.

Second, objectives should be *measurable*; they should provide quantifiable indicators for success. This means they should indicate the amount of change expected and focus on outcomes that can be reliably and validly assessed. For example, all five variables identified in our short-term objectives are based on the health belief model and can be measured using existing scales that have been shown to have strong measurement reliability and validity in numerous studies (e.g., Champion, 1984, 1999; Witte et al., 1996). The same is true for all the behaviors that make up our intermediate objectives (Fishbein & Ajzen, 2010).

Third, objectives should be *achievable*; they should be feasible, realistic, attainable, and easy to put into action. For example, do you have the necessary time, money, and ability to reach each objective? In our case we are hoping to change perceptions (an easier task) by 40% and behavior (a more difficult task) by 20% or 10%. We do not have to maximize everyone's perceptions to be successful (we just must increase them by 40% overall), and we do not have to change everyone's behaviors to be successful (we just must increase it by 20% or 10% overall). Previous theory and research, as well as your formative evaluation results, will go a long way toward helping you set achievable objectives.

Fourth, objectives should be *relevant*; they should be directly related to subsequent objectives or your overarching goal. For example, previous theory and research suggests that our short-term objectives (i.e., changes in severity, susceptibility, benefits, barriers, self-efficacy) should increase the likelihood that individuals will engage in the exercise-related behaviors that make up our intermediate objectives. And, over time, if we meet our intermediate objectives, we increase the chances of reaching our overarching goal, or long-term objective.

Fifth, objectives should be *time-bound*; they should include a time frame or deadline regarding when the objective should be met. In our example we established the end of the fall semester as the specific time frame to meet our short-term objectives, and the end of the spring semester as the specific time frame to meet our intermediate objective and sub-objectives.

## STRATEGIES

*Strategies* describe the specific communication activities (or processes) you will take to accomplish your objectives. As noted in Chapter 1, the term "strategy" is closely related to what people typically mean when they use the words "intervention." In our physical activity example (see Figure 2.2), we outline five specific communication strategies: (1) a presentation, (2) point-of-decision posters, (3) distribution of "personal fitness contracts" or "exercise buddy agreements," (4) social media messages and campus-wide announcements, and (5) campus walking groups and walking events. Each of these message strategies are specifically created and disseminated to help achieve one or more objectives. And, notice how each strategy was derived from formative research with the intended audience. For example, formative evaluation can be used to identify a variety of appropriate settings (e.g., student recreation center, elevators, etc.) and channels (e.g., live presentation, posters, contracts, and social and other electronic media).

Please keep these definitions and examples of goals, objectives, and strategies in mind as you read about the various types of evaluation which will be discussed next.

## TYPES OF EVALUATION

In this section I will provide a definition of evaluation, along with a brief overview of four key types of evaluation that we will be referring to throughout this book: formative, process, outcome, and impact (see Table 2.1).[1] When you *evaluate* something, you are making a judgment about its value or usefulness (Roberto, 2014). More specifically, *intervention evaluation* is a systematic method for collecting, analyzing, and using information to improve or assess the effectiveness of interventions (U.S. Department of Health and Human Services, 2010b). As will be discussed in more detail in Chapters 11 through 13, evaluation research involves studying interventions in a careful, systematic, and rigorous manner to make sure any decisions or conclusions are supported by evidence. As Kreps (2014) notes, poorly conducted research is worse than no research at all, as false or misleading information is worse than no information at all. As you can see in Table 2.1, such evaluations, or judgments, may occur throughout all stages or phases of a public health communication intervention.

To illustrate, formative evaluation is conducted before the intervention is fully designed or implemented, process evaluation is conducted during intervention implementation to make sure the intervention is being implemented as intended, and outcome evaluation and impact evaluation are completed after the intervention has ended. The purpose of outcome evaluation is to determine if the intervention met its specific objectives, whereas the

| **TABLE 2.1    Types of Evaluation** | |
| Evaluation Type | Definition |
| --- | --- |
| Formative Evaluation | Conducted *before* the intervention is designed or implemented to learn about and obtain feedback from the intended audience, and to help ensure the intervention is feasible, appropriate, and acceptable. |
| Process Evaluation | Conducted *during* intervention implementation to make sure all strategies were implemented as planned and to identify unexpected problems while there is still time to adjust and improve the intervention. |
| Outcome Evaluation | Completed *after* the intervention has ended to determine if the intervention led to the desired cognitive and behavioral changes in the intended audience (i.e., objective-based evaluation). * |
| Impact Evaluation | Completed *after* the intervention has ended to determine the broader impact one or more interventions have on a community (i.e., goal-based evaluation). * |

* As a reminder, even though outcome and impact evaluation are completed after an intervention has ended, it is important to plan for them before the intervention begins (e.g., so you can collect pretest data, track potential extraneous variables, etc.).

purpose of impact evaluation is to determine if the intervention met its more general goal. However, even though outcome and impact evaluation are completed after an intervention has ended, it is important to plan for them from the start. For example, you may need to collect pretest data before the intervention begins or keep track of any potential extraneous variables while the intervention is being implemented. There are two general strategies to consider when evaluating interventions: primary and secondary research data.

## PRIMARY AND SECONDARY RESEARCH DATA

First, you can collect *primary research data*, which involves original research conducted by the intervention planner for a specific purpose. For example, intervention planners may conduct qualitative focus groups or in-depth individual interviews with a few community members to obtain a richer understanding of their knowledge, attitudes, and beliefs. Or, intervention planners may collect and statistically analyze quantitative survey data from many members of the intended audience to draw more generalizable conclusions about the whole community.

Second, you can review *secondary research data*, which is existing research that was previously conducted by someone else or for some other purpose. Examples of secondary data include existing federal, state, and local health statistics about the topic or intended audience, medical journals (e.g., *Journal of the American Medical Association*), public health journals (e.g., *American Journal of Public Health*), and communication journals (e.g., *Health Communication* and *Journal of Health Communication*) that publish high-quality studies about a wide variety of health issues and intervention evaluations. Other good sources of secondary data include the *Morbidity and Mortality Weekly Report* (MMWR), the *Behavioral Risk Factor Surveillance System* (BRFSS), and the *Youth Risk Behavior Surveillance System* (YRBSS).

## HEALTHY PEOPLE INITIATIVE

Another important source of secondary data is the Healthy People Initiative (Roberto, 2015). The *Healthy People Initiative* (www.healthypeople.gov) is a comprehensive, nationwide health promotion and disease prevention agenda set by the U.S. Department of Health and Human Services. The overarching goals of the Healthy People Initiative are to: (1) increase *quality of life*, or how happy or fulfilled an individual is with their life; (2) increase *life expectancy*, or how long a person is projected to live; and (3) reduce *health disparities*, or inequalities in the health status among different segments of the population (U.S. Department of Health and Human Services, 2010a). For example, African American men have higher rates of cancer than men or women of any other race/ethnicity. This disproportionately affects their quality of life and life expectancy and represents the type of health disparity the Healthy People Initiative aims to reduce.

*Healthy People 2020* includes over 1,200 objectives for 42 different topics (U.S. Department of Health and Human Services, 2016). Table 2.2 includes a complete list of the 42 different topic areas. Following are just a few of the many topics included in *Healthy People 2020* that are related to physical activity: "cancer," "diabetes," "health-related quality of life and well-being," "heart disease and stroke," "mental health and mental disorders," "nutrition and weight status," "physical activity," and "sleep health."

To provide a more detailed understanding as to why the Healthy People Initiative is such a useful resource for assessing background and the need for a public health communication intervention, we will take a closer look at the "Physical Activity" section (U.S. Department of Health and Human Services, 2016). Each section begins with an overarching goal for the topic. In this case the overarching goal is to improve health, fitness,

| TABLE 2.2 Healthy People 2020 Topic Areas | |
|---|---|
| 1. Access to Health Services | 21. Heart Disease and Stroke |
| 2. Adolescent Health* | 22. HIV |
| 3. Arthritis, Osteoporosis, and Chronic Back Conditions | 23. Immunization and Infectious Diseases |
| 4. Blood Disorders and Blood Safety* | 24. Injury and Violence Prevention |
| 5. Cancer | 25. Lesbian, Gay, Bisexual, and Transgender Health* |
| 6. Chronic Kidney Disease | 26. Maternal, Infant, and Child Health |
| 7. Dementias, Including Alzheimer's Disease* | 27. Medical Product Safety |
| 8. Diabetes | 28. Mental Health and Mental Disorders |
| 9. Disability and Health | 29. Nutrition and Weight Status |
| 10. Early and Middle Childhood* | 30. Occupational Safety and Health |
| 11. Educational and Community-Based Programs | 31. Older Adults* |
| 12. Environmental Health | 32. Oral Health |
| 13. Family Planning | 33. Physical Activity |
| 14. Food Safety | 34. Preparedness* |
| 15. Genomics* | 35. Public Health Infrastructure |
| 16. Global Health* | 36. Respiratory Diseases |
| 17. Healthcare-Associated Infections* | 37. Sexually Transmitted Diseases |
| 18. Health Communication and Health Information Technology | 38. Sleep Health* |
| 19. Health-Related Quality of Life and Well-Being* | 39. Social Determinants of Health |
| 20. Hearing and Other Sensory or Communication Disorders* | 40. Substance Abuse |
| | 41. Tobacco Use |
| | 42. Vision |

Source: U.S. Department of Health and Human Services (2010a).
*Indicates new topic area first added to Healthy People 2020.

and quality of life through daily physical activity. It then goes on to discuss the extent of the problem (i.e., more than 80% of adults do not meet the guidelines for both aerobic and muscle-strengthening activities), and why physical activity is important (i.e., regular physical activity can improve the health and quality of life of Americans of all ages and can lower the risk of early death, heart disease, stroke, high blood pressure, type 2 diabetes, and breast and colon cancer). Further, it provides 48 objectives and sub-objectives that a public health communication intervention might focus on to help achieve this goal. Example objectives include reducing the proportion of adults who engage in no leisure-time physical activity (PA-1); increasing the proportion of adults who meet current federal physical activity guidelines for aerobic physical activity and for muscle-strengthening activity (PA-2); increasing the proportion of physician office visits that include counseling or education related to physical activity (PA-11); increasing the proportion of trips made by walking (PA-13); and increasing the proportion of trips made by bicycling (PA-14).

## FORMATIVE EVALUATION

*Formative evaluation* is conducted before the intervention is fully designed or implemented (i.e., while it is still forming). The aims of formative evaluation are to help improve the design and implementation of your intervention and to give it the greatest chance of success. As the Centers for Disease Control and Prevention (2001) note, formative evaluation helps ensure your intervention is needed, feasible, appropriate, and acceptable before it is fully designed and implemented. In other words, formative evaluation is "designed to make sure that program plans, procedures, activities, materials, and modifications will work as planned" (National Cancer Institute, 2001, p. 247).

As such, formative evaluation is typically conducted when you are designing a new intervention, or when you are adapting, modifying, or revising an existing intervention for a new topic, setting, or intended audience. Formative evaluation incorporates members of the intended audience into the planning process by directly asking them about their lifestyle, culture, motivations, and preferences. It can also let you know if the proposed intervention is needed and how well it will be understood and accepted by the intended audience. For these reasons, both preproduction and postproduction formative research play a critical role in the development of public health communication interventions as they allow you to make modifications before the intervention is fully implemented, which increases the likelihood that you will achieve your objectives and goals.

### Preproduction Formative Evaluation

*Preproduction formative evaluation* seeks to gain insights into and input from the intended audience before messages or materials are developed. A key purpose of preproduction formative evaluation is to better understand the health problem and explore possible ways to prevent it from the perspective of the intended audience. Toward this end, intervention developers go to great lengths to learn as much as possible about the topic and intended audience before specifying goals, objectives, and strategies. Thus, preproduction formative research is a broad activity that includes anything intervention planners do to better understand the health problem or intended audience, segment the intended audience into high-priority subgroups, or specify the cognitive and behavioral changes you want the public health communication intervention to produce (e.g., see sample objectives in Figure 2.2) (Atkin & Freimuth, 1989, 2001; Palmer, 1981; Roberto et al., 2011).

Preproduction formative evaluation can be used to identify general ideas for an intervention, obtain feedback on rough concepts, generate words and phrases that are used by and are meaningful to the intended audience, and select a theory to guide intervention development (Atkin & Freimuth, 1989, 2001). Literature reviews, interviews with subject matter experts, and individual and focus group interviews or surveys with members of the intended audience are common methods intervention planners use to gather the information necessary to make decisions during the preproduction formative evaluation process.

### Postproduction Formative Evaluation

Once you have drafts of your messages and materials you should conduct additional rounds of formative evaluation. *Postproduction formative* seeks input from the intended audience after draft messages and materials have been created but before they are finalized and fully implemented. The goal here is to assess the intended audience's reactions to one or more prototype messages before they are finalized and while changes can still be made. For example, postproduction formative research allows you to assess attention, comprehension, credibility, relevance, and to gauge any sensitive or controversial elements that may alienate or offend the intended audience (Atkin & Freimuth, 1989, 2001; Palmer, 1981).

This can be done via another round of focus groups or individual interviews with members of the intended audience. Alternatively, you could pretest specific intervention strategies by conducting a *pilot test*, or small-scale investigation designed to try out your messages, procedures, and measures before fully implementing them on a larger scale. For example, you could run a small experiment (see Chapter 13) with just a few members of the intended audience to see if the materials are having the anticipated effects on your objectives. Pilot tests are an excellent way to gain important information about an intervention strategy that has not been previously implemented with your intended audience, and to try out measures (i.e., surveys, interview protocol, observational tools, record-keeping systems) that will be used in your process and impact evaluation. Postproduction formative evaluation is an iterative process, which means it should be repeated until your messages and materials communicate the information as intended. Once you have gone through these steps, you can make one final round of revisions to your messages and materials before moving forward.

## PROCESS EVALUATION

The method of documenting an intervention's implementation is called process evaluation. More specifically, *process evaluation* (sometimes called *implementation evaluation*; Centers for Disease Control and Prevention, 2012) is conducted during intervention implementation to make sure it is executed as intended. Process evaluation can use data from many different sources, including individual and focus-group interviews, field observations, naturally collected records, focus groups, and surveys. I will discuss individual and focus group interviews and survey research in detail later in Chapters 11 and 12, respectively. Below I briefly review how field observations and naturally occurring records might be incorporated into a process evaluation plan.

*Field observations* entail watching how people behave in natural settings and situations. Field observations can take on many different forms ranging from covert participation to overt observation (Jorgensen, 1989). A key strength of field observations is that it does not rely on an individual's ability or willingness to report. For example, you might conduct weekly observations to see if any of the posters have been removed or need to be replaced. For the social media component and presentations, you can observe the comments students make to ensure that they are reacting to your message in the way you anticipated. Further, it would be easy and worthwhile to monitor and document how many people joined the campus walking group or attended campus walking events.

*Naturally collected records* (Kreps, 2014) includes data that is normally created as you implement your public health communication intervention. For example, you could use attendance sheets to track how many people attended your presentation or campus walking events. Or, you could use invoices created by the printing company to track how many posters you printed, and maps to document when and where they were posted. Or, you could document how many people like, comment on, or share a given post in the social media portion of your campaign.

It is worth noting that the implementation stage will not always go as planned, and it is common for unexpected problems to occur. Process evaluation helps you identify such issues while there is still time to adjust and improve them. For example, perhaps your activities are not being completed on schedule (in which case you may need to put more resources into your intervention or adjust your timeline). Or, perhaps you are reaching large numbers of people, but very few of them are members of your intended audience (in which case you may need to reevaluate where and when you deliver your intervention). Or perhaps you are reaching your intended audience, but they react negatively or unexpectedly to your messages in some way (in which case you may want to put the intervention on hold, or at least conduct additional interviews or focus groups to determine why—and how to fix it).

A well thought out process evaluation plan provides valuable information about these and many other aspects of your public health communication intervention and allows you to fix such problems as they arise, which further improves your odds of reaching your objectives and goals. As the National Cancer Institute (2001) notes, "there is nothing wrong with altering your plans to fit a changed situation. In fact, you may risk damaging your chances of success if you are not willing to be flexible" (p. 102). Further, when it comes time to assess effectiveness via outcome evaluation, it would be difficult to determine with any certainty what effects your public health communication intervention had if you are not sure it was implemented as intended.

## FIDELITY, COMPLETENESS, EXPOSURE, SATISFACTION, AND REACH

Sanders and colleagues (2005) provide a comprehensive and systematic approach for developing a process-evaluation plan that includes the following components: fidelity, completeness, exposure, satisfaction, and reach. *Fidelity*, or quality, concerns the extent to which the intervention was implemented according to plan (i.e., are you doing what you said you would do, and by when you said you would do it?). For example, in the hypothetical physical activity promotion intervention presented in Figure 2.2, we planned to (1) implement five specific strategies or activities—presentations, posters, contracts/agreements, social and other electronic media, and walking groups/event, and (2) monitor the effects of these efforts as they relate to a variety of objectives and sub-objectives—including behavior and perceptions of severity, susceptibility, benefits, barriers, and self-efficacy. So, fidelity concerns how well we followed this plan.

Completeness, exposure, and satisfaction all focus on the amount of the intervention delivered, and how it was received by the intended audience. *Completeness* concerns how much of the intervention was delivered. For example, we planned to put point-of-decision (or cue-to-action) posters by all campus elevators. Completeness focuses on how well we implemented this strategy (i.e., what percentage of campus elevators had posters placed by them?). *Exposure* concerns how much of the intervention is received by participants, or how often participants have contact with or use intervention messages and materials. In other words, it is not only important to place posters by all campus elevators (completeness), but it is important to display them in such a way that the intended audience sees them before they get on the elevator (and to replace any that may be damaged or removed). Further, while it is important to make sure personal fitness contracts and exercise buddy agreements are distributed to all members of the intended audience (completeness), it is also important to make sure the intended audience actively engages with, interacts with, are receptive to, and use the distributed materials. *Satisfaction* focuses on the intended audience perception of the intervention. For example, you could monitor student reactions to, and questions asked during the mandatory presentation at the student recreation center.

Or, you might ask audience members to complete a short survey to assess how informative, accurate, interesting, useful, and professional (or confusing, misleading, dull, irrelevant, or preachy) they found the presentation to be.

Finally, *reach*, or participation rate, concerns the number or proportion of the intended audience that participates in or is exposed to the intervention. One way to assess reach in our example would be to monitor the number and characteristics of those who attend the presentation or events. Another way would be to conduct a campus-wide survey to determine the percentage of the intended audience that recall being exposed to one or more intervention strategies or activities.

## OUTCOME EVALUATION

*Outcome evaluation* (sometimes called *effectiveness evaluation* or *objective-based evaluation*; Centers for Disease Control and Prevention, 2012) is conducted after the intervention has ended to determine if it met its short-term and intermediate objectives. In other words, outcome evaluation is objective-based, and seeks to answer the question, "what specific effects did the intervention have on the intended audience?" This requires a thorough understanding of intervention planning and evaluation in general, as well as the specific intervention plan. For example, in our hypothetical physical activity intervention, we had a variety of short-term and intermediate objectives (i.e., increase severity, susceptibility, benefits, self-efficacy, and behavior—and decrease barriers—by the end of the fall semester). So, we need to design our outcome evaluation in a manner that allows us to demonstrate whether our intervention led to changes in these outcomes.

Outcome evaluation tests the cause–effect relationship between your public health communication intervention (the cause) and changes in the intended audience on the outcome variables of interest (the effect). This involves demonstrating that any changes in the intended audience are related to the intervention rather than other things going on at the same time. It also involves showing what would have happened had the intervention not occurred. To do this you must typically keep track of what happens to a group of individuals that do receive the intervention, while also keeping track of what happens to a group of individuals that do not receive the intervention (i.e., a control group) or that receive a different intervention (i.e., a comparison group). Surveys (Dillman et al., 2014) and experiments and quasi-experiments (Shadish et al., 2001) are two quantitative research methods that play an important role when conducting an outcome evaluation, and are discussed in detail in Chapters 12 and 13, respectively.

## IMPACT EVALUATION

*Impact evaluation* (sometimes called *goal-based evaluation*; Centers for Disease Control and Prevention, 2012) is conducted after one or more interventions have ended to determine their effect on an overarching goal, or long-term objective. Impact evaluation is goal-based as it seeks to answer the question, "What broader impact did one or more interventions have on a community?" While outcome evaluation is typically conducted immediately or shortly after an intervention is completed, impact evaluation is typically conducted months or years after one or more interventions have ended to determine their lasting effect on the intended audience. In short, impact evaluation focuses on community-level changes and long-term results.

For example, in our hypothetical physical activity intervention, our goal was to improve the health, fitness, and quality of life of the intended audience. However, conducting an impact evaluation to determine if this goal was met is no easy task for at least two reasons. First, a wide variety of genetic, behavioral, or environmental factors can impact health, wellness, and quality of life (Green & Kreuter, 2005); and no single intervention will be able to address all of them. Second, it may take years or decades to observe the impact of behavior on health. To illustrate, the effects of lifestyle choices that colleges students make now may not be apparent until they are in their 40s, 50s, 60s, or beyond. For these and other reasons, impact evaluation is often considered the "holy grail" of intervention evaluation (Crosby & Noar, 2011, p. S15).

## PLANNING MODELS

*Planning models* provide a blueprint, or step-by-step guide, for how to go about building an intervention. Planning models focus more on process than content. So, while planning models provide important structure, they also offer considerable flexibility. In other words, they provide a guideline to follow during the planning process that will help you select appropriate theories, methods, and strategies for your topic and intended audience. However, they do not tell you what those theories, methods, and strategies should be. In the realm of public health communication interventions, there are many different planning tools to choose from. Here are just a few:

- ▶ *Continuous Program Improvement Cycle*, which includes the following four parts: (1) plan, (2) implement, (3) measure and monitor, and (4) evaluate (see Kidder & Chapel, 2018).

- ▶ *Health Communication Program Cycle*, which includes the following four stages: (1) planning and strategy development, (2) developing and pretesting concepts, messages, and materials, (3) implementing the program, and (4) assessing effectiveness and making refinements (National Cancer Institute, 2001).

- ▸ *P.D.C.A. Cycle*, which includes the following four steps: (1) plan, (2) do, (3) check, and (4) act (see Moen & Norman, 2010).

- ▸ *P.E.R.I.E. Process*, which has the following five components: (1) problem, (2) etiology, (3) recommendations, (4) implementation, and (5) evaluation (see Riegelman & Kirkwood, 2015).

- ▸ *PRECEDE-PROCEED Model*, which includes the following eight phases: (1) social assessment, (2) epidemiological assessment, (3) educational and ecological assessment, (4) administrative and policy assessment and intervention alignment, (5) implementation, (6) process evaluation, (7) outcome evaluation, and (8) impact evaluation (Green & Kreuter, 2005).

- ▸ *RE-AIM Framework*, which includes the following 5 dimensions: (1) reach, (2) effectiveness, (3) adoption, (4) implementation, and (5) maintenance (Glasgow et al., 1999).

Notice that while the number of parts, stages, steps, phases, or dimensions may vary, these and similar planning tools generally follow the public health approach that was introduced in Chapter 1, which included (1) defining the problem, (2) identifying risk and protective factors, (3) developing and testing prevention strategies, and (4) assuring widespread adoption. Further, they do not view planning as something you do just once. Instead, all of these approaches view planning as a continuous improvement process using feedback gathered via formative, process, and outcome evaluation to ensure that a public health communication intervention is as appropriate, efficient, and effective as possible at all times.

Regardless of which planning tool is selected, planning models are an essential way to make sure all aspects of the planning process are fully considered. Thus, the balance of Section 2 will review two popular intervention planning tools commonly used to help plan, implement, and evaluate public health communication interventions. Specifically, Chapter 3 will review the Health Communication Program Cycle (National Cancer Institute, 2001), and Chapter 4 will discuss the PREDEDE-PROCEED Model (Green & Kreuter, 2005). As you will see, while there are some notable differences between these two approaches, there are also quite a few similarities. While no process can guarantee success, following the stages or phases in either approach will significantly increase the chances of making your public health communication intervention work.

By way of introduction, a key difference between the two approaches is that the Health Communication Program Cycle adopts more of an individual consumer-based approach; while the PRECEDE-PROCEED Model takes more of an ecological view. The PRECEDE-PROCEED Model's emphasis on the bigger picture is perhaps best captured by the fact

| TABLE 2.3    A Side-by-Side Comparison of the Health Communication Program Cycle and the PRECEDE-PROCEED Model | |
| --- | --- |
| **Health Communication Program Cycle** | **PRECEDE-PROCEED Model** |
| Stage 1:  Planning and Strategy Development | Phase 1:  Social Assessment<br>Phase 2:  Epidemiological Assessment<br>Phase 3:  Educational and Ecological Assessment<br>Phase 4:  Administrative and Policy Assessment and Intervention Alignment |
| Stage 2:  Developing and Pretesting | Phase 4:  Administrative and Policy Assessment and Intervention Alignment (Cont.) |
| Stage 3:  Implementing the Program | Phase 5:  Implementation<br>Phase 6:  Process Evaluation |
| Stage 4:  Assessing Effectiveness and Making Refinements | Phase 7:  Outcome Evaluation *<br>Phase 8:  Impact Evaluation * |

* See Footnote 1 in this chapter for a discussion on the conflicting use of the terms "outcome evaluation" and "impact evaluation" in the literature.

that it includes four planning phases, while the Health Communication Program Cycle includes just one. In terms of similarities, both approaches focus on assessing needs, setting goals and objectives, and how to systematically develop, implement, and evaluate an intervention. More specifically, both approaches (1) include the same steps in one form or another, (2) highlight the importance of conducting evaluation research before (formative evaluation), during (process evaluation), and after (impact and outcome evaluation) a public health communication intervention is designed and implemented, and (3) are cyclical in nature (i.e., information from the final stages or phases provide feedback for future interventions). To better illustrate their similarities and differences, Table 2.3 provides a side-by-side comparison of the two approaches.

## CONCLUSION

Many decisions must be made when planning, implementing, and evaluating public health communication interventions. The importance of using an established planning model to guide the process cannot be overstated, as planning models provide a systematic and rigorous method for making *informed* decisions that will increase the chances of success. The purpose of this chapter was to introduce several basic, yet essential concepts shared by the two intervention planning models covered in this book. Toward this end, this chapter defined and provided examples of goals, objectives, and strategies. It also stressed the value of conducting evaluation research at various points during the intervention planning process to (1) gather information about and feedback from the intended audience, (2) make sure the intervention is being carried out as intended, and (3) determine if the intervention met its specific objectives and general goals. Please keep this information in mind as you read about the Health Communicating Program Cycle in Chapter 3, and the PRECEDE-PROCEED Model in Chapter 4.

## FOOTNOTE

[1] A variety of terms have been used to identify the various types of evaluation discussed in this book. Sometimes this has the positive effect of making the definition of an unfamiliar term easier to remember, such as when the Centers for Disease Control and Prevention (2012) uses "implementation evaluation" as a synonym for "process evaluation," and "effectiveness evaluation" as a synonym for "outcome evaluation."

Sometimes, however, terms are used in conflicting ways, which is a source of confusion. For example, the Centers for Disease Control and Prevention (2012), Kotler and Lee (2008), National Cancer Institute (2001), Weiss (1998), the World Health Organization (2013), and others use "outcome evaluation" to refer to objectives-based evaluation, and "impact evaluation" to refer to goal-based evaluation. Whereas, Green and Kreuter (2005) and DiClemente et al. (2013) and others do the opposite (i.e., they use the "impact evaluation" to refer to objective-based evaluation and "outcome evaluation" to refer to goal-based evaluation). Further, to add to the confusion, "summative evaluation" is a more general term that is sometimes used in place of one or both terms.

Throughout this book, I use the term *outcome evaluation* to refer to the assessment of the specific effects an intervention had on the intended audience (i.e., objective-based evaluation). For example, what effect did the intervention have on an intended audience's beliefs, attitudes, or behavior? I use the term *impact evaluation* to refer to the assessment of the broader effects that one or more interventions had on a community (i.e., goal-based evaluation). For example, how did any changes in beliefs, attitudes, and behaviors ultimately impact the health, social, economic, or environmental conditions for the intended audience?

# REFERENCES

American College Health Association. (2009). American College Health Association—National college health assessment spring 2008 reference group data report (abridged). *Journal of American College Health, 57*(5), 477–488. https://doi.org/10.3200/JACH.57.5.477-488

Atkin, C. K., & Freimuth, V. (1989). Formative evaluation research in campaign design. In R. E. Rice & C. K. Atkin (Eds.), *Public communication campaigns* (2nd ed., pp. 131–150). SAGE.

Atkin, C. K., & Freimuth, V. (2001). Formative evaluation research in campaign design. In R. E. Rice & C. K. Atkin (Eds.), *Public communication campaigns* (3rd ed., pp. 125–145). SAGE.

Berkowitz, J., Orians, C., & Rose, J. (2014). Logic models and program evaluation. In T. L. Thompson (Ed.), *Encyclopedia of health communication* (pp. 80–82). SAGE.

Buckworth, J., & Nigg, C. (2004). Physical activity, exercise, and sedentary behavior in college students. *Journal of American College Health, 53*(1), 28–34. https://doi.org/10.3200/JACH.53.1.28-34

Centers for Disease Control and Prevention. (n.d.). *Developing program goals and measurable objectives.* https://www.cdc.gov/std/program/pupestd/developing program goals and objectives.pdf

Centers for Disease Control and Prevention. (2001). *Program operations guidelines for STD prevention: Program evaluation.* https://www.cdc.gov/std/program/progevaluation.pdf

Centers for Disease Control and Prevention. (2009). *Logic models for planning and evaluation.* https://www.cdc.gov/ncbddd/birthdefects/models/Resource1-Evaluation-Guide-508.pdf

Centers for Disease Control and Prevention. (2012). *Focus the evaluation design.* https://www.cdc.gov/eval/guide/step3/index.htm

Centers for Disease Control and Prevention. (2015). *How to write SMART objectives.* https://www.cdc.gov/cancer/dcpc/pdf/dp17-1701-smart-objectives.pdf

Champion, V. L. (1984). Instrument development for health belief model constructs. *Advances in Nursing Science, 6*(3), 73–85. https://doi.org/10.1097/00012272-198404000-00011

Champion, V. L. (1999). Revised susceptibility, benefits, and barriers scale for mammography screening. *Research in Nursing and Health, 22*(4), 341–348. https://doi.org/10.1002/(sici)1098-240x(199908)22:4<341::aid-nur8>3.0.co;2-p

Crosby, R., & Noar, S. M. (2011). What is a planning model? An introduction to PRECEDE-PROCEED. *Journal of Public Health Dentistry, 71,* S7–S15. https://doi.org/10.1111/j.1752-7325.2011.00235.x

DiClemente, R. J., Salazar, L. F., & Crosby, R. A. (2013). *Health behavior theory for public health: Principles, foundations, and applications.* Jones & Bartlett Learning Company.

Dillman, D. A., Smyth, J. D., & Christian, L. M. (2014). *Internet, mail, and mixed-mode surveys: The tailored design method* (4th ed.). Wiley.

Fishbein, M., & Ajzen, I. (2010). *Predicting and changing behavior: The reasoned action approach.* Psychology Press.

Glasgow, R. E., Vogt, T. M., & Boles, S. M. (1999). Evaluating the public health impact of health promotion interventions: The RE-AIM framework. *American Journal of Public Health, 89*(9), 1322–1327. https://doi.org/10.2105/ajph.89.9.1322

Green, L. W., & Kreuter, M. W. (2005). *Health promotion planning: An educational and ecological approach* (4th ed.). McGraw-Hill.

Gropper, S. S., Simmons, K. P., Connell, L. J., & Ulrich, P. V. (2012). Changes in body weight, composition, and shape: A 4-year study of college students. *Applied Physiology, Nutrition, and Metabolism, 37*(6), 1118–1123. https://doi.org/10.1139/h2012-139

Holm-Denoma, J. M., Joiner, T. E., Vohs, K. D., & Heatherton, T. F. (2008). The "freshman fifteen" (the "freshman five" actually): Predictors and possible explanations. *Health Psychology, 27*(1S), S3–S9. https://doi.org/10.1037/0278-6133.27.1.S3

Huang, T. T.-K., Harris, K. J., Lee, R. E., Nazir, N., Worn, W., & Kaur, H. (2003). Assessing overweight, obesity, diet, and physical activity in college students. *Journal of American College Health, 52*(2), 83–86. https://doi.org/10.1080/07448480309595728

Huhman, M., Heitzler, C., & Wong, F. (2004). The VERB™ campaign logic model: A tool for planning and evaluation. *Preventing Chronic Disease, 1*(3), 1–6. https://www.cdc.gov/pcd/issues/2004/jul/04_0033.htm

Jorgensen, D. L. (1989). *Participant observation: A methodology for human studies.* SAGE.

Kidder, D. P., & Chapel, T. J. (2018). CDC's program evaluation journey: 1999 to present. *Public Health Reports, 133*, 356–359. https://doi.org/10.1177/0033354918778034

Kotler, P., & Lee, N. R. (2008). *Social marketing: Influencing behaviors for good* (3rd ed.). SAGE.

Kreps, G. L. (2014). Evaluating health communication programs to enhance health care and health promotion. *Journal of Health Communication, 19*(12), 1449–1459. https://doi.org/10.1080/10810730.2014.954080

Moen, R. D., & Norman, C. L. (2010). *Circling back: Clearing up myths about the Deming cycle and seeing how it keeps evolving.* http://www.apiweb.org/circling-back.pdf

National Cancer Institute. (2001). *Making health communication programs work.* US Department of Health & Human Services. https://www.cancer.gov/publications/health-communication/pink-book.pdf

Palmer, E. (1981). Shaping persuasive messages with formative research. In R. E. Rice & W. J. Paisley (Eds.), *Public communication campaigns* (pp. 227–238). SAGE.

Pope, L., Hansen, D., & Harvey, J. (2017). Examining the weight trajectory of college students. *Journal of Nutrition Education and Behavior, 49*(2), 137–141. https://doi.org/10.1016/j.jneb.2016.10.014

Racette, S. B., Deusinger, S. S., Strube, M. J., Highstein, G. R., & Deusinger, R. H. (2005). Weight changes, exercise, and dietary patterns during freshman and sophmore years of college. *Journal of American College Health, 53*(6), 245–251. https://doi.org/10.3200/JACH.53.6.245-251

Riegelman, R., & Kirkwood, B. (2015). *Public health 101: Healthy people-healthy populations* (2nd ed.). Jones & Bartlett.

Roberto, A. J. (2014). Evaluation methods, quantitative. In T. L. Thompson (Ed.), *Encyclopedia of health communication* (pp. 456–461). SAGE.

Roberto, A. J. (2015). Healthy people initiative. In G. A. Colditz & G. J. Golson (Eds.), *Encyclopedia of cancer and society* (2nd ed., pp. 533–534). SAGE.

Roberto, A. J., Murray-Johnson, L., & Witte, K. (2011). International health communication campaigns in developing countries. In T. Thompson, R. Parrott, & J. Nussbaum (Eds.), *The Routledge handbook of health communication* (2nd ed., pp. 220–234). Routledge.

Sanders, R. P., Evans, M. H., & Joshi, P. (2005). Developing a process-evaluation plan for assessing health promotion program implementation: A how-to guide. *Health Promotion Practice, 6*(2), 134–147. https://doi.org/10.1177/1524839904273387

Shadish, W. R., Cook, T. D., & Campbell, D. T. (2001). *Experimental and quasi-experimental designs for generalized causal inference.* Houghton Mifflin Company.

U.S. Department of Health and Human Services. (2008). *2008 physical activity guidelines for Americans.* https://health.gov/paguidelines/pdf/paguide.pdf

U.S. Department of Health and Human Services. (2010a). *Healthy People 2020* [Brochure]. U.S. Government Printing Office.

U.S. Department of Health and Human Services. (2010b). *The program manager's guide to evaluation* (2nd ed.). Author.

U.S. Department of Health and Human Services. (2016). *2020 topics and objectives.* https://www.healthypeople.gov/2020/topics-objectives

Weiss, C. H. (1998). *Evaluation: Methods for studying programs and policies* (2nd ed.). Prentice Hall.

Witte, K., Cameron, K. A., McKeon, J. K., & Berkowitz, J. M. (1996). Predicting risk behaviors: Development and validation of a diagnostic scale. *Journal of Health Communication, 1*(4), 317–341. https://doi.org/10.1080/108107396127988

World Health Organization. (2013). *WHO evaluation practice handbook.* Author.

W. P. Kellogg Foundation. (2001). *Using logic models to bring together planning, evaluation, and action: Logic model development guide.* Author.

## CHAPTER 3

# Social Marketing: A Consumer-Based Approach to Health Promotion

## CHAPTER OUTLINE

I. Introduction
II. Social Marketing
    A. Social Marketing Benchmarks
        1. Behavior Change
        2. Audience Research
        3. Audience Segmentation
            a. Generic Messages
            b. Targeted Messages
            c. Tailored Messages
        4. Exchange
        5. The Marketing Mix and "The 4Ps"
            a. Product
                (1) Attributes of Product That Influence Its Rate of Adoption
                    (a) Relative Advantage
                    (b) Compatibility
                    (c) Complexity
                    (d) Trialability
                    (e) Observability
            b. Price
            c. Place
            d. Promotion
        6. Competition
        7. Theory
III. The Health Communication Program Cycle
    A. Stage 1: Planning and Strategy Development
        1. Background and Need
        2. Goals, Objectives, and Strategies
        3. Preproduction Formative Evaluation

## INTRODUCTION

As noted previously, designing effective public health communication interventions requires careful planning based on a wide variety of information. Broadly speaking, there are two general approaches to intervention planning (Collins et al., 2010; Lindridge et al., 2013; Snelling, 2014; Wymer, 2011). One approach focuses on how individual-level variables such as beliefs, attitudes, and intentions influence behavior. This view is traditionally adopted by the social marketing approach to health promotion and is the focus of this chapter. Another approach considers how individual, relationship, community, and societal factors interact to influence behavior. This is the view taken by the ecological approach to health promotion, which is reviewed in Chapter 4. More recently, there have been growing calls to blend the social marketing and ecological approaches to health promotion (Andreasen, 2006; Collins et al., 2010; Kotler & Lee, 2008; Lindridge et al., 2013; Wymer, 2011). This is not surprising; while there are some notable differences between these approaches, they also share much in common (see Chapter 2). However, an important step toward combining these two popular approaches is to first understand them each individually.

With this in mind, I begin this chapter by defining social marketing and reviewing seven benchmarks that represent the hallmark of the social marketing approach. This chapter concludes with an overview of the Health Communication Program Cycle (National Cancer Institute, 2001), which is a four-stage approach to designing, implementing, and evaluating public health communication interventions based on the social marketing framework. In the *next* chapter I will review the ecological approach to health promotion and discuss the PRECEDE-PROCEED Model (Green & Kreuter, 2005) which is a planning model based on the ecological framework.

## SOCIAL MARKETING

*Social marketing* is the use of commercial marketing techniques to design, implement, and evaluate interventions aimed at influencing behaviors in ways that benefit both individuals and society. This definition includes four key components, which are briefly introduced here and discussed in detail throughout this chapter. First, social marketing uses commercial marketing techniques. These include a consumer orientation, audience research, audience segmentation, exchange theory, and the marketing mix or 4Ps (product, price, place, promotion). Second, social marketing is a systematic planning process. That is, it provides several manageable steps that help intervention planners better assess needs, set objectives and goals, and design, implement, and evaluate message strategies to reach these objectives and goals. Third, social marketing focuses on behavior, not just beliefs, attitudes, and intentions. Further, while social marketing traditionally focuses on influencing the voluntary behaviors of individuals, more contemporary efforts have shifted toward influencing various relationship, community, and societal factors that impact individual behavior. Finally, social marketing seeks to improve both the lives of individuals and society as a whole. That is, social marketers target individuals to get them to adopt healthier, safer, or more sustainable practices, which in turn should positively impact public health and safety, the environment, and so forth.

While there are several similarities between commercial marketing and social marketing (including audience research, audience segmentation, exchange theory, and the marketing mix or 4Ps), there are also some notable differences. To illustrate, Kotler and Lee (2008) identify four key distinctions:

1. Traditional marketing is used to sell goods and services, while social marketing is used to sell a desired behavior.

2. The primary goal of traditional marketing is financial gain, whereas the primary goal of social marketing is societal gain.

3. The competition in traditional marketing is usually other organizations offering similar or related goods or services, while the competition in social marketing is the current or preferred behavior of the intended audience.

4. Traditional marketing is less difficult as it typically wields considerable financial resources to sell products or services that customers want or need, whereas social marketing is more difficult as it involves few(er) financial resources and selling behaviors that the customer may not prefer to do.

Please keep these similarities and differences in mind when reading the key social marketing benchmarks in the next section.

## SOCIAL MARKETING BENCHMARKS

A benchmark provides a common point of reference by which something can be evaluated or compared. Thus, *social marketing benchmarks* provide a common standard for assessing the quality of social marketing interventions. The social marketing benchmarks discussed in this section serve at least two important functions. First, they help identify the key elements of social marketing interventions (i.e., what can legitimately be called social marketing; Andreasen, 2002). Second, they identify both a general process that can be employed and specific tasks that can be performed to improve the impact of social marketing interventions (National Social Marketing Centre, 2010). Several different sets of social marketing benchmarks have been advanced (e.g., Almestahiri et al., 2017; Andreasen, 2002; National Social Marketing Centre, 2010; Xia et al., 2016). In this chapter I will focus on the following seven common social marketing benchmarks: (1) behavior change, (2) audience research, (3) audience segmentation, (4) exchange, (5) marketing mix or 4Ps, (6) attention to competing behaviors, and (7) theory.

The first six benchmarks were originally advanced by Andreasen (2002) to identify key elements that can improve the impact of a social marketing intervention. The seventh benchmark was added by the National Social Marketing Centre (2010) to reflect the importance of using theory to guide decision-making during all aspects of the social marketing process. Xia et al. (2016) further subdivided the audience research and marketing mix benchmarks into their component parts to capture the social marketing planning process more fully (see Table 3.1). More specifically, audience research is subdivided into the following five categories: (a) primary preproduction formative evaluation research, (b) secondary formative evaluation research, (c) primary post-production formative evaluation research, (d) process evaluation monitoring research, and (e) outcome or impact evaluation research. Similarly, the marketing mix is subdivided into the following six categories: (a) core product, (b) actual product, (c) augmented product, (d) price, (e) place, and (f) promotion.

Research suggests that the presence of these social marketing benchmarks is indeed associated with intervention success. To illustrate, Xia et al. (2016) assessed the relationship between number and type of social marketing benchmarks and intervention effectiveness. They identified 92 social marketing interventions designed to promote physical activity among adults and coded them using a set of benchmarks and sub-benchmarks similar to those presented in Table 3.1. General results indicated that the number of social marketing benchmarks was positively related to intervention success. More specifically, primary formative research, actual product, core product, augmented product, and attention to competing behaviors each had a significant impact on intervention effectiveness.

In sum, these social marketing benchmarks provide a useful framework for assessing the extent to which an intervention is consistent with the social marketing approach

| | TABLE 3.1 Social Marketing Benchmarks | |
|---|---|---|
| **Benchmark** | **Definition** | |
| 1. | Behavior | Interventions focus on influencing (i.e., shaping, changing, or reinforcing) actual behavior, not just beliefs, attitudes, and intentions. |
| 2a. | Primary Preproduction Formative Evaluation Research | Collection of original data to learn about and better understand the intended audience *before* intervention materials are developed. |
| 2b. | Secondary Formative Evaluation Research | Review past literature to learn about and better understand the health problem or intended audience *before* intervention materials are developed. |
| 2c. | Primary Post-Production Formative Evaluation Research | Collection of original data *after* draft intervention materials are developed (but before they are finalized) to better understand the intended audience's reactions to draft messages. |
| 2d. | Process Evaluation Monitoring Research | Assess whether the intervention strategies were implemented as planned. |
| 2e. | Outcome and Impact Evaluation Research | Assess whether the intervention achieved its objectives and goals. |
| 3. | Segmentation | Divide the population into relatively homogenous subgroups in strategically meaningful ways that allow you to modify your intervention for each subgroup. |
| 4. | Exchange | The central element of any influence strategy involves creating attractive alternatives that encourage healthy behaviors and discourage unhealthy behaviors (typically via the product, price, and place elements from the marketing mix benchmark). |
| 5a. | Product (Actual) | The recommended behavior that you want the intended audience to adopt or "buy." |
| 5b. | Product (Core) | The benefits of adopting or "buying" the recommended behavior. |
| 5c. | Product (Augmented) | Any other intervention components that make the recommended behavior easier or more appealing to perform. |
| 5d. | Price | Any costs or barriers the consumer associates with adopting the recommended behavior (i.e., the actual product). |
| 5e. | Place | Where and when the intended audience will perform the recommended behavior, interact with the intervention, or obtain products and services. |
| 5f. | Promotion | The messages you will use to inform, remind, and persuade the intended audience, and the communication channels you will use to disseminate these messages. |
| 6. | Competition | Acknowledges competing behaviors (and the costs and benefits of competing behaviors) that decrease the likelihood that the intended audience will perform the recommended behavior. |
| 7. | Theory | Social marketing is a planning process that uses theory to inform decisions related to all other social marketing benchmarks. |

Note: 2a–e represents each of the five key elements of the audience research benchmark, and 5a–f represents the six key elements of the marketing mix (or 4Ps) benchmark.
Adapted from Andreasen (2002), Kotler and Lee (2008), National Social Marketing Centre (2010), and Xia et al. (2016).

and identifying opportunities to potentially increase the impact of an intervention (Shams, 2018). Furthermore, research indicates that these benchmarks are associated with intervention success. As you read more about each of the seven benchmarks below, please keep in mind that they work best when considered as a set of integrated concepts rather than individually.

## Behavior Change

The aim of social marketing is to influence behavior; or what people actually do; "simply gaining acceptance of an idea without inducing action is not success" (Andreasen, 2002, p. 7). As a reminder, in this context the word "influence" may mean any or all of the following. First, you might try to get the intended audience to accept a new behavior that did not exist or that they did not know about before (i.e., response shaping). Or, you might try to get them to stop engaging in an unhealthy behavior or to start engaging in a healthy behavior (i.e., response changing). Or, you might try to get them to stay committed or become more committed to a behavior they are already engaging in (i.e., response reinforcing).

The emphasis on behavior represents a notable distinction between health communication and social marketing. That is, while health communication interventions often seek to influence beliefs, attitudes, intentions, or behavior, social marketing programs must also include specific, measurable, achievable, relevant, and time-bound behavioral objectives. In short, the "bottom line" of social marketing is influencing behavior; and providing information and convincing people of the rightness of certain beliefs are only useful in social marketing if they lead to behavior change (Andreasen, 1994).

## Audience Research

As Andreasen (1997) notes, "the essence of the social marketing mind-set is a fanatical devotion to being customer driven" (p. 7). One of the ways this obsession with the consumer manifests itself in social marketing is via continuous audience research. *Audience research* is a systematic way of learning about or gathering information from the target market to improve the planning and effectiveness of your intervention. The purpose of audience research is to find out as much as possible about the intended audience's beliefs, attitudes, intentions, and behaviors with respect to the health issue in general and your intervention in particular. As a reminder, market research can take place before (formative evaluation), during (process evaluation), or after (outcome evaluation) your intervention is designed or implemented.

Also, as you saw in Table 3.1, audience research includes any or all of the following five distinct activities (Xia et al., 2016). The first is *primary preproduction formative evaluation research,* which involves collecting original data to understand the intended audience (typically via individual interviews, focus groups, or surveys). Second, you can conduct *secondary formative evaluation research*, which involves reviewing any existing literature about the health problem or the intended audience (typically using federal, state, or local health statistics or from medical, public health, or communication journals). Third, you can conduct *primary postproduction formative evaluation research*, which involves collecting original data to understand the intended audience's reaction to draft messages (typically via individual interviews, focus groups, and surveys, or a small-scale experiment or pilot test). Fourth, you can conduct *process evaluation monitoring research* to assess whether the intervention strategies were implemented as planned (typically via focus groups, surveys, in-depth individual interviews, field observations, and naturally collected records). Finally, you can conduct *outcome or impact evaluation research*, which will tell you how well the intervention met its objectives and goals (typically via experiments and quasi-experiments).

In sum, social marketers put the customer or intended audience at the center of everything they do. They regularly build partnerships with and seek feedback from the intended audience before, during, and after an intervention is developed and implemented. Social marketers seek to understand where the intended audience is starting from before designing the intervention, how they react during intervention implementation, and how they have changed after the intervention.

### Audience Segmentation

*Audience segmentation* involves dividing a population into relatively similar subgroups in strategically meaningful ways so you can customize your intervention for each subgroup. Selecting the target audience(s) for your intervention is a three-step process that involves (1) segmenting the market, (2) evaluating the segments, and (3) choosing one or more segments to target (Kotler & Lee, 2008). Markets can be segmented using any number or combination of geographic (i.e., region, population density, or climate), demographic (i.e., age, gender, race, ethnicity, income, occupation, or education), psychographic (i.e., beliefs, attitudes, motivations, and lifestyle), or behavioral (i.e., stage of change, usage rate, or usage status) variables. Regardless of which audience segmentation strategy is used, the ultimate goal is to identify subgroups that have something relevant in common; something that will increase the likelihood that they will respond to an intervention in similar ways.

Donovan et al. (1999) present a useful approach for evaluating segments and choosing which segments to target (they use the acronym "TARPARE" to make this approach easier to remember). This approach evaluates the identified segments using the following six criteria:

1. Total number of people in the segment. Larger segments are generally assigned greater priority as even small shifts in large populations can have meaningful benefits. At a minimum, a segment should be large enough to have a potential impact on the problem.

2.  **A**t **R**isk people in the segment. Higher risk segments are generally assigned higher priority as they are more likely to yield a greater return on investments.

3.  **P**ersuasibility of the target audience. Segments that are more likely to change their behaviors are generally assigned a higher priority as they are more likely to be cost-effective.

4.  **A**ccessibility of the target audience. Segments that are easier to reach through various communicating channels are generally assigned a higher priority as this is more likely to lead to effective outcomes.

5.  **R**esources required to meet the needs of the target audience. Segments that can be served by fewer or current financial, human, and structural resources are generally assigned a higher priority as they typically result in a greater return on investment.

6.  **E**quity and social justice considerations. Specific disadvantaged segments may not meet one or more of the above criteria, but they still warrant attention for equity reasons.

In sum, this approach helps programs planners systematically compare, contrast, and prioritize potential target audiences for public health communication interventions. Targeting high scoring segments should lead to greater success and a better return on investment, which is especially important when resources are limited.

Finally, before moving on to the next social marketing benchmark, it is worth noting that developments in technology not only make it easier to target messages to specific subgroups, but it also makes it possible to tailor messages to specific individuals. Given the growing importance of computer tailored messages in virtually every aspect of our lives, a discussion of generic, targeted, and tailored messages follows (and a visual representation of the key differences between these three types of messages is presented in Figure 3.1).

**Generic Messages.** *Generic messages* are designed to reach many individuals in the general population but are not customized to any subgroup or individual within that population (Kreuter et al., 2000; Roberto, 2010). Generic messages "typically aspire to be all things to all people, providing a single comprehensive set of information about a specific content area" (Kreuter et al., 2000, p. 4). In other words, at least some of the information in a generic message will be relevant to everyone, but everyone will have to search through a lot of potentially irrelevant information to find the facts that apply to them.

Outside of a health context, free broadcast television networks such as ABC, CBS, NBC, and PBS are good examples of generic messages. Even the most coveted age group of 18- to 49-year-olds is very broad, and these networks also offer programing for a wide variety of

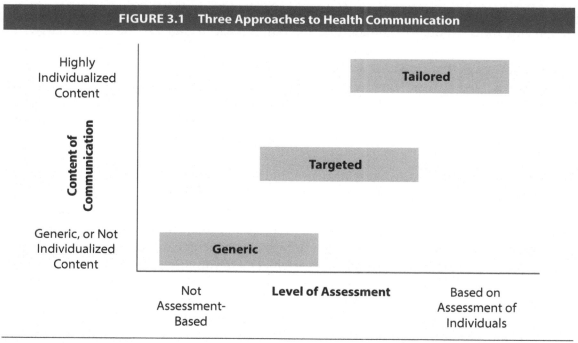

**FIGURE 3.1    Three Approaches to Health Communication**

Adapted from Kreuter et al. (2000).

other audiences throughout the day and week. In short, just about everyone will find some interesting content on broadcast television, but they will also have to sift through a considerable amount of less relevant or interesting shows to find the ones they want to watch.

Bringing the discussion back to public health communication interventions, suppose you wanted to create a fact sheet to encourage people to eat less red and processed meats. There are many good reasons a person might choose to eat less meat, including health, environmental, and animal welfare concerns (Fehrenbach et al., 2016). For example, some people might be motivated by health concerns given that high meat consumption is associated with several chronic health issues such as cardiovascular disease, several types of cancer, and diabetes. Other people may be motivated by environmental concerns given that industrial farm animal production contributes to climate change, resource depletion, and pollution. Other people might be motivated by animal welfare, since today's farm animals are not raised on farms, but rather are raised in industrial production systems where they are cruelly treated and raised in confined living conditions that inhibit natural behaviors. Further, different people may prefer different ways to reduce meat consumption, including eating smaller portions when they do eat meat, skipping meat one day a week as advocated by the "Meatless Monday" campaign, or including meat in one less meal each day. With little information about who might receive your fact sheet, it would be necessary to create a generic message that provided some information about all these concerns to make sure everyone received at least some relevant information that might be motivating to them. Given that space would be limited, you would not be able to provide an in-depth discussion of any of these reasons. Instead, the reader would have to review all the information you did provide to find the information that was worthwhile to them.

**Targeted Messages.** *Targeted messages* use audience segmentation principles to create materials designed to reach a specific subgroup of the general population that is similar in one or more ways (Kreuter et al., 2000; Roberto, 2010). Targeted messages employ some degree of customization to increase the relevance of a message to the subgroup. For example, you might develop targeted messages for a group of people of a certain age, gender, or socioeconomic status (i.e., demographic variables). Or you might develop such messages for a group of people who share the same cultural values or lifestyle (i.e., psychographic variables). According to Kreuter et al. targeted messages are an improvement over generic messages because they take important characteristics of a subgroup into account and use some customization to increase the relevance of the message to individuals within that subgroup. However, targeted messages use a single version of a message to communicate with all members of a subgroup, and therefore do not address important factors that likely vary from person to person.

To continue with our media example from the previous section, cable television offers a wide variety of targeted television choices. Lifetime targets 18- to 49-year-old women, Spike TV targets 18- to 49-year-old men, Nickelodeon targets 8- to 17-year-old children and adolescents, and BET targets African American audiences. If you like sports, you can turn to ESPN and if you like the news you can watch CNN. In short, the goal of each of these channels is to use some degree of customization to attract individuals from various target audiences.

Continuing with our public health communication intervention example, the three motivations for eating less red and processed meats (i.e., health, environment, and animal welfare) would be good ways to target a series of fact sheets to specific intended audiences. Instead of providing generic information about all three of these motivations and distributing to everyone, you could create a separate targeted fact sheet for each of these three audiences. There are likely to be other factors that vary from person to person that your targeted pamphlet cannot consider (such as perceived benefits and barriers, perceptions of threat and efficacy, and readiness for change—see below). However, targeting in this way will allow you to provide a greater amount of more relevant information to the appropriate people.

**Tailored Messages.** *Tailored messages* are intended to reach one specific person based on characteristics that are unique to that person (Kreuter et al., 2000). Tailored messages use a high degree of customization to increase the relevance of a message for the individual. Unlike targeted messages that customize at the group level, tailored messages are designed to focus on the individual. The degree to which messages are customized ranges from "minimal tailoring," meaning the message focuses on just one or two theoretically significant constructs, to complex messages that incorporate multiple demographics psychographic or theoretical variables (Rimer & Kreuter, 2006). Tailored messages are typically created by asking individuals to answer a series of questions (e.g., about their beliefs or behavior), and then using a computer algorithm (i.e., a series of instructions or decision rules) to generate messages that are highly customized to each individual.

To conclude our media examples, many digital media services such as Netflix, Hulu, and Amazon Prime rely heavily on tailored messages in the form of recommendations. To illustrate, they all use a more passive form of tailoring when they make recommendations based on shows you have watched in the past. Further, they all use a more active form of tailoring when they ask you to rate the shows you have watched and adjusts their recommendations based on those you liked and disliked. Most streaming services even allow you to create different profiles for different users in your household, so they can more accurately tailor recommendations to whoever is watching at a given time.

To conclude our public health communication intervention example of trying to convince someone to eat less red and processed meats, in addition to targeting your messages based on the primary reason a person might make this change (i.e., health, environment, or animal welfare), you could also personally tailor your fact sheet in one or more of the following ways. For example, you might begin by asking an individual what they see as the biggest benefits and barriers to making this change (see Health Believe Model in Chapter 6). Then, rather than addressing every benefit and barrier with every person, you could print out a customized fact sheet for each individual that focuses on *just* their motivations. Alternatively, you could tailor messages based on an individual's perceptions of threat and efficacy. Here you would first ask a series of questions to assess an individual's perceived levels of severity, susceptibility, response-efficacy, and self-efficacy (see the Extended Parallel Process Model in Chapter 8), and then print out a fact sheet focusing on just those perceptions that needed to be increased. Further, you could tailor the information you provide based on an individual's readiness for change, which has been shown to be particularly effective (Krebs et al., 2010; Noar et al., 2009; Rimer & Kreuter, 2006). This type of tailoring would first assess a person's stage of change (i.e., precontemplation, contemplation, preparation, action, and maintenance—see the Transtheoretical Model in Chapter 10), and then print out a fact sheet specifically tailored to their current stage of change. Of course, you could also tailor your message based on two or more of these approaches, and these are just a few of the many different possibilities.

In conclusion, computer-tailored messages can be a cost-effective way to reach a large number of individuals with customized content. Further, their on-demand nature has the added potential to reach anyone, anywhere, and at any time if they have the necessary equipment. Finally, computer-tailored messages share some of the benefits of both the mass media and interpersonal communication in that they can reach a large number of individuals with messages that are both interactive and easily adapted.

### Exchange

In social marketing, *exchange* involves creating attractive alternatives that encourage healthy behaviors and discourage unhealthy behaviors. Thus, much of social marketing is rooted in exchange theory, which posits that people behave in ways that will maximize their benefits and minimize their costs (Blau, 1964; Homans, 1958; Thibaut & Kelley, 1959). *Benefits* are the positive aspects or consequences of a given behavior, or anything that makes the behavior easier to perform. Conversely, *costs* are the disadvantages of the behavior, or anything that makes the behavior more difficult to perform. To illustrate using a simple example from traditional marketing, companies typically offer tangible goods or intangible services (the benefit) in exchange for customers' money (the cost).

In social marketing, the voluntary exchange need not be between the intervention developer and the intended audience (though it can be). Instead, the exchange revolves around what the intended audience gets or must give up when adopting a new behavior. For example, "Is the recommended behavior safe and effective?" "Is it convenient, easy, and enjoyable to do?" "Does it save time or money?" "Yes" answers to these and similar questions represent potential benefits—and "No" answers represent potential costs—of engaging in the new behavior. Returning to our physical activity example, individuals who believe that the longer-term benefits of looking and feeling their best (and living a longer, healthier, and happier life) outweigh the shorter-term costs of time and effort spent (or inconvenience or discomfort experienced) will have a positive cost-benefit ratio and therefore be more likely to exercise.

In short, "a key task in social marketing is to develop an 'exchange proposition' that sets out what people have to do and/or the cost of this action in order to get the value that they want" (European Centre for Disease Prevention and Control, 2014, p. 8). At a minimum, perceived benefits should be equal to or greater than perceived costs. Ideally, the benefits will be so great and the costs so minimal that most people will comply (Andreasen, 2002). The concept of exchange is intricately related to product, price, and place elements from the marketing mix benchmark, which is discussed next.

## The Marketing Mix and "The 4Ps"

The phrases "marketing mix" and "the 4Ps" were coined in the 1960s by Neil Borden (1964) and Jerome McCarthy (1964) respectively and adapted for use in social marketing by Kotler and Zaltman (1971). While these two phrases are often used interchangeably, they are somewhat different. The term *marketing mix* is a general term used to describe a set of decisions (social) marketers make to increase the intended audiences' demand for a product or behavior. For example, the original marketing mix presented by Borden (1964) included 12 elements: (1) product planning, (2) pricing, (3) branding, (4) channels of distribution, (5) personal selling, (6) advertising, (7) promotions, (8) packaging, (9) display, (10) servicing, (11) physical handling, and (12) fact finding and analysis. Today, *the 4Ps* (a.k.a., product, price, place, and promotion) represent a common example of a marketing mix.

A marketing mix in general, and the 4Ps in particular, are essential social marketing tools that help ensure that the right product, is offered at the right price, in the right place, and promoted in the right way. However, "the 4Ps in social marketing mix strategies cannot be developed in isolation—it is the 'mix,' or 'synergy,' of the 4Ps that makes a truly successful social marketing campaign possible" (Cheng et al., 2011, p. 9). Please keep this in mind as you read about each element of the 4Ps below.

**Product.** Generally speaking, the product is what you are marketing. In traditional marketing, a product is typically a tangible good or intangible service that a company offers the customer. In the realm of social marketing, however, the term *product* refers to the behavior, and the benefits of the behavior, that you are promoting. In other words, social marketers think of products "as a constellation of benefits" that make engaging in the recommended behavior more enticing (Storey et al., 2015, p. 414). Kotler and Lee (2008) divide products into three levels: core product, actual product, and augmented product. Having a clear understanding and description of each level is an essential part of the social marketing process.

The *core product* refers to the perceived benefits of adopting or "buying" the behavior. In other words, why is the recommended behavior valuable to the intended audience? For example, not only will exercise help you look and feel your best, but it can also lead to a longer, healthier, and happier life. As always, it is important that you emphasize the benefits that will be most appealing to the intended audience, which can be assessed through formative evaluation. The *actual product* refers to the behavior that you want the intended audience to adopt or "buy." This is probably what most people think of when they hear the word "product"; though they probably think of it more in terms of goods and services than in terms of adopting a healthy behavior. The actual product is closely linked to a public health communication intervention's intermediate objective. For example, in Chapter 2, one of the intermediate objectives of our hypothetical intervention was to increases physical activity among college students. In this instance, physical activity represents the actual product for the intervention. Finally, the *augmented product* includes any other intervention components that make the behavior easier or more appealing to perform. For example, our hypothetical physical activity intervention included a number of strategies specifically designed to increase the perceived benefits and decrease the perceived barriers to physical activity, including the creation and promotion of personal fitness contracts, exercise buddy agreements, and campus walking groups. These strategies represent important elements of the augmented product.

***Attributes of Product That Influence Its Rate of Adoption.*** It should come as no surprise to learn that different behaviors (i.e., actual products) are adopted at different rates. Thus, the question becomes, what factors affect a behavior's rate of adoption? Research suggests that rate of adoption is associated with five factors: (1) relative advantage, (2) compatibility, (3) complexity, (4) trialability, and (5) observability (Rogers, 2003). As you read more about each of these factors below, notice how they relate to the discussion of actual, core, and augmented product in the preceding paragraph (as well as the price, place, and promotion elements of the 4Ps that will be discussed later in this section).

*Relative advantage* refers to the perceived benefits of adopting the behavior. Relative advantage might include anything ranging from greater quality, protection, comfort, or prestige, to requiring less time, effort, space, or money. For example, key advantages (or benefits) of the HPV vaccine include protection against genital warts and several types of cancer, including cancer of the mouth, throat, cervix, and penis. The greater a behavior's perceived relative advantage, the quicker its rate of adoption will be.

*Compatibility* is the degree to which a behavior is perceived as being consistent with an individual's life and lifestyle. Is it completely new and different, or is it replacing something the individual already uses or is familiar with? For example, while the HPV vaccine is compatible with most individuals' desire to protect their children, some view it as incompatible with their value of abstinence which has undoubtedly slowed down its rate of adoption despite its many benefits. The greater a behavior's perceived compatibility, the quicker its rate of adoption will be.

Perceived *complexity* refers to how easy or difficult it is to understand or adopt a behavior. For example, a vaccine that requires more doses would be considered more complex than vaccines that need a single dose. The more complex the behavior, the more difficult it will be for potential users to understand or incorporate it into their lives (therefore slowing down its rate of adoption). Hence, to the extent possible, new behaviors should be designed and introduced with simplicity in mind.

*Trialability* is the extent that the behavior can be tested or experimented with on a limited basis before adoption. People usually prefer to see what the behavior can do before committing. This helps reduce uncertainty, and is one reason products come in trial sizes, car dealers let you take test drives, grocery stores give out free samples, and many companies hire representatives to demonstrate new products. The free samples provided by pharmaceutical companies are an easy way to allow both physicians and patients to try out new drugs to learn their benefits and side effects before fully committing to a new treatment. Being able to test or try out a new behavior on a small scale first will increase its rate of adoption.

*Observability* refers to the visible benefits of performing the behavior. For example, behaviors where potential adopters can clearly see how safe and effective the behavior is by first watching someone else do it would be considered high in observability. This is another way to reduce uncertainty, and can be done in many ways including the use of statistics (using large amounts of representative data to show how things are related—e.g., studies have shown that exercise leads to a longer and happier life), side-by-side comparisons (e.g., of two crash test dummies that were and were not using seat belts), before-and-after photos (e.g., of images of individuals who participated in a particular exercise or weight loss program), or testimonials (e.g., a firsthand account from someone whose life was saved by wearing a seat belt during an accident). The more visible the benefits, the faster the behavior's rate of adoption will be.

Unfortunately, Rogers (2003) notes that the relative advantage of many health promotion and disease prevention behaviors are difficult to observe, which can hinder their rate of adoption. According to Rogers, this can happen for at least two reasons. The first reason is that some behaviors improve an individual's long-term health outcomes but have few instant changes or results. For example, you need to exercise and eat well now to prevent heart disease and cancer in the future. The second reason is that sometimes the benefit is a "non-event," or the absence of something that otherwise might have occurred. For example, using a condom can prevent pregnancy and STDs, and getting the HPV vaccine can prevent genital warts and several types of cancers. In both cases you are preventing something harmful from happening, but you do get to observe the outcome in a traditional sense.

**Price.** *Price* refers to any costs or barriers the consumer associates with adopting a behavior (i.e., the actual product). Costs and barriers can take many forms, such as monetary, social, emotional, psychological, or physical. Examples include money, time, effort, inconvenience, peer pressure, embarrassment, fear, physical exertion or discomfort, and so forth. Edgar et al. (2011) note that the process of adopting a healthier behavior is analogous to "a sophisticated game of 'let's make a deal'" (p. 239). That is, consumers will engage in a formal or informal cost-benefit analysis of engaging in the recommended behavior. As a result, social marketers must reframe the behavior in such a way that the anticipated benefits (i.e., the core product) outweigh the perceived costs. Some ways to achieve this include offering monetary and nonmonetary incentives (e.g., discounts or public recognition) or disincentives (e.g., fines or negative publicity) for adopting or not adopting the behavior respectively (Kotler & Lee, 2008).

**Place.** *Place* (a.k.a., distribution channels) refers to where and when the intended audience will perform the recommended behavior, interact with the intervention, or obtain products and services. For example, where and when do we want the intended audience to exercise (i.e., actual product)? Or how will the intended audience obtain the tangible products and services associated with the intervention such as the personal fitness contracts and exercise buddy agreements (i.e., augmented product)? Price and place considerations have much in common, as the primary purpose of both is to make performing the recommended behavior as convenient and pleasant as possible. For example, it is important to make sure (1) the walking group meetings and events are centrally located and as close as possible to the largest number of individuals, (2) the student recreation center schedule is designed to accommodate busy students, and (3) posters are placed where decisions are made (i.e., by elevators to encourage students to take the stairs instead). Kotler and Lee (2008) make an important distinction between distribution channels and communication channels. That is, distribution channels are an important element of the place component of the marketing mix (discussed here), while communication channels are an important element of the promotion component of the marketing mix (discussed next).

**Promotion.** The fourth and final element of the marketing mix is promotion. *Promotion* includes creating the messages you will use to inform, remind, and persuade the intended audience and selecting the communication channels you will use to disseminate these messages. Thus, promotion is closely related to health communication and is typically one of the most visible aspects of any social marketing undertaking. The aim here is to create demand by promoting the product, price, and place features you most want the intended audience to know about. This includes promoting the benefits of the behavior, reducing the barriers to its adoption, and providing information about where and when any tangible products or intangible services can be obtained. It is important to create messages that will resonate with the intended audience, and to distribute them on channels they are most likely to use. For example, in our hypothetical exercise promotion intervention the recommended behavior was promoted using face-to-face (i.e., live presentations), print (i.e., posters), and computer-mediated (i.e., email and social media) channels. As noted throughout this book, getting the word out and creating demand for healthy behaviors is no easy task.

To be successful, you will have to involve the intended audience in all major decisions that are made via extensive preproduction and post-production formative research.

### Competition

*Competition* refers to any behavior (including doing nothing) that decreases the likelihood that the intended audience will perform the recommended behavior. Often this will be the behavior an individual is currently engaged in, such as watching television or playing video games rather than engaging in some form of physical activity. Competition also includes the benefits of rival behaviors, which may be easier or more interesting to perform, or require less time, money, energy, motivation, and so forth. As Andreasen (1994) notes, people "often have very good reasons for maintaining the behavior they have held—often for a lifetime" (p. 48). Therefore, intervention developers must identify both (1) all major competing behaviors and (2) the most important benefits and costs associated with each behavior.

Notice how this potentially doubles the potential number of targets for the cost-benefit exchange discussed earlier in this chapter. That is, not only can intervention developers maximize the benefits and minimize the costs of the recommended behavior, but they can also downplay the benefits and highlight the costs of competing behaviors. In sum, choices do not occur in a vacuum, and every attempt to change behavior faces competition (Andreasen, 1994). Thus, it is important to identify and acknowledge competing behaviors, and to design, implement, and evaluate strategies that will give the health behavior you are promoting a competitive advantage.

### Theory

Social marketing is not a theory; it does not predict or explain how or why people behave in healthy or unhealthy ways (see Chapter 5). Instead, social marketing is a planning process or framework for developing public health communication interventions that are guided by theories from a variety of disciplines including public health, communication, and psychology (Andreasen, 2002; Kotler & Zaltman, 1971). However, the use of theory is intricately related to all other social marketing benchmarks. For example, theory provides guidance about (1) the best ways to understand and change behavior, (2) what questions to ask when conducting audience research, (3) possible ways to segment audiences, (4) potential benefits and barriers essential to the exchange process, (5) the marketing mix, and (6) competing behaviors.

Theories commonly employed by social marketers include the health belief model, social cognitive theory, protection motivation theory or the extended parallel process model, the theory of reasoned action or the theory of planned behavior, and the transtheoretical model (Almestahiri et al., 2017; Andreasen, 1997, 2002; Helmig & Thaler, 2010).

Thus, each of these theories is covered in detail in a chapter included in Section 3 of this book. In sum, predicting, explaining, and changing health behavior is a complex and difficult process. Thus, using existing theory and research to guide intervention planning and evaluation both saves time and money and allows for a more systematic and efficient advancement of science (Witte & Roberto, 2009).

## THE HEALTH COMMUNICATION PROGRAM CYCLE

The *Health Communication Program Cycle* (National Cancer Institute [NCI], 2001) is a four-stage approach to planning, implementing, and evaluating public health communication interventions based on the social marketing framework. The Health Communication Program Cycle includes the following four stages:

Stage 1: Planning and Strategy Development
Stage 2: Developing and Pretesting
Stage 3: Implementing the Program
Stage 4: Assessing Effectiveness and Making Refinements

Table 3.2 provides a brief description of each stage, Figure 3.2 provides a visual representation of these four stages, and a detailed discussion of each of these stages follows.

| TABLE 3.2    Brief Description of the Four Stages of the Health Communication Program Cycle | |
|---|---|
| **Stage** | **Description** |
| Planning and Strategy Development | Create the plan that will serve as the blueprint for your program; includes assessing background and need, creating goals, objectives, and strategies, and conducting formative evaluation. |
| Developing and Pretesting | Determine what messages and materials will be most effective for your topic and intended audience; includes reviewing existing materials, developing the program, and pretesting, revising, and finalizing your messages. |
| Implementing the Program | Implement the communication strategies that were developed for your program and conduct process evaluation to assess how well the implementation is going (and making corrections if needed). |
| Assessing Effectiveness and Making Refinements | Conduct outcome evaluation to determine if the program met its short-term and intermediate objectives; and revising your objectives and creating new communication strategies for current or additional contexts or intended audiences. |

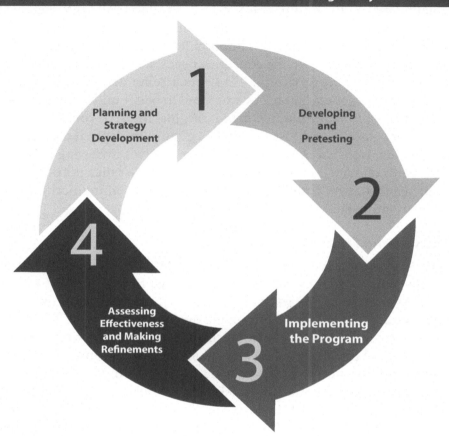

FIGURE 3.2   The Health Communication Program Cycle

Adapted from National Cancer Institute (2001).

## STAGE 1: PLANNING AND STRATEGY DEVELOPMENT

In Stage 1, planning and strategy development, you create the plan that will serve as the blueprint or roadmap for your intervention. Stage 1 consists of three main steps: (1) assessing the background and need regarding the health problem and intended audience; (2) creating goals, objectives, and strategies that allow you to address these needs; and (3) conducting preproduction formative evaluation to learn about the intended audience, and to help you select appropriate settings, channels, and activities to best address the health problem and reach your intended audience (NCI, 2001). A discussion of each of these steps follows.

## *Background and Need*

The better you understand the health issue you want to address and the intended audience you want to target, the better your chances of designing a successful public health communication intervention. Audience analysis is important because it helps you create and refine interventions that are responsive to the concerns, needs, and perspectives of the intended audience that you wish to reach (Kreps, 2014). As a reminder, primary and secondary research data are the two general strategies employed to better understand the health issue and intended audience. *Primary research data* is original research conducted by the intervention planner for a specific purpose (e.g., focus groups, in-depth individual interviews, surveys, experiments, etc.). *Secondary research data* involves reviewing existing research that was previously conducted by someone else or for some other purpose (e.g., federal, state, and local health statistics, medical, public health, and communication journals, the Healthy People Initiative, etc.).

## *Goals, Objectives, and Strategies*

Goals, objectives, and strategies were discussed in detail in Chapter 2, but are briefly reviewed here given they are an essential element of Stage 1 of the Health Communication Program Cycle. As a reminder, (1) *goals* relate to the overall health improvement that you want your intervention to make (e.g., improving quality or quantity of life); (2) *objectives* relate to the specific cognitive and behavioral changes you want your intervention to produce (e.g., changing beliefs, attitudes, intentions, and behavior); and (3) *strategies* are the specific health communication activities you will take to accomplish your objectives (e.g., the intervention's messages and materials). Also, as a reminder, this part of the planning process involves working backward (i.e., you start with your goal and then work backward to develop a plan to reach this goal). Visually, the process will look something like this:

$$(3) \text{ Strategies} \longrightarrow (2) \text{ Objectives} \longrightarrow (1) \text{ Goal}$$

## *Preproduction Formative Evaluation*

A hallmark of social marketing is the use of formative evaluation to increase the chances that an intervention will reach and meet the needs of the intended audience. As a reminder, *formative evaluation* is conducted during the early stages of development to improve the design and implementation of an intervention. Formative evaluation is valuable because health communicators often lack the perspective of the "average" person (Atkin & Freimuth, 1989). Thus, it is important to collect primary research data directly from the intended audience during the program planning process; typically, via individual interviews, focus groups, and survey research.

Also, as a reminder, formative evaluation should take place before (i.e., preproduction formative evaluation) and after (i.e., post-production formative evaluation) intervention messages or materials are developed. Stage 1 of the Health Communication Program Cycle focuses on *preproduction formative evaluation*, which seeks to gain insights into and input from the intended audience before any messages and materials are developed. For example, preproduction formative evaluation is often used to generate ideas for intervention materials, obtain feedback on rough concepts, gather baseline data that will allow you to set realistic objectives, and select a theory to guide the intervention.

## STAGE 2: DEVELOPING AND PRETESTING

By the time you have completed Stage 1 of the Health Communication Program Cycle, planning and strategy development, you should have a better understanding of the problem you plan to address, who it affects, and how to best respond. Stage 2, developing and pretesting, is important because it provides early information about what messages and materials will be most effective for your topic and intended audience (NCI, 2001). During this stage you will (1) review existing materials, (2) develop and refine your intervention, and (3) pretest, revise, and finalize your messages. A discussion of each of these steps follows.

### Review Existing Materials

Developing public health communication interventions is time-consuming and costly. An effective way to save both time and money is to conduct a resource inventory and needs assessment. A *resource inventory* is a systematic process for gathering information about what materials already exist on a topic, and for which intended audiences. For example, a simple Google search will reveal many existing messages designed to increase physical activity, including websites, public service announcements, images, signs, posters, pamphlets, billboards, and more. Also, for example, you can contact the creators of any resources you identify to learn more about these materials and see if they are aware of any other interventions you have not yet identified. A *needs assessment*, or *gap analysis*, reviews existing materials to determine if any gaps exist. For example, have messages been created using some communication channels but not others? Or, do materials exist for some intended audiences but not for other important audiences? In tandem, a resource inventory and needs assessment are important ways to justify the necessity of creating a new public health communication intervention or revising an existing one.

### Develop and Refine Your Intervention

Once you know what you need to include in your intervention, it is time to develop and refine your specific messages and materials, or communication strategies. As always, each message strategy should be guided by preproduction formative evaluation results and developed with previous theory and research in mind. Further, all messages should be specifically designed to help you reach your public health communication intervention's objectives and goals.

### Pretest, Revise, and Finalize Your Messages

After you develop and refine your intervention, it is important to conduct additional formative evaluation research before finalizing your message. Stage 2 of the Health Communication Program Cycle includes *postproduction formative evaluation*, which involves getting feedback from the intended audience after draft messages and materials have been created but before they are finalized and implemented. This typically involves conducting another round of focus groups or individual interviews with members of the intended audience to gather their opinions about draft materials (i.e., are they clear, credible, and interesting?), or a small experiment to try out your messages, procedures, and measures before fully implementing them on a larger scale. Pretesting and revising is an iterative process that should be repeated until your messages and materials communicate the information as intended. Once you have gone through these steps, you can make one final round of revisions to your messages and materials before moving forward to Stage 3 (implementing the program) of the Health Communication Program Cycle.

### STAGE 3: IMPLEMENTING THE PROGRAM

In Stage 3, you implement the communication activities, or strategies, that were developed for your intervention. As the Centers for Disease Control and Prevention (2001) notes, it is important to "assess how well the implementation of the intervention is going and, if needed, to make corrections" (p. E-7). For example, it is important to make sure that all intervention activities take place when and where intended, to monitor the intended audience's exposure and reactions to these activities, and to make any necessary revisions when any issues arise (NCI, 2001). This is the "who," "what," "where," "when," and "how" of intervention evaluation. That is, *who* received the intervention? *What* exactly did they receive? *Where* and *when* did they receive it? And *how* did the intended audience respond? This represents an important way to make sure your intervention was implemented as intended and helps others who want to replicate or adapt your intervention in the future.

### Process Evaluation

As a reminder, the procedures for monitoring and making corrections to an intervention during the implementation stage are collectively referred to as process evaluation. More specifically, *process evaluation* is conducted during intervention implementation to make sure the intervention is executed as intended. Many different methods can provide valuable process-evaluation data. For example, fidelity and completeness are often assessed via naturally collected records or field observations. Exposure and reach can be estimated via naturally collected records or field surveys. Or, satisfaction can be examined using surveys, focus groups, or semi-structured interviews. In short, process evaluation can help you identify problems while there is still time to fix them and provides more confidence when outcome evaluation is conducted during Stage 4 (assessing effectiveness and making refinements) of the Health Communication Program Cycle.

## STAGE 4: ASSESSING EFFECTIVENESS AND MAKING REFINEMENTS

The aims of Stage 4, assessing effectiveness and making refinements, are to determine if an intervention met its objectives and to use this information to determine what changes might be necessary to improve your messages and materials in the future (NCI, 2001). This information can also be used to justify continuing your intervention, or to provide data and insights upon which future interventions can be based. In short, the focus of Stage 4 is outcome evaluation. As a reminder, *outcome evaluation* tests the cause-effect relationship between your health communication intervention (the cause) and changes in the intended audience on the key variables identified in your objectives (the effects). Thus, outcome evaluation relies heavily on *quantitative research methods*, which are those that involve the collection and statistical analysis of numerical data. Surveys and experiments are two quantitative research methods that play an important role when conducting an outcome evaluation and are discussed in detail in Chapters 12 and 13, respectively. Here, I provide a more general overview of Stage 4 of the Health Communication Program Cycle: (1) assessing effectiveness and (2) making refinements.

### Assessing Effectiveness

Even though outcome evaluation occurs during the last stage of the Health Communication Program Cycle, the task actually begins during Stage 1 (planning and strategy development). If you created SMART objectives that were **s**pecific, **m**easurable, **a**chievable, **r**elevant, and **t**ime-bound, you have already taken many important steps toward completing your outcome evaluation plan. For example, you will know who the intended audience is and have already gained access to them. You will have identified what variables you need to measure and perhaps already developed instruments to measure them. Furthermore, you will have selected an evaluation design and may even have collected baseline data before the intervention began that can be compared to the post-intervention data you collect as part of your outcome evaluation.

### Making Refinements

That is not the only connection between Stage 1 and Stage 4 of the Health Communication Program Cycle. As illustrated in Figure 3.2, the Health Communication Program Cycle is circular, which means "the end of Stage 4 is not the end of the process but the step that takes you back to Stage 1" (NCI, 2001, p. 121). For example, if certain objectives were not met, you may need to add new communication strategies (or enhance existing ones) to influence these outcomes. Or, if certain messages or materials had unintended negative consequences, you may have to significantly change or remove them. In fact, even if the intervention met all its objectives, the overarching goal will likely still require attention. As a result, you may have to revise your objectives and create new communication strategies to help improve future interventions (i.e., perhaps for new intended audiences or situations).

## CONCLUSION

This chapter introduced the concept of social marketing and reviewed the four stages of the Health Communication Program Cycle: (1) planning and strategy development, (2) developing and pretesting, (3) implementing the intervention, and (4) assessing effectiveness and making refinements. Social marketing uses commercial marketing techniques to improve the circumstances of individuals and society. The Health Communication Program Cycle is a planning process that is explicitly guided by the social marketing framework.

Social marketing traditionally concentrates its efforts on individual-level behavior change (Andreasen, 1994, 2006). This is metaphorically called *downstream social marketing*, as it directly targets individuals who are engaging in a problem behavior (as one might try to rescue people from drowning downstream, after they have fallen into a dangerous river). More recently, however, there has been a call for social marketers to focus on behavior in context rather than in isolation (Andreasen, 2006; Wallack, 2002). This is metaphorically called *upstream social marketing*, as it targets the environmental factors that impact the problem behavior (as one might try to address the problem upstream, before people fall into the dangerous river in the first place). In other words, public health communication interventions are most likely to obtain and maintain meaningful change by focusing on individual (e.g., beliefs, attitudes, intentions, and behavior), relationship (e.g., norms and relationships with important others), community (e.g., the physical environment; school, work, faith-based, business, and health care organizations), and societal (e.g., local, state, and national laws; cultural beliefs, norms, and values; the mass media) factors that impact behavior. Thus, instead of just trying to convince people to exercise (downstream social marketing), social marketers must also target the individuals, organizations, community leaders, and policy makers that are able to create an environment where the recommended behavior is little easier or more likely (upstream social marketing).

In conclusion, it is essential that public health communication interventions also focus "attention upstream to protect health rather than just trying to save people by pulling them out of the river downstream" (Wallack, 2002, p. 26). Unfortunately, social marketers rarely tap into this upstream potential (Andreasen, 2006; Almestahiri et al., 2017). However, there is another approach that does. It is called the ecological model, and it is the subject of the next chapter of this book.

## REFERENCES

Almestahiri, R., Rundle-Thiele, S., Parkinson, J., & Arli, D. (2017). The use of major components of social marketing: A systematic review of tobacco cessation programs. *Social Marketing Quarterly, 23*(3), 232–248. https://doi.org/10.1177/1524500417704813

Andreasen, A. R. (1994). Social marketing: Its definition and domain. *Journal of Public Policy and Marketing, 13*(1), 108–114. https://doi.org/10.1177/074391569401300109

Andreasen, A. R. (1997). Challenges for the science and practice of social marketing. In M. E. Goldberg, M. Fishbein, & S. E. Middlestadt (Eds.), *Social marketing: Theoretical and practical perspectives* (pp. 3–19). Lawrence Erlbaum Associates.

Andreasen, A. R. (2002). Marketing social marketing in the social change marketplace. *Journal of Public Policy and Marketing, 21*(1), 3–13. https://doi.org/10.1509/jppm.21.1.3.17602

Andreasen, A. R. (2006). *Social marketing in the 21st century.* SAGE.

Atkin, C. K., & Freimuth, V. (1989). Formative evaluation research in campaign design. In R. E. Rice, & C. K. Atkin (Eds.), *Public communication campaigns* (2nd ed., pp. 131–150). SAGE.

Blau, P. M. (1964). *Exchange and power in social life.* John Wiley.

Borden, N. H. (1964). The concept of the marketing mix. *Journal of Advertising Research, 4*, 2–7.

Centers for Disease Control and Prevention. (2001). *Program operations guidelines for STD prevention: Program evaluation.* https://www.cdc.gov/std/program/progevaluation.pdf

Cheng, H., Kotler, P., & Lee, N. R. (2011). Social marketing and public health: An introduction. In H. Cheng, P. Kotler, & N. R. Lee (Eds.), *Social marketing and public health: Global trends and success stories* (pp. 1–30). Jones & Bartlet.

Collins, K., Tapp, A., & Pressley, A. (2010). Social marketing and social influences. Using social ecology as a theoretical framework. *Journal of Marketing Management, 26*, 1181–1200. https://doi.org/10.1080/0267257X.2010.522529

Donovan, R. J., Egger, G., & Francas, M. (1999). TARPARE: A method for selecting target audiences for public health interventions. *Australian and New Zealand Journal of Public Health, 23*(3), 280–284. https://doi.org/ 10.1111/j.1467-842x.1999.tb01256.x

Edgar, T., Volkman, J. E., & Logan, A. M. B. (2011). Social marketing: Its meaning, use, and application for health communication. In T. Thompson, R. Parrott, & J. Nussbaum (Eds.), *The Routledge handbook of health communication* (2nd ed., pp. 235–251). Routledge.

European Centre for Disease Prevention and Control. (2014). *Social marketing guide for public health programme managers and practitioners.* ECDC. https://doi.org/10.2900/41449

Fehrenbach, K. S., Righter, A. C., & Santo, R. (2016). A critical examination of the available data sources for estimating meat and protein consumption in the USA. *Public Health Nutrition, 19,* 1358–1367. https://doi.org/10.1017/S1368980015003055

Green, L. W., & Kreuter, M. W. (2005). *Health promotion planning: An educational and ecological approach* (4th ed.). McGraw-Hill.

Helmig, B., & Thaler, J. (2010). On the effectiveness of social marketing—What do we really know? *Journal of Nonprofit & Public Sector Marketing, 22*(4), 264–287. https://doi.org/10.1080/10495140903566698

Homans, G. C. (1958). Social behavior as exchange. *American Journal of Sociology, 63,* 597–606. https://doi.org/10.1086/222355

Kotler, P., & Lee, N. R. (2008). *Social marketing: Influencing behaviors for good* (3rd ed.). SAGE.

Kotler, P., & Zaltman, G. (1971). Social marketing: An approach to planned social change. *Journal of Marketing, 35*(3), 3–12. https://doi.org/10.2307/1249783

Krebs, P., Prochaska, J. O., & Rossi, J. S. (2010). A meta-analysis of computer-tailored interventions for health behavior change. *Preventive Medicine, 51*(3-4), 214–221. https://doi.org/10.1016/j.ypmed.2010.06.004

Kreps, G. L. (2014). Evaluating health communication programs to enhance health care and health promotion. *Journal of Health Communication, 19,* 1449–1459. https://doi.org/10.1080/10810730.2014.954080

Kreuter, M., Farrell, D., Olevitch, L., & Brennan, L. (2000). *Tailoring health messages: Customizing communication with computer technology.* Lawrence Erlbaum Associates.

Lindridge, A., MacAskill, S., Gnich, W., Eadie, D., & Holme, I. (2013). Applying an ecological model to social marketing communications. *European Journal of Marketing, 47*(9), 1399–1420. https://doi.org/10.1108/EJM-10-2011-0561

McCarthy, J. E. (1964). *Basic marketing. A managerial approach.* Irwin.

National Cancer Institute (NCI). (2001). *Making health communication programs work.* US Department of Health & Human Services.

National Social Marketing Centre. (2010). *Social marketing benchmark criteria.* https://www.thensmc.com/file/234/download?token=P9Vz-7GO

Noar, S. M., Black, H. G., & Pierce, L. B. (2009). Efficacy of computer technology-based HIV prevention interventions: A meta-analysis. *AIDS, 23,* 107–115. https://doi.org/10.1097/QAD.0b013e32831c5500

Rimer, B. K., & Kreuter, M. W. (2006). Advancing tailored health communication: A persuasion and message effects perspective. *Journal of Communication, 56*(S1), S184–S201. https://doi.org/10.1111/j.1460-2466.2006.00289.x

Roberto, A. J. (2010). Computer tailored messages. In S. Priest (Ed.), *Encyclopedia of science and technology communication* (pp. 176–178). SAGE.

Rogers, E. M. (2003). *Diffusions of Innovation* (5th ed.). Free Press.

Shams, S. (2018). Social marketing for health: Theoretical and conceptual considerations. In M. Haider & H. N. Platter (Eds), *Selected issues in global health communications* (pp. 43–56). IntechOpen.

Snelling, A. M. (2014). *Introduction to health promotion.* John Wiley & Sons.

Storey, D. J., Hess, R., & Saffitz, G. (2015). Social marketing. In K. Glanz, B. K. Rimer, & K. Viswanath (Eds.), *Health behavior: Theory, research, & practice* (5th ed.). Jossey-Bass.

Thibault, J. W., & Kelley, H. H. (1959). *The social psychology of groups.* John Wiley.

Wallack, L. (2002). Public health, social change, and media advocacy. *Social Marketing Quarterly, 8*(2), 25–31. https://doi.org/10.1080/15245000212549

Witte, K., & Roberto, A. J. (2009). Fear appeals and public health: Managing fear and creating hope. In L. R. Frey & K. N. Cissna (Eds.), *Handbook of applied communication research* (pp. 584–610). Routledge.

Wymer, W. (2011). Developing more effective social marketing strategies. *Journal of Social Marketing, 1*(1), 17–31. https://doi.org/10.1108/20426761111104400

Xia, Y., Deshpande, S., & Bonates, T. (2016). Effectiveness of social marketing interventions to promote physical activity among adults: A systematic review. *Journal of Physical Activity and Health, 13*(11), 1263–1274. https://doi.org/ 10.1123/jpah.2015-0189

## CHAPTER 4

# The PRECEDE-PROCEED Model: An Ecological Approach to Health Promotion

## CHAPTER OUTLINE

## INTRODUCTION

As noted in the previous chapter, social marketing traditionally takes an individual consumer-based approach to promoting behavior change. However, health behavior is usually affected by numerous contextual factors beyond a person's control, and "many of the challenges that we face . . . are simply too complex to be solved by concentrating solely on the individual" (Collins et al., 2010, p. 1182). To bridge this gap, social marketers have begun to incorporate concepts from the ecological model, which focuses on how individual, relationship, community, and societal factors interact to influence behavior. In short, the ecological model takes a broader view of health promotion and disease prevention in an effort to increase the likelihood that public health communication interventions will obtain and sustain impactful behavior change. This chapter will begin with an overview of ecological models in general and provide definitions and examples of the various levels in such models. This will be followed by a discussion of the PRECEDE-PROCEED Model, which is "a practically useful, widely applied, and easy-to-follow example of a planning model" based on the ecological approach (Crosby & Noar, 2011, p. S8).

## ECOLOGICAL MODELS

*Ecological models* view behavior as part of a larger system and explore how individual and environmental factors interact to produce behavior. Ecological models typically include

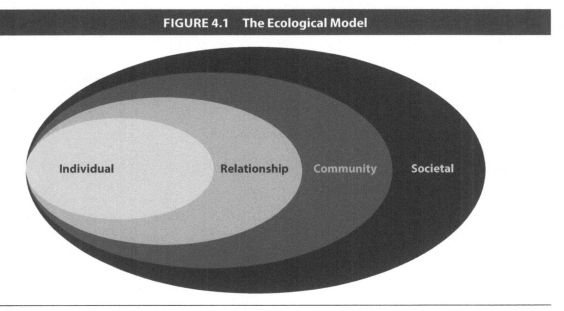

**FIGURE 4.1    The Ecological Model**

Source: Centers for Disease Control and Prevention (2011).

between four and seven nested levels that mutually influence each other (Bronfenbrenner, 1977; Green & Kreuter, 2005; McLeroy et al., 1988; Sallis & Owen, 2015; Simons-Morton et al., 2012). The key differences between the various iterations of ecological models are the number and names of the included environmental factors. For the practical purpose of intervention planning, four levels should suffice. Thus, this section will focus on the four levels commonly used by the Centers for Disease Control and Prevention (2011b) to inform public health communication interventions. According to this approach, public health communication interventions will be most effective when they focus on the connections between individual, relationship, community, and societal factors. Figure 4.1 provides a visual representation of the ecological model, Table 4.1 provides a brief description of each level, and Table 4.2 summarizes five key principles of ecological models.

| TABLE 4.1    Ecological Model Levels of Influence | |
| --- | --- |
| **Concept** | **Definition** |
| Individual Level | How characteristics of the person—such as beliefs, attitudes, and intentions—influence behavior. |
| Relationship Level | How connections to others—such as intimate partners, family, friends, and coworkers—influence behavior. |
| Community Level | How characteristics of the setting—such as the physical environment and school, work, or other institutions—influence behavior. |
| Societal Level | How broad, macro-level factors—such as public policy, cultural norms, and mass media—influence behavior. |

| TABLE 4.2    Five Principles of the Ecological Model |
| --- |
| **Principle** |
| 1. There are multiple levels of influence on health behaviors. |
| 2. Environmental contexts are significant determinants of health behaviors. |
| 3. Influences on health behaviors interact across levels. |
| 4. Multilevel interventions should be most effective in changing health behaviors. |
| 5. Ecological models should be behavior-specific. |

Source: Sallis and Owen (2015).

## INDIVIDUAL FACTORS

*Individual factors* (a.k.a., intrapersonal factors) refer to the characteristics of a person that influence the likelihood that they will engage in each behavior. To illustrate, the theories reviewed in Chapters 6 through 10 focus mainly on how individual factors such as beliefs, attitudes, and intentions influence behavior. For example, individuals are more likely to exercise if they think that managing their weight is important and that exercise is an effective way to do so (beliefs), if they feel positively about exercising (attitude), and if they plan to exercise (intentions). Thus, changing these and similar individual factors are common objectives for public health communication interventions. Other examples of individual factors include demographic variables such as gender, age, race, education, and income, as well as psychographic variables like knowledge, skills, lifestyle, and values. Individual factors make up the core of all ecological models.

## RELATIONSHIP FACTORS

*Relationship factors* (a.k.a., interpersonal factors) explore how interactions with others influence behavior. To illustrate, the theories discussed in Chapters 6 through 10 include explicit social or normative components. For example, social cognitive theory highlights the importance of observational learning (i.e., learning that occurs by watching the behavior of others) and role models (i.e., people you look up to and try to imitate) in the behavior change process. Also, for example, the reasoned action approach predict that individuals are more likely to exercise if they believe others would approve of their doing so (injunctive norms), and if they believe others are also exercising (descriptive norms). Relationships with intimate partners, family, friends, classmates, coworkers, neighbors, and even acquaintances can influence exercise behavior. For example, exercising with an intimate partner or friend can increase both motivation and accountability. With this in mind, public health communication interventions targeting relationship factors might provide or promote exercise classes, groups, clubs, or buddy system exercise options.

## COMMUNITY FACTORS

*Community factors* focus on how characteristics of the setting, such as the physical environment or organizational factors, influence behavior. Some versions of the ecological model divide this factor into two or three different levels (McLeroy et al., 1988; Simons-Morton et al., 2012), but for our purpose the community level will also include both the physical environment and organizational factors. The physical environment includes things like access to nearby sidewalks, bike paths, recreational areas, or fitness centers; all of which are likely to affect exercise behavior. Organizational factors include school, work, faith-based, business, health care, and other institutions, as well as the relationships and communication between them. For example, public health communication intervention planners might work with health insurers and employers to reimburse gym membership fees, or with fitness centers to offer discounted gym memberships. Or they might work with city officials to identify or create walking trails, bike paths, or ask nearby malls to open early so folks can "mall walk" when it may be too hot or too cold to do so outside.

## SOCIETAL FACTORS

*Societal factors* look at how large-scale or macro-level public policies and cultural norms can facilitate or impede behavior. Again, some versions of the ecological model divide this factor into two different levels (Simons-Morton et al., 2012), but for this chapter the societal level includes both policy and culture components. To illustrate, this level includes local, state, and national laws—and their enforcement. For example, according to the National Association for Sports and Physical Education (2016), only 38 states require kindergarten through 12th grade students to take physical education classes, and only six states require schools to provide the nationally recommended amount of time for physical education. Hence, public health communication programmers might work with state policy makers interested in making sure students are getting the recommended amount of exercise. This level also includes shared cultural beliefs, norms, and values, which have also been shown to influence exercise behavior (e.g., D'Alonzo & Fischetti, 2008). Finally, societal factors include mass media, which plays a significant role in shaping, changing, or reinforcing behaviors in the viewing or listening audience (Rubens & Shehadeh, 2014).

## SUMMARY

In sum, the ecological model illustrates that influencing behavior is no easy task. It suggests that healthy behaviors will be maximized when environmental factors support healthy choices, and individuals are persuaded to make those choices (Sallis & Owen, 2015). To understand and successfully influence behavior we must consider individual, interpersonal, community, and societal factors, and the interrelationships between these factors. For example, it makes little sense to try to change individual factors when the requisite environmental factors are not present. To illustrate, "media campaigns that encourage people to walk will be ineffective in communities where there are no or poorly maintained walking paths or where safety is an issue" (Victorian Curriculum and Assessment Authority, 2016). Thus, all four factors are potential targets for public health communication interventions, which broaden the options available to intervention planners.

## PRECEDE-PROCEED MODEL

The *PRECEDE-PROCEED Model* (PPM) is an eight-phase logic model guided by the ecological approach to health promotion that was introduced above. **PRECEDE** stands for **P**redisposing, **R**einforcing, and **E**nabling **C**onstructs in **E**ducational/Environmental **D**iagnosis and **E**valuation. **PROCEED** stands for **P**olicy, **R**egulation, and **O**rganizational **C**onstructs in **E**ducation and **E**nvironmental **D**evelopment. The most recent version of the PRECEDE-PROCEED Model (PPM) includes the following eight phases (Green & Kreuter, 2005):[1]

- ► Phase 1: Social Assessment
- ► Phase 2: Epidemiological Assessment
- ► Phase 3: Educational and Ecological Assessment
- ► Phase 4: Administrative and Policy Assessment and Intervention Alignment
- ► Phase 5: Implementation
- ► Phase 6: Process Evaluation
- ► Phase 7: Outcome Evaluation
- ► Phase 8: Impact Evaluation

A vital aspect of all phases of the PRECEDE-PROCEED Model is *community-based participatory research*, which is a collaborative approach to research that equitably involves community members or recipients of interventions in all phases of the research process (Green & Mercer, 2001). Table 4.3 provides a brief description of each phase, Figure 4.2 provides a visual representation of these eight phases, and a detailed discussion of each of these phases follows.

| Phase | Description |
|---|---|
| **TABLE 4.3** | **Brief Description of the Eight Phases of the PRECEDE-PROCEED Model** |
| Social Assessment | Work with the community to determine what problems impact its health and quality of life. This will serve as the basis for the program's overarching goal(s), or long-term objective(s), that will be assessed during the impact evaluation (Phase 8). |
| Epidemiological Assessment | Identifying the health problem, and the behavioral and environmental factors associated with the health problem. The health problem will serve as another basis for the program's overarching goal(s) which will be assessed during the impact evaluation (Phase 8). Also, the behavioral and environmental factors will serve as the program's intermediate objectives which will be assessed during the outcome evaluation (Phase 7). |
| Educational and Ecological Assessment | Identifying the predisposing, reinforcing, and enabling determinants of the behavioral and environmental factors identified during the epidemiological assessment phase (Phase 2). This will serve as the basis of your short-term objectives that will also be assessed during the outcome evaluation (Phase 7). |
| Administrative and Policy Assessment and Intervention Alignment | Involves making sure all necessary components are present to develop, implement, and evaluate your program; and developing theory- and research-based strategies that will eventually be implemented (Phase 5) and serve as the basis of your process evaluation (Phase 6). |
| Implementation | Putting the program's strategies and evaluation plan into action, and making sure procedures are in place to conduct quality process evaluation (Phase 6), outcome evaluation (Phase 7), and impact evaluation (Phase 8). |
| Process Evaluation | A type of quality assurance conducted during program implementation (Phase 5) that involves monitoring program activities, providing a preliminary assessment of how well the intervention is working (Phase 3), providing corrective feedback, and documenting any changes that were made to your initial plans and why. |
| Outcome Evaluation | Assessing the success of your program at reaching the short-term and intermediate objectives that were developed during the educational and ecological assessment (Phase 3) and epidemiological assessment (Phase 2) phases respectively. |
| Impact Evaluation | Assesses if the program met the goal(s), or long-term objective(s), identified in the social assessment and epidemiological assessment phases (Phases 1 and 2). In other words, did the program improve the health and quality of life of the community? |

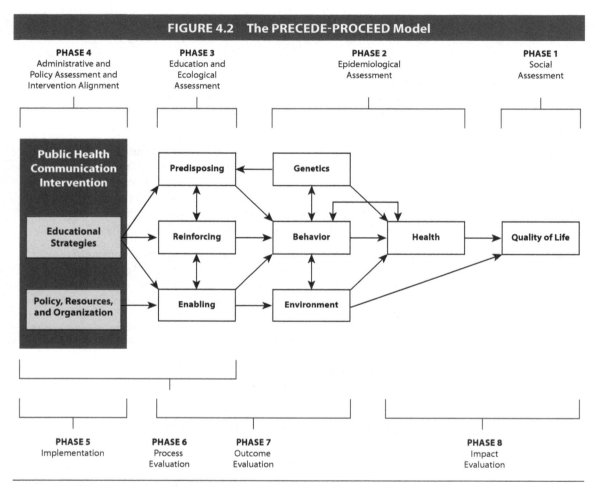

FIGURE 4.2    The PRECEDE-PROCEED Model

Image adapted from Green and Kreuter (2005).
See Footnote 1 for a discussion on the conflicting use of outcome evaluation and impact evaluation in the literature.

The PPM has four planning phases (Phases 1 through 4), one implementation phase (Phase 5), and three evaluation phases (Phases 6 through 8). As you can see in Figure 4.2, the first four phases make up the PRECEDE portion of the model. This portion of the model is dedicated to identifying the most important and changeable behavioral and environmental factors that relate to the health outcome you hope to achieve. This includes the diagnosis and planning steps necessary to develop goals and objectives and culminates in the development of the specific strategies you will implement for your public health communication intervention. This information not only provides a prioritized list of potential variables you might target for change, it can also help you select and appropriate theory to use as the intervention's foundation. The last four phases make up the PROCEED portion of the model. This includes both intervention enactment and evaluation, or putting your plans into actions and monitoring, assessing, and adjusting. A detailed discussion of all eight phases follows.

## PHASE 1: SOCIAL ASSESSMENT

*Social assessment* involves gathering information from or about the intended audience. Here, the aim is to understand the health issues that are most important to the community, and how serious those issues are. One key purpose of this step is to identify and develop an overarching goal (or long-term objective) of the intervention, or the overall health improvement or outcome that you hope to achieve. Another purpose is to get community input on how to best address these issues to determine what health interventions might be most needed or effective. Thus, this phase represents an excellent opportunity to build existing relationships within the community, or to establish new ones.

Using a combination of community voices and statistical data leads to a more comprehensive and complementary approach to social assessment (Snelling, 2014). During the social assessment phase, intervention planners typically collect primary data (i.e., original research conducted by the intervention planner for a specific purpose) and review secondary data (i.e., existing research that was previously conducted by someone else or for some other purpose). As a reminder, examples of the primary data can range from qualitative focus groups or in-depth individual interviews with a few community members to obtain a richer understanding of their beliefs or opinions, to quantitative surveys from many community members to draw more generalizable conclusions about the community. Also, as a reminder, examples of secondary data include research from government offices, or studies published in medical, public health, or communication journals.

## PHASE 2: EPIDEMIOLOGICAL ASSESSMENT

*Epidemiology* is the study of how often health outcomes (e.g., diseases, injuries, etc.) occur in different groups of people and why (Coggon et al. 2003). Thus, *epidemiological assessment* involves identifying the genetic, behavioral, and environmental factors associated with a health problem. One key purpose of this phase is to better understand the magnitude and seriousness of a health problem using epidemiological data. This information can then be used to identify the risk factors that will ultimately serve as the basis for the intervention's intermediate objectives, or the interim changes in behaviors that provide a sense of progress toward reaching one's goal, or long-term objectives.

### Genetic, Behavioral, and Environmental Factors

As a reminder, Figure 4.1 provided an overview of the four levels included in the behavioral ecological model (i.e., individual, relationship, community, and societal). These levels are directly related to activities included in the epidemiological assessment phase of the PPM. To illustrate, genetic and behavioral factors are most closely associated with the individual level, whereas environmental factors would focus more on the relationship, community, and societal levels. Since most health issues are caused by a combination of genetics, lifestyle choices, and the environment, a brief discussion of each of these factors follows.

**Genetic Factors.** *Genetic factors* refer to inherited influences on health outcomes. Many health issues, including heart disease, hypertension, Alzheimer's disease, diabetes, cancer, and alcoholism, have all been shown to have a key genetic component (Centers for Disease Control and Prevention, 2011a). With this in mind, genetic factors were added to the most recent iteration of the PPM to acknowledge "the rapid strides being made to isolate the genetic predispositions associated with various illnesses, risk factors, and biological conditions" (Green & Kreuter, 2005, pp. 13–14). However, Green and Kreuter go on to note that "the science is not yet developed sufficiently for widespread application" (p. 14). As a result, and for the time being, behavioral and environmental factors remain the primary focus of the epidemiological assessment phase.

**Behavioral Factors.** *Behavioral factors* refer to actions taken by individuals or groups that exert a strong influence on health. In other words, what lifestyle factors protect or put an individual at risk for a given health problem (Green & Kreuter, 2005)? For example, physical activity, diet, tobacco use, and alcohol consumption are all behavioral factors that have a great effect on an individual's quality and quantity of life (U.S. Department of Health and Human Services, 2016).

**Environmental Factors.** *Environmental factors* refer to the effects of a person's surroundings on their behavior or health. In other words, what outside factors can be influenced to promote health or healthy behavior? Many environmental factors are beyond the control of any given individual but might be more amenable to change with community or societal involvement and support. For example, air and water quality, homes and communities, access to healthy or unhealthy foods, recreational resources, and medical care all represent important environmental factors that have a great effect on health (U.S. Department of Health and Human Services, 2016).

## PHASE 3: EDUCATIONAL AND ECOLOGICAL ASSESSMENT

Phase 3, *educational and ecologic assessment*, involves identifying the determinants of the behavioral and environmental factors identified during the previous epidemiological assessment phase. In other words, what causes or contributes to the identified risk factors. These risk factors are further subdivided into predisposing, enabling, and reinforcing factors, and will serve as the basis of your short-term objectives, or the most immediate changes you expect the intervention to have on your target audience. A discussion of each type of factor is provided next.

### Predisposing Factors

*Predisposing factors* are individual factors that impact how motivated an individual is to engage in a behavior. A few common examples include an individual's beliefs, attitude, and intention regarding the behavior. To illustrate using familiar variables from the health belief model, individuals who believe that physical *in*activity has serious negative consequences (i.e., high perceived severity) and that those consequences are likely to happen to them (i.e., high perceived susceptibility) should be more motivated to exercise; and vice versa. The individual-level theories discussed in Chapters 6 through 10 provide excellent insights regarding how to appropriately address these and similar predisposing factors.

### Enabling Factors

*Enabling factors* refer to individual or environmental factors that impact behavior. An example of an individual enabling factor from the health belief model is self-efficacy. That is, individuals believe they are able to exercise under various challenging circumstances (i.e., high self-efficacy) are more likely to do so; and vice versa. Examples of external enabling factors include things like availability and accessibility of resources. That is, the presence and proximity of sidewalks, bike paths, recreational areas, or fitness centers are all likely to impact exercise behavior.

### Reinforcing Factors

*Reinforcing factors* relate to the feedback or rewards an individual receives after performing a behavior. An example of an internal reward would be the feeling of accomplishment that comes with setting, monitoring, and achieving a fitness goal. An example of an external reward would include the positive reinforcement provided by an exercise buddy. Other examples include subjective norms, normative beliefs, and motivation to comply from the reasoned action approach (see Chapter 9) (i.e., do important others approve or disapprove of the behavior?). In short, our perception regarding what is expected or supported by others can serve as a reinforcing factor for behavior. For example, how your doctor or other health care providers, best friend or other peers, and parents feel about a behavior can be an important reinforcing factor.

## PHASE 4: ADMINISTRATIVE AND POLICY ASSESSMENT AND INTERVENTION ALIGNMENT

The first three phases of the PPM help you identify and set specific, measurable, achievable, relevant, and time-bound (SMART) goals and objectives (Centers for Disease Control and Prevention, 2015). The ultimate purpose of Phase 4, *administrative and policy assessment and intervention alignment*, is to identify, select, and design the specific strategies necessary to reach the intervention's goals and objectives. That is, while Phases 1 through 3 help you determine what predisposing, enabling, and reinforcing behavioral and environmental factors need to change, Phase 4 focuses on how and what is needed to best change them. This phase serves as a "reality check" (Jack et al., 2010, p. 74) to make sure all necessary components are present to develop, implement, and evaluate your intervention. A key task during this phase is the selection and application of a theory or theories that will promote the necessary changes identified in the previous phases. Thus, by the time you are done with this Phase 4, you will have selected and created the theory- and research-based program components that will be implemented in Phase 5 and evaluated in Phases 6 through 8. This phase's two components—(1) administrative and policy assessment, and (2) intervention alignment—are discussed next.

### *Administrative and Policy Assessment*

The *administrative and policy assessment* portion of Phase 4 involves determining if you have what you need to develop and successfully implement the intervention. In other words, "does the program have the policy, organizational, and administrative capabilities and resources to make this program work" (Green & Kreuter, 2005, p. 15)? For example, what policies exist or need to be developed to support the intervention (e.g., what is the organization's mission, and what internal and external rules and regulations must the organization follow)? What aspects of the organization can help or hinder intervention implementation (e.g., location, staff commitment and values, access to the intended audience, community trust and involvement, etc.)? And do you have the necessary resources to successfully implement the intervention (e.g., time, personnel, money)? The answer to this last question involves putting the finishing touches on your formal plan with a timetable, assignment of responsibilities, and a budget. For example, what staff do you already have, who else do you need to hire, and how will you train and supervise them?

### Intervention Alignment

The *intervention alignment* portion of Phase 4 involves selecting and developing intervention strategies that match the predisposing, enabling, and reinforcing behavioral and environmental factors you plan to change. In other words, "what program components and interventions are needed to affect the changes specified in the previous phases" (Green & Kreuter, 2005, p. 15). This process involves (1) intervention matching, mapping, pooling, and patching, (2) formative evaluation, and (3) pilot testing (a.k.a., pretesting). As a reminder, formative evaluation and pilot testing are conducted before the intervention is fully designed or implemented to test or try out one or more components of your public health communication intervention on a smaller scale to make sure it is feasible, appropriate, and acceptable. Both formative evaluation and pretesting were discussed in detail in the Introduction to Planning and Evaluation chapter (Chapter 2). Next I will discuss intervention matching, mapping, pooling, and patching.

**Matching, Mapping, Pooling, and Patching.** Matching, mapping, pooling, and patching are important tools for bridging theory and practice when planning, selecting, and developing intervention components. *Matching* involves identifying which potential strategies and activities affect which ecological levels. As a reminder, the ecological model views behavior as part of a larger system, and that individual, relationship, community, and societal level factors interact to produce behavior. The idea here is to explicitly select and connect each intervention strategy or activity to the appropriate ecological level. *Mapping* involves connecting each intervention strategy or activity to each predisposing, enabling, and reinforcing behavioral and environmental factor based on previous theory, research, and practice. For example, it is important to include strategies that are specifically designed to change the relevant variables in the theory you select to guide the intervention.

*Pooling* involves identifying and examining relevant prior interventions and community-preferred interventions. As Green and Kreuter (2005) note, "a program never starts from scratch . . . other attempts elsewhere and here should be considered resources and guides" (pp. 201–202). This is analogous to conducting a *resource inventory,* which was defined earlier as a systematic process for gathering information about what materials already exist on a topic, and for which intended audiences (see, for example, Goei et al., 2003). *Patching* involves identifying and filling in the gaps in evidence-based best practices. This is analogous to conducting a *needs assessment*, or *gap analysis*, which consists of reviewing existing interventions, campaigns, and programs to determine if any gaps exist. Using or slightly revising existing messages or materials not only saves time and money, but it also allows you to focus on designing, implementing, and evaluating new strategies to fill existing needs and gaps.

## PHASE 5: IMPLEMENTATION

*Implementation*, the first phase of the PROCEED part of the model, involves putting the intervention's strategies and evaluation plan into action. Up to this point, the focus has been on finalizing the intervention plan and selecting and designing specific strategies and activities. Here the focus shifts to executing the plan. This includes providing the necessary support (i.e., policy, organizational/administrative, and resources) to successfully implement the intervention, and taking the steps necessary to properly evaluate the intervention. For example, it is imperative to put procedures into place to track and assess the fidelity, completeness, exposure, satisfaction, and reach of your intervention (discussed next under process evaluation). It is also important to collect baseline data that will allow you to assess the effects of your intervention on your short-term and intermediate objectives (see outcome evaluation); and perhaps even your goal or long-term objective (see impact evaluation).

## PHASE 6: PROCESS EVALUATION

*Process evaluation* is conducted during intervention implementation. Process evaluation is closely related to Phase 5 (implementation) as it asks, are you doing what you planned to do? In other words, process evaluation is more concerned with procedures than outcomes. Process evaluation is a type of quality assurance that involves monitoring intervention activities, providing corrective feedback, and documenting any changes that were made to your initial plans and why. As Sanders et al. (2005) note, process evaluation is important because "it aids in understanding the relationship between specific program elements and program outcomes" (p. 134). While process evaluation focuses primarily on whether or not program activities are being implemented as intended, it can also be used to monitor and provide *preliminary* information regarding how well the intervention is working (e.g., whether the intervention appears to be making progress toward short-term objectives identified in Phase 6), while there is still time for adjustments to be made (Centers for Disease Control and Prevention, n.d.; Green & Kreuter, 2005). Process evaluation can use data from many different sources, including naturally collected records and field observations, surveys, and occasionally even individual and focus group interviews.

## PHASE 7: OUTCOME EVALUATION

*Outcome evaluation* involves assessing the initial success of your efforts (i.e., has the intervention met its short-term and intermediate objectives?). Outcome evaluation tests the cause-effect relationship between an intervention (the cause) and changes in the intended audience on key variables of interest (the effects). Thus, outcome evaluation relies heavily on practical experimental design (see Chapter 13), which allow an intervention's developer to confidently determine what changes can be attributed to the intervention, and what would have happened without the intervention.

A properly conducted outcome evaluation allows for evidence-based decision-making as it lets you know if and how well an intervention worked, what did not work, and, when accompanied by proper planning and strong process evaluation components, why it worked or did not work. While outcome evaluation is primarily concerned with how well the intervention met its short-term and intermediate objectives and sub-objectives (i.e., its intended consequences), it can also provide important information about any other positive or negative unintended consequences (Cho & Salmon, 2007; Salmon & Murray-Johnson, 2001).

Outcome evaluation typically focuses on short-term or intermediate objectives as they are easier to measure and more prone to change (i.e., perceptions and behavior), as opposed to long-term objectives or goals which focus on health outcomes that may take years or decades to achieve (i.e., improved health, fitness, and quality of life). Thus, outcome evaluation is closely related to Phase 2 (epidemiological assessment) and Phase 3 (educational and ecological assessment) as it asks if the short-term and intermediate behavioral and environmental objectives and sub-objectives identified in these steps were met. Recall that the behavioral and environmental factors identified in Phase 2 will serve as the basis for our intermediate objective, and the predisposing, reinforcing, and enabling factors identified in Phase 3 will serve as the basis of our short-term objectives and intermediate sub-objectives. Also recall that these short-term and intermediate objectives and sub-objectives should be theory-based (i.e., see Chapters 6 through 10), so changes in the short-term objectives should lead to changes in the intermediate objectives and sub-objectives, which, in turn, should eventually lead to improvements in our long-term objective or goal.

## PHASE 8: IMPACT EVALUATION

The purpose of *impact evaluation* is to determine if the intervention met the goal(s), or long-term objective(s), identified in Phase 1 (social assessment) and Phase 2 (epidemiological assessment). In other words, did the intervention reduce morbidity and mortality (Phase 2) and improve quality of life (Phase 1) of the community? Even if you do exactly what you planned (process evaluation) and achieved your short-term and intermediate objectives (outcome evaluation), it is still important to monitor these broader issues to determine if they were achieved (impact evaluation). As noted in Chapter 2, this is no easy task given the number of different factors that affect health and the fact that it may take years or decades to observe health impacts.

## CONCLUSION

This chapter introduced the ecological approach to behavior change, which highlights the importance of considering individual and environmental factors when developing public health communication interventions. In other words, ecological models stress the need for considering individual, relationship, community, and societal factors when attempting to influence health behavior. This chapter also reviewed the PRECEDE-PROCEED Model, which takes an ecological approach to program planning. Its four planning phases assess the behavioral and environmental risk factors associated with a health problem and targets these factors with theory- and research-based interventions. Further, its four implementation and evaluation phases involve putting the intervention's strategies and evaluation plan into action and making sure that the intervention is implemented as intended and having the anticipated effects. In tandem, the ecological approach and the PRECEDE-PROCEED Model for those planning and evaluation public health communication interventions since "multilevel interventions should be most effective in changing health behaviors" (Sallis & Owen, 2015, p. 49).

## FOOTNOTE

[1] As noted in Chapter 2, in the PRECEDE-PROCEED Model, Phase 7 is traditionally labeled "impact evaluation" and Phase 8 is traditionally labeled "outcome evaluation." But this is not consistent with how these terms are defined in this book, so they have been switched throughout this chapter to reflect the definitions presented in Chapter 2. However, while the labels of the last two phases have been changed, the content of these phases remains the same.

In this book, I use the term *outcome evaluation* to refer to the assessment of the specific effects an intervention had on the intended audience (i.e., objective-based evaluation). For example, what effect did the intervention have on an intended audiences' beliefs, attitude, or behavior? I use the term *impact evaluation* to refer to the assessment of the broader effects that one or more interventions had on a community (i.e., goal-based evaluation). For example, what effect did any changes in beliefs, attitudes, and behavior have on the health and quality of life of the community?

# REFERENCES

Bronfenbrenner, U. (1977). Toward an experimental ecology of human development. *American Psychologist, 32*, 513–531. https://doi.org/10.1037/0003-066X.32.7.513

Centers for Disease Control and Prevention. (n.d.). *Types of evaluation.* https://www.cdc.gov/std/Program/pupestd/Types of Evaluation.pdf

Centers for Disease Control and Prevention. (2011a). *Genomics and disease.* https://www.cdc.gov/health communication/toolstemplates/entertainmented/tips/Genomics.html

Centers for Disease Control and Prevention. (2011b). *The social-ecological model: A framework for violence prevention* (NIH Publication No. 11-7782). https://www.cdc.gov/violenceprevention/pdf/sem_frame wrk-a.pdf

Centers for Disease Control and Prevention. (2015). *How to write SMART objectives.* https://www.cdc.gov/cancer/dcpc/pdf/dp17-1701-smart-objectives.pdf

Cho, H., & Salmon, C. T. (2007). Unintended effects of health communication campaigns. *Journal of Communication, 47*, 293–317. https://doi.org/10.1111/j.1460-2466.2007.00344.x

Coggon, D., Rose, G., & Barker, D. J. P. (2003). *Epidemiology for the uninitiated* (5th ed.). BMJ Publishing Group.

Collins, K., Tapp, A., & Pressley, A. (2010). Social marketing and social influences: Using social ecology as a theoretical framework. *Journal of Marketing Management, 26*, 1181–1200. https://doi.org/10.1080/0267 257X.2010.522529

Crosby, R., & Noar, S. M. (2011). What is a planning model? An introduction to PRECEDE-PROCEED. *Journal of Public Health Dentistry, 71*, S7–S15. https://doi.org/ 10.1111/j.1752-7325.2011.00235.x

D'Alonzo, K. T., & Fischetti, N. (2008). Cultural beliefs and attitudes of Black and Hispanic college-age women toward exercise. *Journal of Transcultural Nursing, 19*, 175–183. https://doi.org/10.1177/1043659607313074

Goei, R. C., Meyer, G., & Roberto, A. J. (2003). An assessment of violence prevention and intervention programs in Michigan: Policy and programmatic insights and implications. *Criminal Justice Policy Review, 14*, 306–321. https://doi.org/10.1177/0887403403252666

Green, L., & Mercer, S. (2001). Community-based participatory research: Can public health researchers and agencies reconcile the push from funding bodies and the pull from communities? *American Journal of Public Health, 91*, 1926–1929. https://doi.org/ 10.2105/ajph.91.12.1926

Green, L. W., & Kreuter, M. W. (2005). *Health promotion planning: An educational and ecological approach* (4th ed.). McGraw-Hill.

Jack, L., Grim, M., Gross, T., Lynch, S., & McLin, C. (2010). Theory in health promotion programs. In C. I. Fertman, & D. D. Allensworth (Eds.), *Health promotion programs: From theory to practice* (pp. 57–90). Jossey-Bass.

McLeroy, K. R., Bibeau, D., Steckler, A., & Glanz, K. (1988). An ecological perspective on health promotion programs. *Health Education Quarterly, 15*, 351–377. https://doi.org/ 10.1177/109019818801500401

National Association for Sports and Physical Education. (2016). *Shape of the nation: Status of physical education in the USA.* http://www.shapeamerica.org/advocacy/son/2016/upload/Shape-of-the-Nation-2016_web.pdf

Rubens, M., & Shehadeh, N. (2014). Gun violence in the United States: In search for a solution. *Frontiers in Public Health, 2*, 1–4. https://doi.org/10.3389/fpubh.2014.00017

Sallis, J. F., & Owen, N. (2015). Ecological models of health behavior. In K. Glanz, B. K. Rimer, K. Viswanath, (Eds.), *Health behavior: Theory, research, and practice* (5th ed., pp. 43–64). Jossey-Bass.

Salmon, C. T., & Murray-Johnson, L. (2001). Communication campaign effectiveness: Critical distinctions. In R. E. Rice & C. K. Atkin (Eds.), *Public communication campaigns* (3rd ed., pp. 168–180). SAGE.

Sanders, R. P., Evans, M. H., & Joshi, P. (2005). Developing a process-evaluation plan for assessing health promotion program implementation: A how-to guide. *Health Promotion Practice, 2*, 134–147. https://doi.org/ 10.1177/1524839904273387

Simons-Morton, B. G., McLeroy, K. R., & Wendel, M. L. (2012). *Behavior theory in health promotion and research*. Jones & Bartlett.

Snelling, A. M. (2014). *Introduction to health promotion*. John Wiley & Sons.

U.S. Department of Health and Human Services. (2016). *2020 topics and objectives*. https://www.healthy people.gov/2020/topics-objectives

Victorian Curriculum and Assessment Authority. (2016). *Social-ecological model*. Author.

# SECTION 3

## Theories and Models
## of Health Behavior Change

## CHAPTER 5

# Introduction to Theory and Meta-Analysis

**CHAPTER OUTLINE**

## INTRODUCTION

Few experts would disagree with the premise that public health communication interventions should be theory-based. This is not surprising given that theory-based programs generally outperform those that are atheoretical (Bluethmann et al., 2017; Glanz & Bishop, 2010; Noar et al., 2007; Webb et al., 2010). Further, theories help you determine what questions to ask when conducting formative evaluation, what to track and observe during process evaluation, and what variables to measure for your outcome evaluation.

While many different theories of health behavior change have been developed, only a small number have been widely used (Glanz et al., 2015). This section of the book reviews five theories that are commonly used to plan, implement, and evaluate public health communication interventions: (1) the health belief model, (2) social cognitive theory, (3) the extended parallel process model, (4) the theories of reasoned action and planned behavior, and (5) the transtheoretical model. All five of the chapters in this section of the book will follow the same general outline. That is, each of the theory chapters in this section will:

1. describe a theory;

2. provide conceptual and operational definitions for all key constructs in the theory; and

3. review seminal meta-analyses results regarding the theory.

The purpose of this chapter is to provide the background information necessary to understand the material presented in subsequent chapters in this section. Toward this end, this chapter will answer the questions: What is a theory? What are conceptual and operational definitions? And what is a meta-analysis?

## WHAT IS A THEORY?

A *theory* is a systematic explanation of how something works. For example, a common goal of all the theories discussed in this section is to explain why people behave in healthy or unhealthy ways. That is, they identify the major factors that influence health behavior, as well as the relationship between those factors. As Rimer and Glanz (2005) note, "a theory presents a systematic way of understanding events or situations. It is a set of concepts, definitions, and propositions that explain or predict these events or situations by illustrating the relationships between variables" (p. 4). In the context of public health communication interventions, theories suggest more effective ways to change behavior, and provide a conceptual link between a program's goals, objectives, and strategies.

For example, social cognitive theory (see Chapter 7) posits that self-efficacy (i.e., beliefs about one's ability to perform the recommended behavior) has both a direct and indirect effect on behavior. In terms of the direct relationship between self-efficacy and behavior, social cognitive theory predicts that individuals are more likely to engage in a behavior when they are confident in their ability to do so. Further, social cognitive theory also predicts that self-efficacy has an indirect influence on behavior through outcome expectations (i.e., the anticipated costs or benefits of engaging in the behavior), goals (i.e., what you plan or intend to do), and sociostructural factors (i.e., other issues that help or hinder the desired behavior such as social support or the environment) (Bandura, 2004).

The main goals of all the theories described in this section are to predict and explain (health) behavior. Several additional criteria for evaluating theories grounded in the scientific method have been advanced, including scope, parsimony, falsifiability, internal consistency, heuristic value, and practical utility (Chaffee & Berger, 1987; Glanz et al., 2015; Griffin et al., 2019; Shoemaker et al., 2004). Definitions for all eight criteria for evaluating theory are presented in Table 5.1. As you will see in subsequent chapters, the theories reviewed in this book generally score fairly high along most or all of these criteria.

| TABLE 5.1 Criteria for Evaluating Theory | |
|---|---|
| **Criteria** | **Definition** |
| Predictive Power | Good theories accurately forecast future observations (e.g., they predict the probability that people will engage in a given behavior). |
| Explanatory Power | Good theories provide plausible (causal) explanations for observations regarding its subject matter (i.e., they explain why). |
| Scope (a.k.a., Comprehensiveness) | Good theories predict and explain a range of observations (i.e., they are applicable to a variety of topics and intended audiences). |
| Parsimony (a.k.a., Simplicity) | Good theories are as simple as possible (i.e., they contain a manageable number of constructs and are no more complex than they need to be). |
| Falsifiability (a.k.a., Testability) | Good theories are testable and capable of being proved false (i.e., there should be a way to disprove a prediction if it is wrong). |
| Internal Consistency (a.k.a., Logic) | Good theories do not contradict themselves (i.e., they make sense, and their predictions are compatible with each other). |
| Heuristic Value | Good theories generate new research questions and hypotheses (i.e., they stimulate new thinking and provide directions for future research). |
| Practical Utility | Good theories are useful (e.g., they provide effective advice for improving messages and changing behavior). |

## THEORY VS. MODEL

The terms "theory" and "model" are often used synonymously. For example, we refer to the health belief model (see Chapter 6) and the extended parallel process model (see Chapter 8), which are both theories (Bartholomew & Mullen, 2011; Skinner et al., 2015; Witte, 1992). Further, the integrative model of behavior (see Chapter 9) and the transtheoretical model (see Chapter 7) are *meta-theories*, as they integrate or provide an overarching structure for multiples theories (Bartholomew & Mullen, 2011; Prochaska et al., 2015; Willis, 2010).

The fact that these two terms are often used interchangeably is not surprising given their close relationship to each other and the fact that both terms share several common elements. To illustrate, both theories and models provide possible explanations for phenomena, though they do so in different ways. A *theory* is a set of interrelated concepts, definitions, and propositions that explain how something works. So, theories tend to be more abstract, and advance their key arguments via formal propositions or mathematical formulas. A *model*, on the other hand, is a simplified graphic depiction of a process or theory. A model is a representation of the original. So, models tend to be more concrete and practical.

All the theories discussed in Chapters 6 through 10 have a corresponding model. For example, Witte (1992) provided 11 formal propositions regarding fear appeal messages. This process culminated in the extended parallel process model (see Chapter 8), which provides a step-by-step guide for creating effective health risk messages. Also for example, one part of the theory of planned behavior (see Chapter 9) predicts that a person's intention (i.e., what they are motivated to do) is a joint function of attitude (i.e., how the person feels about the behavior), subjective norms (i.e., the person's perception of the behavior expected by others), and perceived behavioral control (i.e., beliefs about their ability to perform the behavior) (Fishbein & Ajzen, 2010). Mathematically, this portion of the theory is expressed as follows:

$$I = A + SN + PBC$$

However, this part of the theory is more commonly expressed using the following model, or graphical representation of this formula:

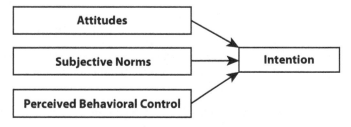

In sum, a theory is a conceptual framework for explaining a process, whereas a model provides a visual representation of that process. The purpose of a theory is to predict and explain, the purpose of a model is to describe and imagine (Shoemaker et al., 2004). Further, as was mentioned throughout the previous section on program planning, both theories and models play an important role in the planning, implementation, and evaluation of public health communication interventions.

## THE ROLE OF THEORY IN PUBLIC HEALTH COMMUNICATION INTERVENTIONS

As noted in previous chapters, theory plays an important role in all stages of the Health Communication Program Cycle (National Cancer Institute, 2001), and in all phases of the PRECEDE-PROCEED model (Green & Kreuter, 2005). More specifically, Bartholomew and Mullen (2011) identify five key roles theory may play when planning, evaluating, and reporting public health communication interventions. A brief discussion of each role follows.

First, theory helps identify the key determinants of behavior. In other words, theory can help us understand why people behave the way they do, or how a behavior is created and maintained. The more one knows about the determinants of a behavior, the more likely one can develop effective strategies to shape, change, or reinforce that behavior.

Second, theory provides a causal model for changing behavior that is essential for creating specific, measurable, achievable, relevant, and time-bound (SMART) objectives. This not only makes it possible to order your objectives based on their anticipated time sequence (e.g., beliefs → attitude → intention → behavior), it also allows you to estimate the amount of expected change, which will generally be "greater in proximal indicators, such as change in beliefs, than in more distal indicators, such as change in behavior" (Green, 2000, p. 127).

Third, theory should inform the selection, development, and implementation of feasible intervention strategies to maximize potential effects. This helps ensure that an intervention is complete, addresses all important variables, and provides a benchmark by which you can assess whether the intervention was properly implemented.

Fourth, theory guides all aspects of evaluation and provides guidelines for measuring success. This includes the developing of research questions and hypotheses, selecting a research design (including what to measure and how to measure it), collecting and analyzing data, and interpreting results.

Finally, theory can help describe the intervention and report results. This includes clearly articulating how theory directly and indirectly informed an intervention and reporting the essential elements of the intervention so it can be replicated.

In sum, the quality of an intervention and its evaluation are affected by how well a developer attends to theoretical concerns during all stages or phases of the process. Theory helps intervention developers make assumptions explicit and examine the logic of their ideas (Bartholomew & Mullen, 2011). Theory helps summarize knowledge and guide research.

When it comes to planning, implementing, and evaluating effective public health communication interventions, "nothing is as practical as a good theory" (Lewin, 1945, p. 129).

### Theory Coding Scheme

Michie and Prestwich (2010) provide a formal and systematic framework for assessing the role of theory in program planning, implementation, and evaluation. Their theory coding scheme provides an excellent tool for program developers as it asks six key questions that will help them more clearly describe the role of theory in their public health communication interventions. The six questions are:

1. Is theory mentioned (even if the intervention is not based on the mentioned theory)?
2. How did theory directly inform the intervention (i.e., are the relevant theoretical constructs targeted)?
3. How did theory indirectly influence the intervention (e.g., is the theory used to select recipients likely to benefit from the intervention or to individually tailor the intervention)?
4. Are the relevant theoretical constructs measured (and reliability and validity information reported)?
5. Is theory tested (e.g., is theory used to explain intervention outcomes and impacts)?
6. Are evaluation results used to extend or refine theory?

Notice how these six questions nicely parallel the stages and phases of the program planning process discussed in Section 2. Recall that key purposes of program planning include selecting an appropriate theory to use as the program's foundation (Question 1), to develop SMART objectives and effective strategies (Questions 2 and 3), and evaluate the program (Question 4). At first glance, testing and refining theory (Questions 5 and 6) may seem beyond the scope of most public health communication interventions. In their purest form these can indeed be complex tasks that require a special skillset to complete. But, practically, this does not have to be the case.

To illustrate, while there may be sound theoretical reasons to create low-threat/low-efficacy messages to test the extended parallel process model (Witte, 1992; see Chapter 8), there are few practical reasons to do so given that such messages are known to be less effective (Peters et al., 2013; Sheeran et al., 2015; Tannenbaum et al., 2015). However, outcome evaluation results can help you determine if you successfully manipulated the targeted theoretical constructs, and if these constructs had the expected impact on behavior (Question 5), which speaks to the theories of predictive and explanatory power. Further, outcome evaluation can provide insight into whether the theory was effective for a new topic and intended audience (Question 6), which can extend or limit the scope of the theory.

Unfortunately, many program planners often fail to fully consider or answer such questions during the planning and evaluation process. Consider, for example, Bluethmann et al.'s (2017) recent application of the theory coding scheme to 14 behavior-change programs. This study shows the role of theory in public health communication interventions varies widely from superficial to central. To illustrate, of the 14 programs assessed in their review, 12 mentioned theory (Question 1), 12 targeted relative theoretical constructs (Question 2), three used theory to tailor the program to different subgroups (Question 3), nine presented some evidence of reliability for all theory-based measures (Question 4), three discussed results in relation to theory (Question 5), and none used results to refine theory (Question 6). This is practically problematic given that this study also found that more extensive use of theory was associated with enhanced intervention effectiveness.

In sum, the theory coding scheme encourages "more careful consideration of what constitutes theory-based interventions and how they can be most usefully developed and evaluated" (Michie & Prestwich, 2010, p. 7). Such questions make it easier to fully articulate the role of theory in your own program, and to assess the role of theory in other programs. This is important given the myriad of roles that theory plays in the planning, implementation, and evaluation of public health communication interventions, and given that theory-based programs are more likely to succeed than those that are not based on theory.

## WHAT ARE CONCEPTUAL AND OPERATIONAL DEFINITIONS?

### CONCEPTS, CONSTRUCTS, AND VARIABLES

Concepts, constructs, and variables are the basic building blocks of theory (Turner, 2013). The terms "concept" and "construct" are often used interchangeably, but for our purposes there is a small but important difference between the two. A *concept* is an abstract label or representation of a general idea. A *construct* is a concept that is developed or adopted for a special scientific purpose (i.e., for use in a theory). For example, "self-efficacy" (i.e., an individual's beliefs about their ability to perform a behavior) is an important construct in all of the theories reviewed in this book.

A *variable* is a construct that can have two or more values. For example, one program strategy might be to generate different messages for individuals who are low, moderate, or high in self-efficacy. Another program objective might be to increase self-efficacy regarding some behavior (i.e., from lower to higher). To achieve either strategy or objective, however, you must be able to measure the construct. When you describe how you are going to measure a construct, you are creating a variable. In short, concepts and constructs are more abstract and general, while variables are more concrete and specific. However, in the realm of public health communication interventions, concepts, constructs, and variables are inextricably linked through their conceptual and operational definitions, which will be discussed next.

## CONCEPTUAL DEFINITION

A *conceptual definition* describes what a concept means by relating it to other terms or ideas. For example, consider the following conceptual definition of "efficacy:"

> Efficacy refers to the thoughts a person has about the effectiveness and ease with which a recommended response can prevent a threat.

Here, the concept of "efficacy" is being related to the concepts of "effectiveness" and "ease." Conceptual definitions are like dictionary definitions in the sense that they "strive to communicate a uniform meaning to all those who use them" (Turner, 2013, p. 8). However, conceptual definitions are typically more precise when developing or testing theory. To illustrate, Table 5.2 includes conceptual definitions for eight theoretical constructs common to many of the theories discussed in this book. Further, Table 5.3 shows how each of these key terms (or their approximate equivalents) relates to the health behavior change theories discussed in this section. This list of key variables includes severity, susceptibility, response-efficacy, self-efficacy, norms, attitudes, intentions, and behavior.

| TABLE 5.2    Conceptual Definitions for Common Theoretical Constructs | |
|---|---|
| **Construct** | **Conceptual Definition** |
| Severity | Beliefs about the significance, magnitude, or seriousness of a health threat (e.g., how serious are the short- or long-term consequences of the threat?). |
| Susceptibility | Beliefs about the likelihood or chances that one will experience a health threat (e.g., how likely is it that a threat will occur?). |
| Self-Efficacy | Beliefs about one's ability to perform a behavior under various challenging circumstances (e.g., do the necessary skills and resources exist to engage in the behavior?). |
| Response-Efficacy | Beliefs about the safety or effectiveness of the recommended behavior (e.g., is it an effective way to prevent the threat?). |
| Attitude | How favorably or unfavorably a person feels toward the behavior. |
| Norms | Perceived social pressure to perform a behavior. |
| Intention | A person's readiness, motivation, or plans to perform a behavior in the future. |
| Behavior | What a person does or the way a person acts in a particular situation. |

| TABLE 5.3 | A Comparison of Five Health Behavior Change Theories | | | | |
|---|---|---|---|---|---|
| **Construct** | **HBM** | **SCT** | **EPPM** | **RAA** | **TTM** |
| Severity | ✓ | Outcome Expectations and Facilitators/ Impediments | ✓ | Outcome Evaluation | Decisional Balance |
| Susceptibility | ✓ | Outcome Expectations and Facilitators/ Impediments | ✓ | Behavioral Beliefs | Decisional Balance |
| Response-Efficacy | Benefits and Barriers | Outcome Expectations and Facilitators/ Impediments | ✓ | Behavioral Beliefs | Decisional Balance |
| Self-Efficacy | ✓ | ✓ | ✓ | Perceived Behavioral Control | Confidence & Temptation |
| Norms | Cues to Action | Outcome Expectations and Facilitators/ Impediments | | ✓ | Social Liberation Process of Change |
| Attitudes | Benefits and Barriers | Outcome Expectations and Facilitators/ Impediments | Danger Control | ✓ | Decisional Balance (Pros & Cons) |
| Intentions | Goals | Goals | Danger Control | ✓ | Preparation, Contemplation, & Preparation Stages [1] |
| Behavior | ✓ | ✓ | Danger Control | ✓ | Action and Maintenance Stage [1] |

HBM = Health Belief Model; SCT = Social Cognitive Theory; EPPM = Extended Parallel Process Model; RAA = Reasoned Action Approach; TTM = Transtheoretical Model

Note: A check mark (✓) indicates that the theory explicitly lists the variable in question. Otherwise, when available, the approximate equivalent for a variable is provided. If a cell has been left blank, it means the theory does not include the variable in any form.

[1] Vilicer et al. (2000) note that the stages before behavior change occurs are conceptualized as behavioral intention, and that the stages after behavior change occurs are conceptualized as behavior.

## OPERATIONAL DEFINITION

One interesting aspect of all the concepts defined in Table 5.2 is that they are difficult to observe or are completely unobservable. For example, it is not possible to directly observe an individual's beliefs or attitudes. So, to evaluate the effects a program has on these and other important theoretical concepts, we must find a way to assess them in the real world. Toward that end, an *operational definition* defines a concept by specifying the procedures used to measure it. An operational definition is a "how-to manual" or "step-by-step guide" that tells the program evaluator what to do and how to do it. Unfortunately, developing reliable and valid measures for such abstract concepts is no easy task. The good news is that all the variables discussed in this section have established operational definitions you can use to measure these variables.

So, how do you measure a belief or other construct that you cannot see? The most common way to operationalize such variables is with a series of survey items designed to measure the otherwise unobservable construct. For example, perceived efficacy regarding regular physical activity can be measured with the following set of items:

| | Strongly Disagree | Disagree | Neither Disagree or Agree | Agree | Strongly Agree |
|---|---|---|---|---|---|
| I am able to engage in regular physical activity. | ❑ | ❑ | ❑ | ❑ | ❑ |
| I can engage in regular physical activity. | ❑ | ❑ | ❑ | ❑ | ❑ |
| It is easy for me to engage in regular physical activity. | ❑ | ❑ | ❑ | ❑ | ❑ |
| Regular physical activity is an effective way to prevent heart disease. | ❑ | ❑ | ❑ | ❑ | ❑ |
| Regular physical activity is a good way to prevent heart disease. | ❑ | ❑ | ❑ | ❑ | ❑ |
| If I regularly engage in physical activity, I am less likely to get heart disease. | ❑ | ❑ | ❑ | ❑ | ❑ |

In tandem, these six items measure perceived efficacy as it was defined in the previous section. That is, the first three items focusing on the "ease" portion of this definition (a.k.a., self-efficacy), and the last three items focusing on the "effectiveness" portion of the definition (a.k.a., response-efficacy).

Each item serves as an indicator of a person's beliefs about efficacy, and the resulting score is used to represent the construct of interest. Measurement reliability and validity help us determine the quality of our operational definition by telling us how consistently and accurately we measured what we intended to measure. Given how complex many public health communication variables are, you often need multiple items to measure them fully and accurately. For a variety of statistical reasons that will not be presented here, each variable should be measured with a minimum of three items, and preferably four or more items. Please keep this rule of thumb in mind when creating your own operational definitions or evaluating those presented throughout this book and elsewhere.

### Measurement Reliability

*Measurement reliability* refers to the extent to which an instrument consistently measures whatever it measures. One key aspect of measurement reliability is *internal consistency*, or the extent to which the items used to measure a variable give the same or similar results. The most common way to assess internal consistency is using Cronbach's alpha (sometimes denoted simply using the Greek letter for alpha, or α). *Cronbach's alpha (α)* tells you how connected or related a set of items are. Cronbach's alpha is expressed as a number ranging from 0.00 to 1.00, with higher numbers indicating better internal consistency. The higher the internal consistency, the more confidence we have that the set of items measure the same concept or variable. When evaluating measures for public health communication interventions, the following represents a generally accepted interpretation of Cronbach's alpha:

> .80 to 1.00 = very strong internal consistency
> .70 to  .79 = strong internal consistency
> .60 to  .69 = weak internal consistency
> .00 to  .59 = unacceptable or very weak internal consistency

Note that it is impossible to assess internal consistency with a single item as there would be nothing to compare it to, or no point of reference.

### Measurement Validity

*Measurement validity* refers to the extent to which an instrument fully and accurately measures the construct it is designed to measure. Three key techniques for assessing measurement validity include (1) content validity, (2) factor analysis, and (3) criterion-related validity.

**Content validity.** *Content validity* (sometimes referred to as *face validity* or *conceptual fit*) concerns the match between the conceptual definition of a variable and the operational definition used to measure it. That is, in your opinion (or in the opinion of other relevant experts), does the measure seem like a good translation of the conceptual definition (Trochim, 2001). For example, if your goal is to create a measure of efficacy in general and you included just the first three self-efficacy items provided above, you would have low content validity since self-efficacy is just one of two important aspects of perceived efficacy—the other being response-efficacy (Witte, 1992; Witte et al., 1996). So, for a measure of perceived efficacy to have a strong fit between its conceptual and operational definition, it must measure both self-efficacy and response-efficacy. Content validity is an important but less rigorous way to assess a measure's validity.

**Factor analysis.** Factor analysis is a powerful statistical technique used to assess measurement reliability and validity (Bandalos, 2018). Put simply, the word "factor" is another word for construct or variable. So, *factor analysis* is used to determine how well a set of survey items measures the construct(s) they were designed to measure. It does this by analyzing the relationships between survey items and indicating which items belong together. This allows you to collapse responses to a large number of survey items into a more manageable number of variables. Notably, factor analysis can be used to find or verify relationships between survey items.

*Exploratory factor analysis* (EFA) is used to find underlying patterns or relationships among survey items. EFA is most appropriate when you are uncertain about which survey items measure which construct, which will sometimes be the case when developing new measures for new constructs. For example, imagine that you are the first person to attempt to measure efficacy. You start by developing a set of items similar to those presented earlier in this chapter. Next you administer the survey to members of your intended audience. Finally, you statistically analyze their responses using EFA to organize items into constructs. As it turns out, your results indicate that these survey items measure not one, but two different variables. Upon closer inspection, you realize that one set of items focuses on effectiveness while the other set of items focuses on ease. Thus, you label these constructs response-efficacy and self-efficacy, respectively. I will provide a few examples of EFA in action when I discuss early attempts to measure some of the theoretical constructs included in this book.

*Confirmatory factor analysis* (CFA) is used to verify that the expected items measure the same underlying constructs. CFA is more appropriate when you have a good idea of which survey items measure which construct, as will often be the case when adapting existing measures for new topics or intended audiences. For example, imagine you want to adapt an existing efficacy measure for use with a new topic or intended audience. Based on previous theory and research you expect these items to measure two different types of efficacy (i.e., response-efficacy and self-efficacy). You also expect that the items emphasizing effectiveness will be part of the response-efficacy measure, whereas the items that emphasize ease will be part of the self-efficacy measure. To test this hypothesis, you administer these survey items to members of your intended audience, and statistically analyze their responses using CFA to confirm or reject your supposition that the expected items measure the expected construct. All of the theories reviewed in this book have been applied to a wide variety of topics and intended audiences over the past several decades. Thus, CFA is commonly used to assess the reliability and validity of these constructs.

**Criterion-related validity.** *Criterion-related validity* involves comparing the performance of your measure to some external standard or criteria. For example, *convergent validity* assesses the degree to which a measure is related to (i.e., converges with) other measures in theoretically meaningful ways (Trochim, 2001). To illustrate, the extended parallel process model suggests that measures of self-efficacy and response-efficacy should be more strongly related to each other than to measures of severity or susceptibility—which comprise perceived threat (Witte, 1992; Witte et al., 1996). Similarly, the health belief model suggests that self-efficacy will be positively related to perceived benefits and negatively related to perceived barriers (Skinner et al., 2015). So, if you administered a survey measuring these variables to participants and observed the expected pattern of results, you would have evidence of convergent validity. Also, for example, *predictive validity* concerns how well a measure predicts something it should theoretically be able to predict (Trochim, 2001). To illustrate, social cognitive theory (Bandura, 2004) predicts that increasing an individual's perceptions of self-efficacy regarding a given behavior will increase the likelihood that they will engage in that behavior. Thus, if you find a strong correlation—or better yet, a causal relationship—between your self-efficacy measure and behavior, you will have evidence of predictive validity for this measure.

In sum, those with less experience in the ways of program evaluation often ask, "why do you keep asking the same question over and over again?" Now you know why. First, none of the items are actually the same (i.e., they may be similar, but they are not identical). Second, this is done on purpose and for two very important reasons: to assess measurement reliability and measurement validity. Strong conceptual and operational definitions allow others to judge and replicate your evaluation procedures. Further, just as multiple items provide one good way to judge the reliability and validity of a measure, multiple studies provide a good way to judge the predictive power and practical utility of a theory (especially when a theory generates the same or similar results across a wide variety of topics, intended audiences, messages, etc.). This brings us to the final topic of this chapter: meta-analysis.

## WHAT IS A META-ANALYSIS?

A *meta-analysis* is a quantitative research method used to succinctly combine, compare, and summarize the results of a collection of primary research studies on a topic. When conducting a meta-analysis, a researcher collects all available studies on a subject, calculates an effect size for each study, and produces an average effect size for the topic under investigation. Combining studies in this way provides a more accurate estimate of the topic under investigation. Chapters 6 through 10 will include a summary of seminal meta-analyses related to the theory discussed in each chapter. Thus, a general overview of meta-analysis is presented here.

The goal of most meta-analyses is to answer two major questions: (1) what is the main effect of some independent variable on one or more dependent variables, and (2) do any other variables moderate this effect (Noar, 2006)? Thus, meta-analyses offer a useful point of reference to which you can compare your study's results and provide valuable information for conducting a *power analysis* (i.e., to determine what sample size is required to confidently detect an effect of a given size) for research and grant proposals. A typical meta-analysis will include the following six steps (Cooper, 2017; Del Re & Flückiger, 2016; Durlak, 1995; Hunter et al., 1982; Noar, 2006; Tanner-Smith et al., 2017).

*Step 1* involves formulating the research question or hypothesis. The goals here are to set the boundary conditions for your study by identifying what literature you will review, and to advancing formal research questions and hypotheses about this body of research. *Step 2* entails searching the literature selected in Step 1. This step focuses on how articles are identified, how many articles are identified, and how many articles were ultimately included in the manuscript. Figure 5.1 outlines the meticulous process of identifying, assessing, and selecting studies for a meta-analysis. *Step 3* consists of gathering the information necessary to conduct the meta-analyses from studies selected in Step 2. This includes gathering the data necessary to compute effect sizes, including both main effects and moderator effects (more will be said about effect sizes, main effects, and moderator effects below). *Step 4*

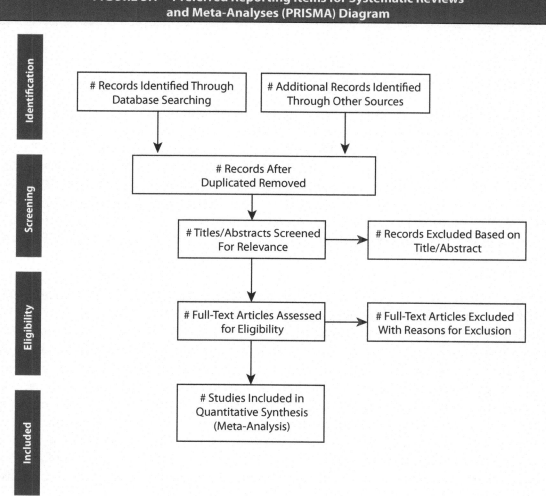

**FIGURE 5.1    Preferred Reporting Items for Systematic Reviews and Meta-Analyses (PRISMA) Diagram**

Adapted from Moher et al. (2009).

entails calculating effect sizes using the the data gathered during Step 3. *Step 5* involves analyzing data for main effects and moderator effects. The goal here is to determine the average effect size across all the studies in the meta-analysis, as well as what descriptive, conceptual, and methodological moderators are associated with stronger effects. Finally, *Step 6* concludes the process by presenting and interpreting the results using the thresholds for effect sizes included in Table 5.4.

| TABLE 5.4    Threshold for Interpreting Effect Sizes | | | | |
|---|---|---|---|---|
| Test | Small | Medium | Large | Very Large |
| Standardized Mean Difference (*d, g*) | .20 | .50 | .80 | 1.30 |
| Correlation (*r*) | .10 | .30 | .50 | .70 |

Adapted from Cohen (1988) and Rosenthal (1996).

Each of these steps has its own set of detailed instructions that are extremely important for those who want to conduct a meta-analysis, but that are less important for occasional readers of meta-analyses. So, Table 5.5 contains a "Meta-Analysis Worksheet" that I adapted from these steps to help occasional readers more easily keep track of and assess the quality of the most important information presented in a meta-analysis. Most of the steps for conducting a meta-analysis will be familiar to those who have taken a research methods class. However, some important aspects of Step 4 (effect sizes) and Step 5 (main effects and moderator effects) may be less familiar, so a brief introduction to these two steps follows.

## EFFECT SIZE

*Effect size* represents a standardized way of quantifying the magnitude of a relationship between two variables or a difference between two groups (Del Re & Flückiger, 2016). For example, suppose you conduct an experiment to assess the effects of a public health communication campaign on behavior (i.e., you compared a treatment group that was exposed to the campaign to a no treatment control group that was not). An effect size would tell you if there were a small, medium, or large difference between these two groups (i.e., those who were and were not exposed public health communication campaign). Also, for example, suppose you conduct an experiment to assess the effects of threatening communication on behavior (i.e., you compared a treatment group that received a threatening message to a no treatment control group that did not). Here, the effect size would tell how much of an effect the independent variable (i.e., threatening communication) had on the dependent variable (i.e., behavior).

Effect sizes have been called the "common currency" of meta-analyses, as they allow researchers to convert results from different studies into the same metric and make it possible to compare results across studies (Becker, 2000; Durlak, 1995; Tanner-Smith et al., 2017). Coe (2002) notes that effect sizes are especially valuable for determining the effectiveness of public health communication interventions. Further, given that effect size estimates are independent of sample size, "it allows us to move beyond the simplistic, 'Does it work or not?' to the far more sophisticated, 'How well does it work?'" (Coe, 2002).

As is the case with many statistics, there are several different ways to calculate effect size depending on the nature of the data being studied. A few of the most common include

| TABLE 5.5     Meta-Analysis Worksheet |
|---|

**Step 1:  Formulate the Research Question or Hypothesis**
- ▶  What literature was reviewed? What were the key research questions or hypothesis?

**Step 2:  Search the Literature (see Figure 5.1)**
- ▶  What were the inclusion/exclusion criteria (i.e., what criteria did a study have to meet to be included in the meta-analysis)?
- ▶  How were articles/manuscripts identified (i.e., computer search, references from obtained articles, etc.)?
- ▶  How many articles/manuscripts were initially identified (were unpublished studies included)?
- ▶  How many articles/manuscripts were ultimately included in the meta-analysis (were unpublished manuscripts included)?
- ▶  How many datasets were included in the meta-analysis (i.e., sometimes a single article may include multiple relevant tests or studies)?
- ▶  How many total participants were included in the meta-analysis?

**Step 3:  Gather Information From Studies (Study Coding)**
- ▶  What descriptive, conceptual, or methodological moderators were studied in the meta-analysis?
- ▶  What coding procedures were used? Was inter-coder reliability assessed and reported?

**Step 4:  Calculate Effect Sizes**
- ▶  What effect size was used (i.e., typically *d*, *g*, or *r*)?

**Step 5:  Analyze Data for Main Effects and Moderator Effects**
- ▶  What were the main effects for the phenomenon under investigation? What was the average effect size across all the studies in the meta-analysis?
- ▶  Were there any moderator effects? What descriptive, conceptual, or methodological features were associated with stronger study outcomes (i.e., larger effect sizes)?

**Step 6:  Present and Interpret Results**
- ▶  Would you classify these effect sizes as small, medium, large, or very large (see Table 5.4)?

Cohen's *d*, Hedges' *g*, and Pearson's *r*. Table 5.4 presents the conventional thresholds for interpreting each type of effect size as small, medium, large, or very large. As you can see from this table, all four effect sizes serve a similar purpose. However, there are some differences in how they are calculated and when they are used. For example, Pearson's *r* is used when both the independent variable and dependent variable are continuous (i.e., when both variables are measured along some continuum, such as a seven-point scale). Cohen's *d* and Hedge's *g*, on the other hand, are used when the independent variable is dichotomous (i.e., has only two levels, such as a treatment group and a control group) and the dependent variable is continuous (Del Re & Flückiger, 2016). Also, for example, Cohen's $d$ works well with larger sample sizes but has a slight bias with smaller samples sizes, whereas Hedge's $g$ provides a correction for small sample sizes (Bornstein et al., 2009). Though there are many ways to calculate effect sizes, it should be sufficient for occasional readers of meta-analyses to know the most common effect sizes and how they are interpreted. Readers desiring more information about effect sizes are referred to Becker (2000), Coe (2002), Wilson (2013), and Bornstein et al. (2009).

## MAIN EFFECTS AND MODERATOR EFFECTS

As noted above, meta-analyses typically assess both main and moderator effects. A *main effect* is the impact of one independent variable on the dependent variable, ignoring the effects of all other variables. For example, Snyder and colleagues (2002, 2004, 2009) conducted a series of meta-analyses to assess the impact of public health communication campaigns on behavior. Their 2002 meta-analysis included 48 studies and 168,362 participants. Results from this meta-analysis indicate that public health communication campaigns tended to have a small and significant main effect on behavior ($r = .09$). Also, for example, a meta-analysis by Peters et al. (2013) assessed the effects of threatening communication on behavior. They found that threatening communication had a small but insignificant main effect ($d = .11$) on behavior across the six randomized control trials included in their meta-analysis.

A *moderator* is a third variable that changes the strength of the relationship between two variables. In addition to determining the main effect of an independent variable on the dependent variable, a meta-analysis allows a researcher to test whether these effects are influenced by other variables. For example, Snyder et al. (2002) examined whether the effect of public health communication campaigns on behavior was moderated by the presence or absence of an enforcement component (e.g., the enforcement of a law regarding seat belt use). Results indicate that campaigns with an enforcement component ($r = .17$) were more successful than campaigns without an enforcement component ($r = .05$). Also, for example, Peters et al. (2013) examined whether the effect of threatening communication on behavior was moderated by efficacy messages. That is, were high threat/high efficacy messages more effective at influencing behavior than high threat/low efficacy messages? The answer was clearly yes. High threat/high efficacy messages had a significant effect of $d = .31$, while high threat/low efficacy messages had an insignificant effect of $d = -.31$. In other words, threatening communication only worked when accompanied with an efficacy message. This is a perfect example of the potential importance of a moderator variable. It would be tempting to conclude from the small and insignificant main effect reported above that threatening communication does not work. However, that would not be a completely accurate conclusion, as including efficacy as a moderator tells a different story (i.e., threatening communication does work when it is also accompanied by a high efficacy message).

### *Descriptive, Theoretical, and Methodological Moderators*

Potential moderators can be classified into three main categories. *Descriptive moderators* typically include the demographic or psychographic characteristics of the samples being studied, or some basic features of the included studies themselves. Some common descriptive moderators that you will read about in this book include gender, age, study topic, publication status, and so on. *Theoretical moderators* focus on the concepts included in, and the relationships predicted by, the theory or theories under investigation. For example, are messages guided by certain theories more or less effective at changing behavior than messages guided by other theories? Or does the presence or absence of certain variables increase or decrease the theory's effectiveness at predicting behavior in expected ways? Efficacy is a perfect example of a theoretical moderator that was assessed in the Peters et al. (2013) meta-analysis discussed above (Witte, 1992). *Methodological moderators* concern the procedures used to conduct the study or collect the data. For instance, intervention duration, time between pretest and posttest (or between the intervention and posttest), study setting (e.g., lab vs. field), and type of behavior measure used (i.e., objective vs. self-report) are just a few of the common methodological moderators that may be investigated in a meta-analysis.

In sum, meta-analysis is a valuable way to analyze and integrate data from multiple studies on a topic. A meta-analysis quantifies the magnitude of a relationship between two variables or difference between two groups and identifies if the main effect is influenced (i.e., moderated) by a variety of descriptive, theoretical, or methodological factors. While meta-analysis does have a few limitations (Bornstein, 2009; Del Re & Flückiger, 2016), when carefully conducted it is a valuable tool for evaluating public health communication theories and the effectiveness of programs guided by these theories. For example, Tanner-Smith et al. (2017) note that "such research summaries are critical for informing evidence-based practices and policies" (p. 134). Thus, all five chapters included in this section will provide a review of recent meta-analysis results regarding the theory in question.

## CONCLUSION

The main goal of this chapter was to review three key topics you will want to keep in mind as you read the remainder of the chapters in this section of the book: theory, conceptual and operational definitions, and meta-analysis. In short, theories provide systematic explanations for how to change behavior, conceptual and operational definitions describe what the constructs in the theory mean and how to measure them, and meta-analysis provides a concise way to summarize the results of many studies on a specific topic or guided by a theory. All three topics represent indispensable tools that provide essential information during the planning, implementation, and evaluation of public health communication interventions.

## REFERENCES

Bandalos, D. L. (2018). *Measurement theory and applications for the social science.* Guilford Press.

Bandura, A. (2004). Health promotion by social cognitive means. *Health Education & Behavior, 31*(2), 143–164. https://doi.org/10.1177/1090198104263660

Bartholomew, L. K., & Mullen, P. D. (2011). Five roles for using theory and evidence in the design and testing of behavior change interventions. *Journal of Public Health Dentistry, 71*(S1), S20–S33. https://doi.org/10.1111/j.1752-7325.2011.00223.x

Becker, L. A. (2000). *Effect sizes (ES).* http://www.uccs.edu/lbecker/effect-size.html

Bluethmann, S. M., Bartholomew, L. K., Murphy, C. C., & Vernon, S. W. (2017). Use of theory in behavior change interventions: An analysis of programs to increase physical activity in posttreatment breast cancer survivors. *Health Education & Behavior, 44*(2), 245–253. https://doi.org/10.1177/1090198116647712

Bornstein, M., Hedges, L. V., Higgins, J. P. T., & Rothstein, H. R. (2009). *Introduction to meta-analysis.* John Wiley & Sons.

Chaffee, S. H., & Berger, C. R. (1987). What communication scientists do. In C. R. Berger & S. H. Chaffee (Eds.), *Handbook of communication science* (pp. 99–122). SAGE.

Coe, R. (2002). *It's the effect size, stupid: What effect size is and why it is important.* https://www.leeds.ac.uk/educol/documents/00002182.htm

Cohen, J. (1988). *Statistical power analysis for the behavioral sciences* (2nd ed.). Laurence Erlbaum Associates.

Cooper, H. (2017). *Research synthesis and meta-analysis: A step-by-step approach* (5th ed.). SAGE.

Del Re, A. C., & Flückiger, C. (2016). Meta-analysis. In J. C. Norcross, G. R. VandenBos, D. K. Freedheim, & B. O. Olatunji, (Eds.), *APA handbook of clinical psychology: Theory and research* (Vol. 2, pp. 479–491). American Psychological Association. https://doi.org/10.1037/14773-022

Durlak, J. A. (1995). Understanding meta-analysis. In L. G. Grimm & P. R. Yarnold (Eds.), *Reading and understanding multivariate statistics* (pp. 319–352). American Psychological Association.

Fishbein, M., & Ajzen, I. (2010). *Predicting and changing behavior: The reasoned action approach.* Psychology Press.

Glanz, K., & Bishop, D. B. (2010). The role of behavioral science theory in development and implementation of public health interventions. *Annual Review of Public Health,* 31, 339–418. https://doi.org/10.1146/annurev.publhealth.012809.103604

Glanz, K., Rimer, B. K., & Viswanath, K. (2015). Theory, research, & practice in health behavior. In K. Glanz, B. K. Rimer, & K. Viswanath (Eds.), *Health behavior: Theory, research, and practice* (5th ed.). Jossey-Bass.

Green, J. (2000). The role of theory in evidence-based health promotion practice. *Health Education Research, 15*(2), 125–129. https://doi.org/10.1093/her/15.2.125

Green, L. W., & Kreuter, M. W. (2005). *Health promotion planning: An educational and ecological approach* (4th ed.). McGraw-Hill.

Griffin, E., Ledbetter, A., & Sparks, G. (2019). *A first look at communication theory.* McGraw-Hill.

Hunter, J. E., Schmidt, F. L., & Jackson, G. B. (1982). *Meta-analysis: Cumulating research findings across studies.* SAGE.

Lewin, K. (1945). The Research Center for Group Dynamics at Massachusetts Institute for Technology. *Sociometry, 8*(2), 126–136. https://doi.org/10.2307/2785233

Michie, S., & Prestwich, A. (2010). Are interventions theory based? Development of a theory coding scheme. *Health Psychology, 29*(1), 1–8. https://doi.org/10.1037/a0016939

Moher, D., Liberati, A., Tetzlaff, J., Altman, D. G., & The PRISMA Group. (2009). *Preferred Reporting Items for Systematic Reviews and Meta-Analyses: The PRISMA statement. Annals of Internal Medicine, 151*(4), 264–269. https://doi.org/10.7326/0003-4819-151-4-200908180-00135

National Cancer Institute .(2001). *Making health communication programs work.* US Department of Health & Human Services. https://www.cancer.gov/publications/health-communication/pink-book.pdf

Noar, S. M. (2006). In pursuit of cumulative knowledge in health communication: The role of meta-analysis. *Health Communication, 20*(2), 169–175. https://doi.org/10.1207/s15327027hc2002_8

Noar, S. M., Benac, C., & Harris, M. (2007). Does tailoring matter? Meta-analytic review of tailored print health behavior change interventions. *Psychological Bulletin, 133*(4), 673–693. https://doi.org/10.1037/0033-2909.133.4.673

Peters, G. J. Y., Ruiter, R. A., & Kok, G. (2013). Threatening communication: A critical re-analysis and a revised meta-analytic test of fear appeal theory. *Health Psychology Review, 7*(S1), S8–S31. https://doi.org/10.1080/17437199.2012.703527

Prochaska, J. O., Redding, C. A., & Evers, K. E. (2015). The transtheoretical model and stages of change. In K. Glanz, B. K. Rimer, & K. Viswanath (Eds.), *Health behavior: Theory, Research, and Practice* (5th ed., pp. 125–148). Jossey-Bass.

Rimer, B. K., & Glanz, K. (2005). *Theory at a glance: A guide for health promotion practice* (2nd ed.) National Cancer Institute, U.S. Department of Health and Human Services. National Institutes of Health.

Rosenthal, J. A. (1996). Qualitative descriptors of strength of association and effect size. *Journal of Social Service Research, 21*(4), 37–59. https://doi.org/10.1300/J079v21n04_02

Sheeran, P., Harris, P. R., & Epton, T. (2014). Does heightening risk appraisals change people's intentions and behavior? A meta-analysis of experimental studies. *Psychological Bulletin, 140*(2), 511–543. https://doi.org/10.1037/a0033065

Shoemaker, P. J., Tankland, J. W., & Lasorsa, D. L. (2004). *How to build social science theories.* SAGE.

Skinner, C. S., Tiro, J., & Champion, V. L. (2015). The health belief model. In K. Glanz, B. K. Rimer, & K. Viswanath (Eds.), *Health behavior: Theory, research, and practice* (5th ed., pp. 75–94). Jossey-Bass.

Snyder, L. B., & Hamilton, M. A. (2002). A meta-analysis of U.S. health campaign effects on behavior: Emphasize enforcement, exposure, and new information, and beware the secular trend. In R. C. Hornik (Ed.), *Public health communication: Evidence for behavior change* (pp. 357–383). Lawrence Erlbaum Associates.

Snyder, L. B., Hamilton, M. A., & Huedo-Medina, T. (2009). Does evaluation design impact communication campaign effect size? A meta-analysis. *Communication Methods and Measures, 3*(1–2), 84–104. https://doi.org/10.1080/19312450902809722

Snyder, L. B., Hamilton, M. A., Mitchell, E. W., Kiwanuka-Tondo, J., Fleming-Milici, F., & Proctor, D. (2004). A meta-analysis of the effect of mediated health communication campaigns on behavior change in the United States. *Journal of Health Communication, 9*(S1), 71–96. https://doi.org/10.1080/10810730490271548

Tannenbaum, M. B., Hepler, J., Zimmerman, R. S., Saul, L., Jacobs, S., Wilson, K., & Albarracín, D. (2015). Appealing to fear: A meta-analysis of fear appeal effectiveness and theories. *Psychological Bulletin, 141*(6), 1178–1204. https://doi.org/10.1037/a0039729

Tanner-Smith, E. E., Lipsey, M. W., & Durlak, J. A. (2017). Meta-analysis: Potentials and limitations for synthesizing research in community psychology. In M. A. Bond, I. Serrano-García, C. B. Keys, & M. Shinn (Eds.), *APA handbook of community psychology: Methods for community research and action for diverse groups and issues* (Vol. 2, pp. 123–137). American Public Health Association. https://doi.org/10.1037/14954-008

Trochim, W. M. K. (2001). *The research methods knowledge base.* Atomic Dog Publishing.

Turner, J. H. (2013). *Contemporary sociological theory* (3rd ed). SAGE.

Velicer, W. F., Prochaska, J. O., Fava, J. L., Rossi, J. S., Redding, C. A., Laforge, R. G., & Robbins, M. L. (2000). Using the transtheoretical model for population-based approaches to health promotion and disease prevention. *Homeostasis in Health & Disease, 40*(5), 174–195.

Webb, T. L., Joseph, J., Yardley, L., & Michie, S. (2010). Using the internet to promote health behavior change: A systematic review and meta-analysis of the impact of theoretical bias, use of behavior change techniques, and mode of delivery on efficacy. *Journal of Medical Internet Research, 12*(1), e4. https://doi.org/10.2196/jmir.1376

Willis, S. E. (2010). Toward a science of metatheory. *Integral Review, 6*(3), 73–120. https://integralreview.org/issues/vol_6_no_3_wallis_toward_a_science_of_metatheory.pdf

Wilson, D. B. (2013). *Practical meta-analysis effect size calculator.* http://cebcp.org/practical-meta-analysis-effect-size-calculator/

Witte, K. (1992). Putting the fear back into fear appeals: The extended parallel process model. *Communication Monographs, 59*(4), 329–349. https://doi.org/10.1080/03637759209376276

Witte, K., Cameron, K. A., McKeon, J. K., & Berkowitz, J. M. (1996). Predicting risk behaviors: Development and validation of a diagnostic scale. *Journal of Health Communication, 1*(4), 317–341. https://doi.org/10.1080/108107396127988

# Health Belief Model

**CHAPTER OUTLINE**

## INTRODUCTION

The health belief model (HBM) represents one of the earliest attempts to predict and explain health behavior. Rosenstock (1966, 1990) notes that the original HBM was developed in the 1950s by a group of social psychologists at the U.S. Public Health Service. At the time, they sought to better understand why so few people were participating in programs designed to prevent, detect, or diagnose disease and illness—even when these services were offered in convenient locations and free of charge. In short, their findings suggested that whether or not an individual engages in a health behavior is a function of two overarching factors: perceived threat and outcome expectations. In other words, individuals who believe they are susceptible to a health issue that has severe consequences (perceived threat) will be more likely to take an action that they believe will reduce the threat (outcome expectations).

With this in mind, I will begin this chapter with an overview of the original HBM, which was designed to describe the relationships between health behavior and (1) demographic and psychographic variables, (2) four individual health beliefs, and (3) cues to action. Two proposed extensions of the HBM are also discussed in this section. Next, I will review how to reliably and validly measure all key constructs in this model and provide sample survey items for each variable. Finally, I review results from three meta-analyses on the HBM. Before continuing, however, please consider the following background information about breast cancer, which will serve as the running example for this chapter.

Generally speaking, cancer is a disease where abnormal cells in the body grow out of control and have the ability to infiltrate and destroy normal body tissue (Mayo Clinic, 2021a). When cancer starts in the breast, it is called breast cancer. Breast cancer affects millions of individuals each year, either through one's own diagnosis or the diagnosis of a family member or friend. In the US, nearly 250,000 cases (245,000 women and 2,200 men) of breast cancer are diagnosed, and nearly 42,000 people (41,000 women and 460 men) die from breast cancer every year (Centers for Disease Control and Prevention, 2019a).

According to the Centers for Disease Control and Prevention (CDC; 2018a), being female and getting older are the two biggest risk factors for breast cancer. Other risk factors can include family history, lack of physical activity, poor diet, being overweight or obese, and drinking alcohol. The National Breast Cancer Foundation (2016) notes that one in eight women and 1 in 1,000 men will be diagnosed with breast cancer in their lifetime. And, while male breast cancer is rare, "men carry a higher mortality than women do, primarily because awareness among men is less and they are less likely to assume a lump is breast cancer, which can cause a delay in seeking treatment." Also, while most breast cancers are found in women who are 50 or older, about 11% of all new cases affect women younger than 45 years of age (CDC, 2019b). The National Cancer Institute (2018) notes that breast cancer is one of the most common types of cancer among 25- to 39-year-olds. Further, young women generally face more aggressive breast cancers and lower survival rates than their older counterparts (Anders et al., 2008; Anders et al., 2011). Thus, it is important for women and men of all ages to be aware of the potential signs of breast cancer.

Unfortunately, breast cancer cannot be prevented. But there are steps you can take to increase your chances of finding breast cancer early, which provides the best chance of effective treatment (Mayo Clinic, 2021b). First, be aware of potential breast-cancer warning signs and symptoms. Examples include a lump in the breast or armpit, thickening or swelling of part of the breast, nipple discharge other than breast milk, any change in the size or shape of the breast, or pain in any area of the breast (CDC, 2018b). The second is breast self-awareness, which involves being familiar with the look and feel of your breasts, so you know what is normal for you (Torborg, 2018). If you notice any changes, you should contact your health care provider as soon as possible to determine if these symptoms are the result of breast cancer or some other condition. Third, schedule a regular mammogram, which is an x-ray of the breast. The CDC (2018c) notes that "mammograms are the best test doctors have to find breast cancer early, sometimes up to three years before it can be felt." The American Cancer Society recommends that all women should begin yearly mammograms at age 45; though women at higher risk may need mammograms earlier or more often (Oeffinger et al., 2015). Please keep this information in mind as I discuss the HBM in the following sections.

## HEALTH BELIEF MODEL

The original HBM looked at the direct effects of four health beliefs—susceptibility, severity, benefits, barriers—on preventive behaviors. It viewed demographic and psychographic variables as modifying factors that indirectly influence behavior by moderating the effects of individual beliefs. Finally, it viewed cues to action as having both a direct and indirect influence on behavior. Figure 6.1 provides a visual representation of the HBM, and Table 6.1 provides conceptual definitions for each component of the HBM. Next, I discuss the original components of the HBM, followed by some suggested extensions to the model.

**FIGURE 6.1    The Health Belief Model[1]**

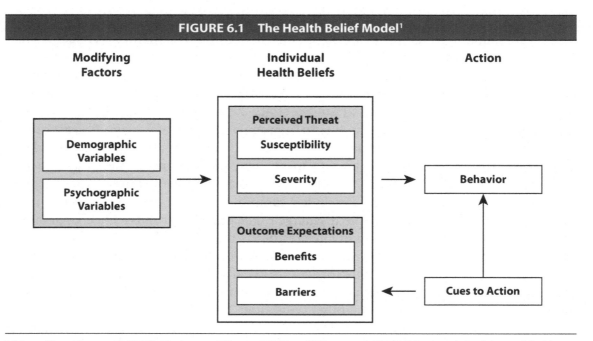

[1] Adapted from Rosenstock (1990), Abraham and Sheeran (2015), and Skinner et al. (2015). Other iterations of the model add general health motivation (Abraham & Sheeran, 2015; Becker, 1974) or self-efficacy (Rosenstock, 1990; Rosenstock et al., 1988; Skinner et al., 2015) to the health beliefs box.

## MODIFYING FACTORS: DEMOGRAPHIC AND PSYCHOGRAPHIC VARIABLES

The first part of the HBM includes any demographic and psychographic variables that might influence health beliefs. *Demographic variables* divide people into groups based on basic characteristics of a population. Age, gender, ethnicity, and socioeconomic status (which can be further subdivided into things like occupation, education, and income) are all examples of demographic variables. Other examples include marital status, family size, religion, home ownership, location, sexual orientation, and so forth. *Psychographic variables* divide people into groups based on lifestyle, personality, or other psychological factors. For example, those interested in maintaining a healthy lifestyle are more likely to exercise and eat well, and less likely to drink alcohol in excess or to use tobacco products. Other psychological factors include things like innovativeness (i.e., how early or late the person is in adopting a new idea, practice, or product; Rogers, 2003) and sensation seeking (i.e., the search for experiences that are varied, novel, complex, and intense, often regardless of the risks involved; Zuckerman, 1994). In sum, demographic variables describe who your intended audience is, whereas psychographic variables help explain why they do or do not engage in a particular behavior.

| TABLE 6.1 | Conceptual Definitions for Health Belief Model Constructs |
|---|---|
| **Construct** | **Conceptual Definition** |
| Demographic Variables | Divide people into groups based on basic characteristics of a population (e.g., age, gender, socioeconomic status, etc.). |
| Psychographic Variables | Divide people into groups based on lifestyle, personality, or other psychological factors. |
| Perceived Threat | Thoughts a person has about a danger that exists in the environment. |
| Severity | Beliefs about the significance, magnitude, or seriousness of a health threat. |
| Susceptibility | Beliefs about the likelihood or chances that one will experience a health threat. |
| Outcome Expectations | One's subjective estimate regarding the likelihood that a specific behavior will lead to a particular consequence. |
| Benefits | Any benefits or advantages that help or encourage a person to engage in a behavior. |
| Barriers | Any cons or disadvantages that hinder or discourage a person from engaging in a behavior. |
| Self-Efficacy | Beliefs about one's ability to perform a behavior under various challenging circumstances. |
| General Health Motivation | One's overall state of readiness to be concerned about health matters. |
| Cues to Action | Internal or external prompts that cause people to change or want to change their beliefs or behavior. |
| Behavior | What a person does or the way a person acts in a particular situation. |

Demographic and psychographic variables are referred to as modifying factors by the HBM as they do not influence behavior directly. Instead, they influence health beliefs (discussed below), which in turn have a direct impact on behavior. For example, gender likely moderates the relationship between perceived susceptibility and breast cancer detection behaviors since women typically know they can get breast cancer, whereas men may not even be aware that males can also get breast cancer. The same would likely be true for any health problem that disproportionately impacts people of different ages, races, sexual orientations, lifestyles, and so forth.

## INDIVIDUAL HEALTH BELIEFS

Again, the original HBM predicted that people will be more likely to engage in a healthy behavior if they believe that (1) they are susceptible to a health issue, (2) the issue has severe consequences, and that (3) the benefits of the recommended behavior outweigh (4) the costs of engaging in the behavior. As indicated in Figure 6.1, susceptibility and severity may be combined to form *perceived threat*, the belief that a health issue will negatively impact one's lifestyle. And, benefits and barriers can be combined to form *outcome expectations*, or one's subjective estimate regarding the likelihood that a specific behavior will lead to a particular consequence (Lippke, 2017; Rosenstock et al., 1988, 1994).

Unfortunately, the original HBM did not provide clear guidelines for calculating perceived threat or outcome expectations (Abraham & Sheeran, 2015). Skinner et al. (2015) suggest calculating perceived threat by multiplying perceived susceptibility by perceived severity (i.e., threat = susceptibility × severity), so that if either component is zero, perceived threat would also be zero. Others suggest calculating that outcome expectations by subtracting perceived barriers from perceived benefits (i.e., outcome expectations = barriers – benefits; Janz & Becker, 1984; Rosenstock, 1974). Unfortunately, the best way to calculate perceived threat and outcome expectations remain largely unresolved to this day (Abraham & Sheeran, 2015; Skinner et al. 2015). Thus, the HBM is typically investigated as a series of separate independent variables that potentially impact health behaviors (Abraham & Sheeran, 2015). With this in mind, the balance of this section will define and provide examples for the four variables that make up the original "health belief box" (i.e., susceptibility, severity, benefits, and barriers).

### Perceived Susceptibility

*Perceived susceptibility* refers to beliefs about the likelihood or chances that one will experience a health threat (i.e., how likely is it that a negative health outcome will occur?). For example, individuals who believe that there is a good possibility that they will get breast cancer sometime during their life would be higher in perceived susceptibility than individuals who did not hold such beliefs (Champion, 1999). To provide another example, individuals who eat red or processed meats more than a few times a week, are not physically active, or use tobacco products are often aware that they are more susceptible to heart disease and a wide variety of cancers than those who eat lots of vegetables and whole grains, are physically active several times a week, and do not smoke.

### Perceived Severity

*Perceived severity* refers to one's beliefs about the significance, seriousness, or magnitude of a health threat (i.e., how dangerous are the short- or long-term consequences of the threat?). Most people view any type of cancer as severe. For example, most successful cancer treatments involve some combination of surgery, chemotherapy, or radiation, all of which have considerable side effects. And, when treatment is not successful, the mental and physical impact of cancer itself (up to and including death) are also very serious. So, there is typically little need to spend much time convincing people that cancer is severe (Champion, 1999). But, what about something as simple and common as a mosquito bite?

Normally mosquito bites cause only minor itching or discomfort for a short period of time (i.e., low severity). However, a few years before this book was written there were serious concerns about the spread of the Zika virus in parts of the US. The Zika virus can cause serious birth defects (high severity) if passed from an infected mother to her fetus and was spreading at an alarming rate in parts of Florida (high susceptibility). Given this, the Centers for Disease Control and Prevention (CDC) issued a historic travel warning to one northern Miami community; it was "the first time the CDC has warned people not to travel to an American neighborhood for fear of catching an infectious disease" (LaMotte, 2016). In sum, the HBM model predicts that when both susceptibility and severity are high, perceived threat will be high, and individuals will be more likely to engage in a recommended behavior that reduce this threat.

## Perceived Benefits

*Perceived benefits* are any advantages that help or encourage a person to engage in a behavior (i.e., the "pros" of the behavior). Typically, perceived benefits focus on the value or usefulness of a behavior in reducing the health threat (i.e., does it reduce the susceptibility to or severity of a threat?). For example, do you believe that mammograms can detect breast cancer early? Or, that eating more vegetables and whole grains, being physically active, and tobacco-free living help prevent heart disease and a wide variety of cancers? Or that getting vaccinated against the human papillomavirus (HPV) will provide protection against genital warts and cervical cancer? If you answered yes to one or more of these questions, your perceived benefits for that behavior would be considered high (Champion, 1984, 1999). Other common examples of benefits include lowering costs, saving time, increasing convenience or ease, or improving quality and length of life.

## Perceived Barriers

*Perceived barriers* (a.k.a., *perceived costs*) are any disadvantages that hinder or discourage a person from engaging in a behavior (i.e., the "cons" of the behavior). For example, some people believe that getting a mammogram is embarrassing, painful, or takes too much time, while others may simply be afraid of getting a positive result (Champion, 1999). Some people find eating healthier to be expensive or inconvenient, engaging in physical activity to be uncomfortable or time-consuming, and the side effects of quitting smoking to be especially difficult. Further, a vaccine that requires just a single dose at one point in time has fewer barriers than one that requires multiple doses over a longer period of time. A lack of health insurance is also a barrier as treatment without insurance is often cost-prohibitive or difficult to obtain. Further, lack of knowledge or skills are barriers making it more difficult to know what to do or how to do it. In sum, the HBM model predicts that behaviors with greater benefits and fewer barriers are more likely to be adopted than behaviors with fewer benefits and greater barriers.

## CUES TO ACTION

Finally, the HBM suggests that individual health beliefs and behaviors are also influenced by *cues to action*, or internal or external prompts that cause people to change or want to change their beliefs or behavior. *Internal cues to action* usually involve noticing some sort of physical or mental change in yourself. It could be something as simple as noticing you've gained some weight (the cue) and deciding it is time to adjust your diet or start exercising (the action). Or, you might realize that you have been feeling depressed or anxious lately (the cue) and decide to seek help from a mental health professional (the action). Or, you might notice a lump or soreness on your breast (the cue) and decide to get screened for breast cancer (the action).

*External cues to action* include a wide variety of environmental factors that might trigger behavior change. For example, seeing a friend or family member deal with an illness (the cue) may trigger a desire to get screened or take steps to prevent experiencing the health problem yourself (the action). Recommendations from doctors or other health professionals also serve as external cues to action (as do the reminder calls, texts, or emails that doctors, dentists, and other health professionals send to remind you about an upcoming appointment). Also, many grocery stores and pharmacies have prominently located point-of-purchase displays (often near the checkout register) that serve as cues to action. Finally, the media is filled with entertainment programming, public service announcements (PSA), health communication interventions, and news stories that can serve as cues to action. For example, singer Sheryl Crow, actress Christina Applegate, and comedian Wanda Sykes are just a few of the many famous women to publicly announce their breast cancer diagnoses in an effort to raise awareness of the disease. Also, for example, many men had no idea that males could get breast cancer until Peter Criss (the original drummer for the band Kiss) was diagnosed with the disease in 2008. He talked about his battle with breast cancer during an interview in 2009 and shared this message for men who noticed a painful lump in their chest: "Don't sit around playing Mr. Tough Guy. Don't say 'It's going to go away.' It's just important, just go get it checked out" (Rolling Stone, 2009).

Unfortunately, even though cues to action is an original component of the HBM, it remains relatively understudied to this day. For example, Zimmerman and Vernberg

(1994) note that only 4 of the 30 studies in their meta-analysis included cues to action. On a related note, Harrison et al. (1992) and Carpenter (2010) did not include cues to action in their meta-analyses given that so few of the studies included cues to action. Finally, it is worth noting that individual studies often report nonsignificant relationships between cues to action and behavior (e.g., Gabrie et al., 2018; McClenahan et al., 2006). Abraham and Sheeran (2015) note this is likely because cues to action can refer to very different factors for different topics and intended audiences, making it difficult to measure or successfully target cues to action during an intervention.

## ADDITIONS TO THE HEALTH BELIEF MODEL

Perceived severity, susceptibility, benefits, and barriers, represent the four major components of the health belief box in the HBM. However, the HBM has since been revised to include one or two other variables; namely general health motivation (Abraham & Sheeran, 2015; Becker, 1974) and self-efficacy (Rosenstock et al., 1988; Skinner et al., 2015). And, while these variables are sometimes included in HBM studies today, they tend to be included less frequently than the four original HBM variables. To illustrate, Zimmerman and Vernberg (1994) note that only 6 of the 30 studies in their meta-analysis included general health motivation, and only 2 of the 30 studies included self-efficacy. More recently, the Carpenter (2010) meta-analysis opted to focus on just the four original HBM variables given that so few HBM studies included general health motivation and self-efficacy. Nonetheless, one or both of these variables represent potentially important extensions to the HBM that are sometimes included in HBM research (e.g., Champion, 1984; Gabriel et al., 2018; McClenahan et al., 2006). Thus, brief discussions of general health motivation and self-efficacy follow.

### General Health Motivation

Becker (1974) argued that some individuals are more predisposed than others to be concerned about health and respond to cues to action. This predisposition has been labeled *general health motivation*, which refers to an individual's overall state of readiness to be concerned about health matters. Individuals high in general health motivation have a greater desire to maintain health and avoid illness. So, they are more likely to engage in a range of healthy behaviors, including eating a well-balanced diet, exercising regularly, getting regular physical or dental exams, following medical advice, and so forth (Champion, 1984). While no HBM meta-analysis to date has looked at the effects of general health motivation, results from several individual HBM studies typically report small but significant relationships between general health motivation and behavior (e.g., Champion, 1984; Gabriel et al., 2018; McClenahan et al., 2006).

## Self-Efficacy

Finally, self-efficacy was added to the HBM after research guided by Bandura's (1977, 1997, 2004) social cognitive theory demonstrated its impact on behavior and behavior change (Rosenstock et al., 1988; Skinner et al., 2015). Given that social cognitive theory is the subject of the next chapter of this book, here I will simply define and provide a few examples of self-efficacy. *Self-efficacy* refers to a person's beliefs about their ability to perform the behavior needed to prevent a health threat. For example, a person who is confident they would get a mammography would be higher in self-efficacy and therefore be more likely to do so. Alternatively, a person who noticed a change in their breast but did not feel they had the time or money to visit a health care professional would be lower in self-efficacy and would therefore be less likely to schedule such a visit. As you can imagine, a variety of factors can impact how easy or difficult a person perceives a behavior to be, including time, money, knowledge, skills, experience, and so forth. In short, individuals who feel more efficacious, or capable, of engaging in a given behavior are more likely to do so. While no HBM meta-analysis to date has examined the individual effects of self-efficacy on behavior, results from individual HBM studies typically find that self-efficacy is one of the strongest predictors of behavior (e.g., Gabriel et al., 2018; McClenahan et al., 2006). These results are further corroborated by research regarding social cognitive theory, which will be reviewed in detail in the next chapter in this book.

### SUMMARY

In sum, the HBM was among the earliest frameworks to include many of the individual beliefs that we will see in subsequent theories in this book. And, while there is evidence that the HBM can predict health-related behavior, its predictive power is often lower than other theories (Zimmerman & Vernberg, 1994). A key reason is that while the HBM provides a list of potentially important variables for influencing health behavior, it does not provide a specific rationale regarding how these variables relate to or interact with each other or to behavior change (Abraham & Sheeran, 2015; Skinner et al., 2015). Three of the other theories discussed in this book—social cognitive theory, the extended parallel process model, and the reasoned action approach—incorporate many of these same constructs, but more clearly articulate the types of relationships missing from the HBM.

### OPERATIONAL DEFINITIONS

Numerous studies have assessed the validity and reliability of health belief model measures for a wide variety of topics and intended audiences. In this section I will review in detail a series of studies conducted to assess the reliability and validity health belief model scales focused on breast self-examinations and mammography utilization (Champion 1984,

1999; Champion et al., 2005). When considered together, this series of studies nicely illustrates (1) how to measure most of the variables that were a part of the health belief model at one time or another, and (2) how the health belief model evolved and changed over time. To illustrate, Champion (1984) developed measures for severity, susceptibility, benefits, barriers, and general health motivation. However, when these measures were revised by Champion (1999), general health motivation was no longer included. And, Champion et al. (2005) eventually developed a self-efficacy scale that could be included in subsequent health belief model studies. So, as was the case for the theory itself, health motivation was eventually dropped, and self-efficacy was added to the HBM.

Sample survey items for key health belief model variables are presented in Table 6.2. Items for severity, susceptibility, benefits, barriers, general health motivation, and self-efficacy were taken or adapted from one or more of the studies conducted by Champion and colleagues (1984, 1999, 2005). Unfortunately, cues to action were not measured in any of these studies. So, instead, sample cues to action items from other studies on other topics were adapted for this table (Gabriel et al., 2018; Ross et al., 2010). With this in mind, a discussion of measurement validity and reliability follow.

## MEASUREMENT VALIDITY

### Champion (1984)

As a reminder, measurement validity refers to the extent to which a scale fully and accurately measures the variable it is designed to measure. To assess the validity of her HBM scales, Champion (1984) began by writing 20 to 24 items each for five of the HBM variables (i.e., severity, susceptibility, benefits, barriers, and general health motivations). Content validity was assessed by asking eight faculty and doctoral students who had studied the HBM to match each item to one of these five HBM concepts. Items were selected for inclusion if at least 75% of the judges concurred on a category. These and other procedures resulted in a 39-item HBM survey that included 12 severity items, 6 susceptibility items, 5 benefits items, 8 barriers items, and 8 general health motivation items. These 39 items, along with items measuring other variables of interest, were administered to 301 women between the ages of 17 and 82 using both mail and in-person surveys.

Exploratory factor analysis was conducted to organize the items into constructs (also known as variables or factors). Results supported the prediction that each sub-scale measured a mutually exclusive HBM construct. Predictive validity was assessed by testing how well the five HBM variables predicted breast self-examination behavior. Overall, the HBM explained 26% of the variance for this behavior. However, only barriers and general health motivation (but not severity, susceptibility, and benefits) accounted for a significant amount of the variance explained. Taken together, Champion (1984) interpreted these results as supporting the construct validity of her HBM measures.

| TABLE 6.2 | Sample Operational Definitions for Health Belief Model Contructs | | |
|---|---|
| **Construct** | **Operational Definition[1]** |
| Severity[2] | ▶ Breast cancer is a hopeless disease. |
| | ▶ If I had breast cancer, my whole life would change. |
| | ▶ Breast cancer is more serious than other diseases. |
| | ▶ My financial security would be endangered if I got breast cancer. |
| Susceptibility[2] | ▶ It is likely that I will get breast cancer. |
| | ▶ My chances of getting breast cancer in the next few years are great. |
| | ▶ I feel I will get breast cancer sometime during my life. |
| | ▶ There is a good possibility that I will get breast cancer. |
| Benefits[2] | ▶ Having a mammogram will help me find breast lumps early. |
| | ▶ If I find a lump through a mammogram, my treatment for breast cancer may not be as bad. |
| | ▶ Having a mammogram is the best way for me to find a very small lump. |
| | ▶ Having a mammogram will decrease my chances of dying from breast cancer. |
| Barriers[2] | ▶ Having a mammogram is too embarrassing. |
| | ▶ Having a mammogram is too painful. |
| | ▶ Having a mammogram takes too much time. |
| | ▶ I have other problems more important than getting a mammogram. |
| Self-efficacy[2] | ▶ I can get a mammogram even if I am worried. |
| | ▶ I can make an appointment for a mammogram. |
| | ▶ I know for sure I could get a mammogram if I really wanted to. |
| | ▶ I can find a place to have a mammogram. |
| General Health Motivation[2] | ▶ I exercise at least three times a week. |
| | ▶ I eat a well-balanced diet. |
| | ▶ I have regular checkups even when I am not sick. |
| | ▶ Maintaining good health is extremely important to me. |
| Cues to Action[3] | ▶ During the past year, a doctor or health care professional has recommended that I get a mammogram. |
| | ▶ During the past year, I recall seeing print ads (i.e., magazine, newspaper, etc.) about the importance of getting a mammogram. |
| | ▶ During the past year, I recall seeing TV commercials about the importance of getting a mammogram. |
| | ▶ During the past year I received a post card or other form of reminder from my doctor reminding me it was time to get a mammogram. |
| Behavior[2] | ▶ Have you had a mammography in the last 12 months? ❑ No    ❑ Yes |

[1] Unless otherwise noted, all items are measured using five-point Likert scales ranging from "strongly disagree" to "strongly agree."
[2] Taken or adapted from Champion (1984), Champion (1999), Champion et al. (2005), or Saadat et al. (2016).
[3] Adapted from McClenahan et al. (2006), Ross et al. (2010), and Gabriel et al. (2018).

### Champion (1999)

Champion revised her original susceptibility, benefits, and barriers scales for mammography screening. Notice that the perceived severity and general health motivation have been dropped from this version of the instrument. Champion (1999) notes severity was dropped because just about everyone perceives breast cancer to be a serious and dangerous disease; thus, susceptibility alone is used to estimate perceived threat. No explanation is provided for why general health motivation was dropped, but its absence is consistent with the fact that general health motivation was also dropped from the most recent iterations of the model (Rosenstock et al., 1988; Skinner et al., 2015). Content validity was assessed via two focus groups with women age 50 and over. This led to minor changes in wording for some items, the deletion of three susceptibility items, and the addition of three barriers items. The final survey contained 19 items, including three susceptibility items, five benefits items, and 11 barriers items. These 19 items, along with items measuring other variables of interest, were administered to 618 women between the ages of 50 and 85 and who were members of a local health maintenance organization (HMO) or general medicine clinic.

Next, Champion (1999) conducted exploratory and confirmatory factor analyses to organize items into constructs and to ensure that the expected items measured the same underlying constructs. Results were consistent with the prediction that the susceptibility, benefits, and benefits items measured their respective variables. To assess predictive validity, Champion analyzed the relationship between scale scores and stage of mammography compliance (i.e., precontemplation, contemplation, action—see transtheoretical model in Chapter 10). All three scales successfully differentiated between women who were at different stages of mammography compliance in theoretically meaningful ways (e.g., those in the action stage reported significantly greater benefits and significantly fewer barriers than those in the precontemplation or contemplation stages). In tandem, Champion interprets these results as supporting the construct validity of the revised susceptibility, benefits, and barriers measures, and also notes that these measures represent an improvement over the earlier versions of these scales.

### Champion, Skinner, and Menon (2005)

Finally, and as noted previously, given that self-efficacy proved to be a useful predictor of behavior (Bandura, 1977), it was eventually added to the HBM (Rosenstock et al., 1988; Skinner et al., 2015). So, Champion et al. (2005) developed a self-efficacy scale that could be included in subsequent HBM studies. The content validity of the 20 potential items was assessed by asking five content experts whether or not each item measured self-efficacy. These experts included "a psychometrician, a behavioral scientist working in breast cancer screening, two researchers who had used Bandura's theory extensively, and Dr. Bandura" (p. 331). Items were kept when at least 80% agreement was achieved, which resulted in a

10-item self-efficacy scale. These 10 items, along with items measuring other variables of interest, were administered to 1,244 women aged 50 or over who were members of a local HMO or general medicine clinic.

Next, Champion et al. (2005) conducted confirmatory factor analysis to test the prediction that these 10 items measured the same underlying constructs. Results were consistent with this prediction. To assess predictive validity, they analyzed the relationship between self-efficacy and mammography adherence. As predicted, women with higher self-efficacy scores were more likely to have received a mammogram than women with lower self-efficacy scores. In short, the researchers concluded that the mammography self-efficacy scale demonstrated satisfactory content and construct validity.

## MEASUREMENT RELIABILITY

As a reminder, measurement reliability refers to the extent to which the items in a scale consistently measure the intended measure. As a reminder, Cronbach's alpha ($\alpha$) is commonly used to assess measurement reliability; with an alpha of .70 or higher indicating strong reliability. With this in mind, and as you can see from the sample reliability estimates presented in Table 6.3, Cronbach's alphas ($\alpha$) for each of the health belief model scales are typically well above the .70 threshold. This holds true for a wide variety of topics, ranging

| Study (Year) | Topic | Severity | Susceptibility | Benefits | Barriers | Self-Efficacy | Cues to Action | Health Motivation |
|---|---|---|---|---|---|---|---|---|
| Champion (1984) | Breast Self-Exam | .78 | .77 | .61 | .76 | – | – | .60 |
| Champion (1999) | Mammography Screening | – | .87 | .75 | .88 | – | – | – |
| Champion et al. (2005) | Mammography Screening | – | – | – | – | .87 | – | – |
| McClenahan et al. (2006) | Testicular Self-Exam | .85 | .85 | .75 | .85 | .71 | .72 | .79 |
| Ross et al. (2010)[1] | Bicycle Helmets | .80 | .80 | .86 | .87 | – | .80 | – |
|  |  |  |  | .84 | .75 |  | .90 |  |
|  |  |  |  |  |  |  | .70 |  |
| Gabriel et al. (2018) | Injury Prevention | .85 | .95 | .86 | .81 | .81 | .84 | .80 |

**TABLE 6.3    Sample Alpha ($\alpha$) Coefficients for Health Belief Model Constructs**

[1] Ross et al. (2010) assessed two types of benefits (i.e., emotional and safety), two types of barriers (i.e., personal vanity/discomfort and cost), and three types of cues to action (friends/family, parent rules in childhood, and media). Thus, separate alpha coefficients are presented for each of these types.

from fairly general behavioral categories such as exercise-related injury prevention, which may include many different types of activities (e.g., Gabriel et al., 2018) to very specific behaviors such as breast self-examinations (Champion, 1984), mammography utilization (Champion, 1999; Champion et al., 2005), testicular self-examinations (McClenahan et al., 2006) and bicycle helmet use (Ross et al., 2010). High reliability are also common when the HBM scales are translated into a wide variety of different languages including Korean (Lee et al., 2002), Persian (Saadat et al., 2016), Spanish (Medina-Shepherd & Kleier, 2010), and Turkish (Secginli & Nahcivan, 2004). These examples represent just a few of the many different topics, intended audiences, and languages for which these scales have been successfully adapted.

## THE HEALTH BELIEF MODEL: ADVANCES THROUGH META-ANALYSIS

As noted at the outset of this chapter, the health belief model represents one of the earliest efforts to predict and explain health behavior. It has also been the subject of three meta-analyses; two of which examined the effects of each health belief on behavior (Carpenter, 2010; Harrison et al., 1992), and one of which assessed the ability of the HBM as a whole to predict behavior (Zimmerman & Vernberg, 1994). This section will examine (1) the main effects for each health belief on behavior, (2) the factors that moderate the strength of the relationships between health beliefs and behavior, and (3) how well the HBM as a whole predicts behavior.

### MAIN EFFECTS: RELATIONSHIPS BETWEEN HEALTH BELIEFS AND BEHAVIOR

Table 6.4 summarizes the relevant information from the Carpenter (2010) and Harrison et al. (1992) meta-analyses, including the number of subjects ($N$), number of studies ($k$), and the effect sizes for the four HBM variables on behavior (i.e., severity, susceptibility, benefits, and barriers). As a reminder, when reporting effect sizes using correlations, or $r$, as is done in Table 6.4, values of .10, .30, .50 are considered small, medium, and large effects respectively (Cohen, 1988). So, the main effects for severity and susceptibility on behavior tend to be small in size, and the main effects for benefits and barriers on behavior tend to be small to medium in size.

### MODERATOR EFFECTS

As a reminder, a moderator variable changes the strength of the relationship between two other variables. This section looks at three factors that potentially strengthen or weaken the relationships between each health belief and behavior.

| Study | N (k)[1] | Severity | Susceptibility | Benefits | Barriers |
|---|---|---|---|---|---|
| **TABLE 6.4    Effect Sizes (r) Between Health Belief Model Variables and Behavior** | | | | | |
| Harrison et al. (1992)—Various Health Behaviors | 3,515 (17) | .08* | .15* | .13* | −.21* |
| Carpenter (2010)[2]—Various Health Behaviors | 2,702 (18) | .15 | .05 | .27* | −.30* |

*p < .05.

[1] N = total number of participants included in the meta-analysis. k = total number of studies or independent samples included in the meta-analysis.

[2] Carpenter (2010) originally reverse coded the correlation between perceived barriers and behavior to obtain a positive correlation. Here, it has been reversed back to maintain consistency with predictions of the health belief model and previous meta-analysis results.

### Time Interval Between the Measurement of Beliefs and Behavior

The Carpenter (2010) meta-analysis assessed how the time interval between the measurement of health beliefs and the measurement of behavior influenced the strength of the relationship between these variables. Results indicate that time interval negatively impacted the severity-behavior, susceptibility-behavior, and benefits-behavior relationships (i.e., longer time intervals lead to weaker relationships between these beliefs and behavior). However, time interval did not impact the barriers-behavior relationship. Carpenter notes this is likely because severity, susceptibility, and benefits tend to be based on perceptions of possible future outcomes that are more likely to change over time (e.g., cues to action can cause someone to adopt a behavior despite their original perceptions). Barriers, on the other hand, tend to be based on current problems that prevent adopting a behavior that are less likely to change over time (e.g., access to medical care).

### Prospective Versus Retrospective Studies

The Harrison et al. (1992) meta-analysis assessed the impact of measuring behavior prospectively versus retrospective. *Prospective studies* look forward and attempt to predict *future* behavior. For the health belief model this typically involves measure severity, susceptibility, benefits and barriers at one point in time, and measuring behavior at a second, later point it time. *Retrospective studies* look back and attempt to "postdict" *past* behavior after the fact. This typically involves collecting cross-sectional data that measures health beliefs and behavior at a single point in time. Note that under these circumstances you are measuring health beliefs *after* the behavior has already happened.

Harrison et al. (1992) report that that the correlations between both benefits and barriers and *future* behavior were significantly lower than correlations between benefits and barriers and *past* behavior. However, the opposite pattern was observed for severity. That is, the correlations between severity and *future* behavior were significantly higher than correlations between severity and *past* behavior. The strength of the susceptibility-behavior relationship was unaffected by when behavior was measured. While Harrison et al. do not offer any explanation for these findings, results from other meta-analyses testing other theories discussed elsewhere in this book suggest the most likely explanation is that past behavior exerts a strong influence on our beliefs (Albarracin et al., 2001), thereby changing the strength of the relationship between these variables.

### Type of Behavior

Finally, the Carpenter (2010) meta-analysis examined whether or not type of behavior moderated the strength of the relationships between health beliefs and behavior. To illustrate, he compared (1) behaviors that focused on the *treatment* of an illness—such as gum disease or sleep apnea to (2) behaviors that focused on the *prevention* of an illness—such as quitting smoking or getting an influenza vaccine. Carpenter concludes that benefits and barriers are better predictors of prevention rather than treatment behaviors, and that type of behavior does not moderate the severity-behavior or susceptibility-behavior relationships. Carpenter notes that this is not surprising given that the original health belief model "was designed to predict the adoption of preventive measures rather than the treatment for existing diseases or disorders" (p. 667).

### PREDICTING BEHAVIOR

Up to this point the discussion has focused on the relationship between each individual health belief and behavior. Zimmerman and Vernberg (1994) sought to answer the question: How well does the health belief model as a whole fare when it comes to predicting behavior? The answer: When considered together, severity, susceptibility, benefits, barriers, cues to action, general health motivations, and self-efficacy explain 24% of the variance in behavior (which was 10% less than both social cognitive theory [see Chapter 7] and the theory of reasoned action [see Chapter 9]). Unfortunately, none of the identified meta-analyses provide information about which health beliefs do and do not significantly contribute to the prediction of behavior when all of these variables are considered together.

### SUMMARY

In sum, three general conclusions can be drawn about the health belief model based on meta-analyses results. First, perceived severity and susceptibility have small effects on behavior, and perceived benefits and barriers have small to medium effects on behavior.

Second, the strength of these relationships will often be stronger (1) when health beliefs and behavior are measured closer together, (2) when "postdicting" past behavior rather than predicting future behavior, and (3) when the goal is to prevent a negative health outcome before it occurs rather than treat a negative health outcome after it occurs. Finally, when considered together the health belief model explains a small to medium amount of the variance in behavior.

## CONCLUSION

In conclusion, the HBM was one of the earliest attempts to predict and explain health-related behaviors. The original model posits that individuals are more likely to engage in a health behavior when perceived susceptibility, severity, and benefits are high, and when perceived barriers are low. It also highlighted how cues to action can impact both health beliefs and behavior. Subsequent versions of the model added general health motivation or self-efficacy to the health belief box, which nicely illustrates how a theory can evolve and change over time. In addition to describing the HBM, this chapter reviewed how to reliably and validly measure each construct in the model and summarized results from numerous individual studies and meta-analyses indicating that these six variables can have small to medium impacts on behavior. In sum, the HBM provides as a useful point of reference as it introduces several key concepts that will be revisited throughout this section of the book and that remain important targets of public health communication interventions to this day.

## REFERENCES

Abraham, C., & Sheeran, P. (2015). In M. Conner & P. Norman (Eds.), *Predicting health behavior* (3rd ed., pp. 28–80). McGraw-Hill.

Albarracin, D., Johnson, B. T., Fishbein, M., & Muellerleile, P. A. (2001). Theories of reasoned action and planned behavior as models of condom use: A meta-analysis. *Psychological Bulletin, 127*(1), 142–161. https://doi.org/10.1037/0033-2909.127.1.142

Anders, C. K., Fan, C., Parker, J. S., Carey, L. A., Blackwell, K. L., Klauber-DeMore, N., & Perou, C. M. (2011). Breast carcinomas arising at a young age: Unique biology or a surrogate for aggressive intrinsic subtypes? *Journal of Clinical Oncology, 29*(1), e18–e20. https://doi.org/10.1200/JCO.2010.28.9199

Anders, C. K., Hsu, D. S., Broadwater, G., Acharya, C. R., Foekens, J. A., Zhang, Y., Wang, Y., Marcom, P. K., Marks, J. R., Febbo, P. G., Nevins, J. R., Potti, A., & Blackwell, K. L. (2008). Young age at diagnosis correlates with worse prognosis and defines a subset of breast cancers with shared patterns of gene expression. *Journal of Clinical Oncology, 26*(2), 3324–3330. https://doi.org/10.1200/JCO.2007.14.2471

Bandura, A. (1977). Self-efficacy: Toward a unifying theory of behavioral change. *Psychological Review, 84*(2), 191–215. https://doi.org/10.1037/0033-295X.84.2.191

Bandura, A. (1997). *Self-efficacy: The exercise of control.* Freeman.

Bandura, A. (2004). Health promotion by social cognitive means. *Health Education and Behavior, 31*(2), 143–164. https://doi.org/10.1177/1090198104263660

Becker, M. H. (1974). The health belief model and sick role behavior. *Health Education Monographs, 2*(4), 409–419. https://doi.org/10.1177/109019817400200407

Carpenter, C. J. (2010). A meta-analysis of the effectiveness of health belief model variables in predicting behavior. *Health Communication, 25*(8), 661–669. https://doi.org/10.1080/10410236.2010.521906

Centers for Disease Control and Prevention. (2018a). *What are the risk factors for breast cancer?* https://www.cdc.gov/cancer/breast/basic_info/risk_factors.htm

Centers for Disease Control and Prevention. (2018b). *What are the symptoms of breast cancer?* https://www.cdc.gov/cancer/breast/basic_info/symptoms.htm

Centers for Disease Control and Prevention. (2018c). *What is a mammogram?* https://www.cdc.gov/cancer/breast/basic_info/mammograms.htm

Centers for Disease Control and Prevention. (2019a). *Basic information about breast cancer.* https://www.cdc.gov/cancer/breast/basic_info/index.htm

Centers for Disease Control and Prevention. (2019b). *Breast cancer in young women.* https://www.cdc.gov/cancer/breast/young_women/

Champion, V. L. (1984). Instrument development for health belief model constructs. *Advances in Nursing Science, 6*(3), 73–85. https://doi.org/10.1097/00012272-198404000-00011

Champion, V. L. (1999). Revised susceptibility, benefits, and barriers scale for mammography screening. *Research in Nursing and Health, 22*(4), 341–348. https://doi.org/10.1002/(sici)1098-240x(199908)22:4<341::aid-nur8>3.0.co;2-p

Champion, V., Skinner, C. S., & Menon, U. (2005). Development of a self-efficacy scale for mammography. *Research in Nursing and Health, 28*(4), 329–336. https://doi.org/10.1002/nur.20088

Cohen, J. (1988). *Statistical power analysis for the behavioral sciences* (2nd ed.). Laurence Erlbaum Associates.

Gabriel, E. H., Hoch, M. C., & Cramer, R. J. (2018). Health belief model scale and theory of planned behavior scale to assess attitudes and perceptions of injury prevention program participation: An exploratory factor analysis. *Journal of Science and Medicine in Sport, 22*, 544–549. https://doi.org/10.1016/j.jsams.2018.11.004

Harrison, J. A., Mullen, P. D., & Green, L. W. (1992). A meta-analysis of studies of the health belief model with adults. *Health Education Research, 7*(1), 107–116. https://doi.org/10.1093/her/7.1.107

Janz, N. K., & Becker, M. H. (1984). The health belief model: A decade later. *Health Education Quarterly, 11*(1), 1–47. https://doi.org/10.1177/109019818401100101

LaMotte, S. (2016). CDC issues historic travel warning over Miami Zika outbreak. http://www.cnn.com/2016/08/01/health/cdc-miami-florida-zika-travel-warning/

Lee, E. H., Kim, J. S., & Song, M. S. (2002). Translation and validation of Champion's health belief model scale with Korean women. *Cancer Nursing, 25*(5), 391–395. https://doi.org/10.1097/00002820-200210000-00010

Lippke, S. (2017). Outcome expectation. In V. Zeigler-Hill & T. K. Schakelford (Eds.), *Encyclopedia of Personality and Individual Differences* (pp. 1–2). Springer International Publishing.

Mayo Clinic. (2021a). *Cancer.* https://www.mayoclinic.org/diseases-conditions/cancer/symptoms-causes/syc-20370588

Mayo Clinic. (2021b). Breast self-exam for breast awareness. https://www.mayoclinic.org/tests-procedures/breast-exam/about/pac-20393237

McClenahan, C., Shevlin, M., Adamson, G., Bennett, C., & O'Neill, B. (2006). Testicular self-examination: A test of the health belief model and the theory of planned behaviour. *Health Education Research, 22*(2), 272–284. https://doi.org/10.1093/her/cyl076

Medina-Shepherd, R., & Kleier, J. A. (2010). Spanish translation and adaptation of Victoria Champion's health belief model scales for breast cancer screening-mammography. *Cancer Nursing, 33*(2), 93–101. https://doi.org/10.1097/ncc.0b013e3181c75d7b

National Breast Cancer Foundation. (2016). *Helping women now.* https://www.nationalbreastcancer.org/

National Cancer Institute. (2018). *Adolescents and young adults with cancer.* https://www.cancer.gov/types/aya

Oeffinger, K. C., Fontham, E. T., Etzioni, R., Herzig, A., Michaelson, J. S., Shih, Y. C. T., Walter, L. C., Church, T. R., Flowers, C. R., LaMonte, S. J., Wolf, A. M. D., DeSantis, C., Lortet-Tieulent, J., Andrews, K., Manassaram-Baptiste, D., Saslow, D., Smith, R. A., Brawley, O. W., & Wender, R. (2015). Breast cancer screening for women at average risk: 2015 guideline update from the American Cancer Society. *Journal of the American Medical Association, 314*(15), 1599–1614. https://doi.org/10.1001/jama.2015.12783

Rogers, E. M. (2003). *Diffusions of innovation* (5th ed.). Free Press.

Rolling Stone. (2009). *Kiss' Peter Criss reveals breast cancer "nightmare."* https://www.rollingstone.com/music/music-news/kiss-peter-criss-reveals-breast-cancer-nightmare-111393/

Rosenstock, I., Strecher, V., & Becker, M. (1994). The Health Belief Model and HIV risk behavior change. In R. J. DiClemente & J. L. Peterson (Eds.), *Preventing AIDS: Theories and methods of behavioral interventions* (pp. 5–24). Plenum Press.

Rosenstock, I. M. (1966). Why people use health services. *The Milbank Memorial Fund Quarterly, 44*(3), 94–124. https://doi.org/10.1111/j.1468-0009.2005.00425.x

Rosenstock, I. M. (1974). *Historical origins of the health belief model. Health Education Monographs, 2*(4), 328–335. https://doi.org/10.1177/109019817400200403

Rosenstock, I. M. (1990). The health belief model: Explaining health behavior through expectancies. In Glanz, K., Lewis, F. M., & Rimmer, B. K. (Eds.) *Health behavior and health education: Theory, research, and practice* (pp. 39–62). Jossey-Bass.

Rosenstock, I. M., Strecher, V. J., & Becker, M. H. (1988). Social learning theory and the health belief model. *Health Education Quarterly, 15*(2), 175–183. https://doi.org/10.1177/109019818801500203

Ross, T. P., Ross, L. T., Rahman, A., & Cataldo, S. (2010). The bicycle helmet attitudes scale: Using the health belief model to predict helmet use among undergraduates. *Journal of American College Health, 59*(1), 29–36. https://doi.org/10.1080/07448481.2010.483702

Saadat, M., Ghalehtaki, R., Sadeghian, D., Mohammadtaheri, S., & Meysamie, A. (2016). Can we create a reliable and valid short form of Champion Health Belief Model questionnaire? *Archives of Breast Cancer, 3*(1), 19–23. https://doi.org/10.19187/abc.20163119-23

Secginli, S., & Nahcivan, N. O. (2004). Reliability and validity of the breast cancer screening belief scale among Turkish women. *Cancer Nursing, 27*(4), 287–294. https://doi.org/10.1097/00002820-200407000-00005

Skinner, C. S., Tiro, J., & Champion, V. L. (2015). The health belief model. In K. Glanz, B. K. Rimer, & K. Viswanath (Eds.), *Health behavior: Theory, research, and practice* (5th ed., pp. 74–94). Jossey-Bass.

Torborg, L. (2018). Mayo Clinic Q and A: Many women diagnosed with breast cancer don't have signs or symptoms. https://newsnetwork.mayoclinic.org/discussion/mayo-clinic-q-and-a-many-women-diagnosed-with-breast-cancer-dont-have-signs-or-symptoms/

Zimmerman, R. S., & Vernberg, D. (1994). Models of preventive health behavior: Comparison, critique, and meta-analysis. In G. Albrecht (Ed.), *Advances in medical sociology, health behavior models: A reformulation* (pp. 45–67). JAI Press.

Zuckerman, M. (1994). *Behavioral expressions and biosocial bases of sensation seeking.* Cambridge University Press.

# Social Cognitive Theory

## Chapter Outline

## INTRODUCTION

Social cognitive theory (SCT) is a comprehensive theory that has been applied to a wide variety of contexts, including organizational management (Wood & Bandura, 1989), personality (Bandura, 1999), mass communication (Bandura, 2001), and health promotion (Bandura, 2004); the latter being the focus of this chapter. Entire books have been written on SCT, including *Social Learning Theory* (Bandura, 1977b), *Social Foundations of Thought and Action: A Social Cognitive Theory* (Bandura, 1986), and *Self-Efficacy: The Exercise of Control* (Bandura, 1997). Though broad in scope, the impact of SCT on the field of public health communication in particular cannot be overstated. To provide just one example, all of the other theories discussed in this book were strongly influenced by SCT, which is best illustrated by the eventual inclusion of self-efficacy in each of these theories. Given its extensive range, I will not attempt to review SCT in its entirety in this chapter. Instead, this chapter will focus on some key elements that will allow you to effectively apply SCT to the design, implementation, and evaluation of public health communication interventions.

Toward that end, this chapter contains four main sections. Section one introduces the notion of triadic reciprocal causation, which describes how behavioral, environmental, and personal factors interact to produce behavior. Section two focuses on SCT for health promotion, which emphasizes the direct and indirect effect of self-efficacy on health behavior. Section three reviews how to measure key SCT constructs reliably and validly and provides sample survey items for each variable. Finally, section four summarizes results from three sets of meta-analyses that provide useful insights into various aspects of SCT. Before continuing, please consider the following reminders about a healthy diet, which will serve as the running example for this chapter.

A "healthy diet" involves eating a variety of foods that give your body the nutrients it needs to maintain or improve your overall health and well-being (Breastcancer.org, 2020). As noted in Chapter 1, a healthy diet (1) includes a variety of fruits and vegetables, fiber and whole grains, fat-free and low-fat dairy, and a variety of protein foods, and (2) limits saturated fats, added sugars, and sodium (U.S. Department of Health and Human Services and U.S. Department of Agriculture, 2015). Further, healthy eating patterns are associated with a reduced risk of a variety of health conditions, including heart disease and stroke, some types of cancer, neurodegenerative diseases such as Alzheimer's, and depression or depressive symptoms (Firth et al., 2019; Lassale et al., 2019; Loughry et al., 2017; Sofi et al., 2010). Please keep this information in mind as you read about SCT in the sections that follow.

## TRIADIC RECIPROCAL CAUSATION

Bandura (1978, 1986) notes that early theories of behavior emphasized the unidirectional effects of environmental or personal factors. That is, previous explanations viewed context or cognitions—but not both—as causing behavior, and not the other way around. In response, Bandura advanced the notion of *triadic reciprocal causation*, which highlights how behavioral, personal, and environmental factors interact (i.e., they both influence and are influenced by each other; see Figure 7.1). Bandura's notion of triadic reciprocal causation closely parallels the discussion on ecological model presented in Chapter 4, and therefore also highlights the importance of targeting multiple factors when designing public health communication interventions. Next, I review Bandura's conceptualization of this process, define each element in the triad, and identify some of the key factors that impact each element (Bandura, 2004; Kelder et al., 2015). Four of these factors—goals, facilitators and impediments, outcome expectations, and self-efficacy—are also core components of Bandura's (2004) SCT of health promotion. Thus, these four constructs will be introduced here, and discussed in more detail in the Social Cognitive Theory of Health Promotion section that follows.

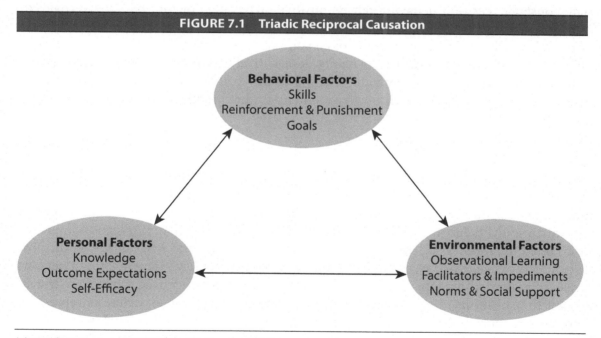

**FIGURE 7.1    Triadic Reciprocal Causation**

**Behavioral Factors**
Skills
Reinforcement & Punishment
Goals

**Personal Factors**
Knowledge
Outcome Expectations
Self-Efficacy

**Environmental Factors**
Observational Learning
Facilitators & Impediments
Norms & Social Support

Adapted from Bandura (1986, 1997) and Kelder et al. (2015).

## BEHAVIORAL FACTORS

*Behavior* refers to what a person does or the way a person acts in a particular situation. This book focuses on behaviors that directly impact health. For example, eating a healthy diet can improve one's health, whereas failure to do so can compromise it. Three common examples of supporting behavioral factors include skills, goals, and reinforcement and punishment.

*Skills* involve having the actual ability or expertise to perform the behavior. For example, individuals wishing to maintain a healthy diet must be capable of finding, selecting, and preparing nutritional foods. Skills acquired via mastery experiences are one of the four key sources of self-efficacy, which will be discussed in more detail below.

*Goals* (a.k.a., intentions) refer to a person's readiness or plans to perform a behavior in the future. Goals reflect a person's motivation and commitment. Thus, people who intend to eat healthy are more likely to do so, and vice versa.

Reinforcement and punishment are based on the notion that every behavior has consequences that impact whether or not it will be repeated in the future. More specifically, *reinforcements* encourage a behavior thereby increasing the likelihood it will reoccur, whereas *punishments* discourage a behavior thereby decreasing the likelihood it will occur again. The consequences of a behavior can be positive or negative or internal or external. For example, feeling more energetic, receiving admiration from friends and family, or promising to buy yourself a new wardrobe once you reach your weight goal represent rewards that might encourage healthy eating habits. Alternatively, feeling more lethargic, receiving criticism from friends and family, or refusing to buy yourself a new wardrobe until you reach your weight goal represent negative outcomes that might discourage unhealthy eating habits.

## ENVIRONMENTAL FACTORS

*Environmental factors* are external influences that facilitate or limit behavior. Three common examples of environmental factors include observational learning, facilitators and impediments, and norms. *Observational learning* involves acquiring knowledge and skills by watching the behavior of others. For example, public health communication interventions often use models to demonstrate the negative effects of unhealthy behaviors, the positive effects of healthy ones, or the transition between the two (e.g., showing how a person's unhealthy diet led to poor health outcomes that ultimately improved when they transitioned to a healthier diet). Observational learning via vicarious experiences represents another key source of self-efficacy which will be discussed in more detail below.

*Facilitators and impediments* are environmental factors that make it easier or more difficult for a person to perform a behavior. Examples include the (un)availability, (un)affordability, or (in)accessibility of healthy food options in one's surroundings (e.g., home, school, work, community, etc.). Facilitators and impediments are also related to norms (reviewed next) and represent key components of the sociostructural factors construct in SCT for health promotion (reviewed later).

*Perceived norms* are what we view as typical or expected in a given situation. This definition highlights two related ideas. The "what is typical" or *descriptive norms* portion of this definition concerns whether or not a person believes a behavior is being performed by others. For example, do you believe that most people who are important to you are themselves eating (or not eating) healthy? The "what is expected" or *injunctive norms* portion of this definition concerns whether or not a person believes a behavior is approved of by important others. For example, do most people who are important to you support (or oppose) eating healthy? Injunctive norms are closely related to the notion of *social support*, which includes both the perceived availability of help and help actually received (Schwarzer & Knoll, 2010). Social support can be practical, informational, or emotional. For example, our family and friends might prepare or order healthy meals when dining with us, provide tips so we can prepare healthier meals for ourselves, or simply remind us that they care about us and want us to be healthy.

## PERSONAL FACTORS

*Personal factors* include any internal or cognitive influences on how a person behaves in various situations. Three common examples of personal factors include knowledge, outcome expectations, and self-efficacy.

In the context of public health communication, *knowledge* involves an awareness of the facts and skills associated with a health issue. This definition distinguishes between two types of knowledge. *Conceptual knowledge* is fact-based; it involves having correct information about a health issue. For example, one must know why eating well is important, be aware of the recommended dietary guidelines, and understand which foods do and do not belong in a healthy diet. *Procedural knowledge* is skills-based; it involves knowing how to correctly perform a health behavior. Bandura (2004) notes that knowledge is a necessary but insufficient precondition for behavior change. For example, knowing what to do (i.e., procedural knowledge) and having the expertise to actually do it (i.e., skills) are two very different things. Nonetheless, knowledge is the foundation upon which all public health communication interventions are built.

However, one must also have the motivation and ability to do something about a health threat. This is why outcome expectations and self-efficacy are important. *Outcome expectations* refers to the perceived consequences of engaging in a behavior. For example, individuals who believe that maintaining a healthy diet will reduce their risk of illness will be more motivated to do so, and vice versa. *Self-efficacy* is a belief about one's ability to perform the recommended behavior. For example, people who are confident they can stick to a healthy diet even under a variety of challenging circumstances are more likely to do so and vice versa. However, it is important to keep in mind that self-efficacy is a perception that may or may not reflect an individual's actual *behavioral capacity*, which is comprised of a person's procedural knowledge and actual skills with respect to that behavior.

In sum, SCT's notion of triadic reciprocal causation posits that "people are actors as well as products of their environment" (Luszczynska & Schwarzer, 2005, p. 128). Given that behavioral, environmental, and personal factors can interact to influence health behaviors in potentially limitless ways, the question becomes, where should you start? Bandura's (2004) SCT for health promotion answers this question by specifying "a core set of determinants, the mechanisms through which they work, and the optimal ways of translating this knowledge into effective health practices" (p. 144).

## SOCIAL COGNITIVE THEORY FOR HEALTH PROMOTION

According to SCT for health promotion (Bandura, 2004), self-efficacy influences behavior both directly and indirectly through outcome expectations, goals, and sociostructurally factors. Figure 7.2 provides a visualization of SCT and Table 7.1 contains conceptual definitions for all SCT's constructs. Next, I review the four key constructs of SCT: (1) self-efficacy, (2) outcome expectations, (3) sociostructural factors, and (4) goals.

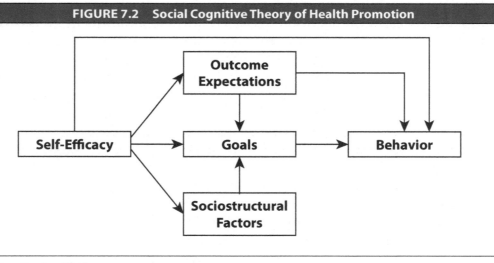

**FIGURE 7.2    Social Cognitive Theory of Health Promotion**

Adapted from Bandura (2004).

| Construct | Conceptual Definition |
|---|---|
| **TABLE 7.1    Conceptual Definitions for Social Cognitive Theory Constructs** ||
| Self-efficacy | Beliefs about one's ability to perform a behavior under various challenging circumstances. |
| Outcome Expectations | The perceived consequences of engaging in a behavior. |
| Outcome Expectancies | The positive or negative assessment of each consequence. |
| Sociostructural Factors | Environmental factors that impact behavior, but that are largely beyond an individual's control. |
| Facilitators | Environmental factors that help or encourage a person to engage in a behavior. |
| Impediments | Environmental factors that hinder or discourage a person from engaging in a behavior. |
| Goals | A person's readiness, motivation, or plans to perform a behavior in the future. |
| Distal Goals | Long-term goals that require an extended period of time to achieve. |
| Proximal Goals | Short-term goals that can be achieved fairly quickly. |
| Behavior | What a person does or the way a person acts in a particular situation. |

## SELF-EFFICACY

*Self-efficacy* refers to a person's belief about their ability to perform the recommended behavior under a variety of challenging circumstances. For example, how confident are you that you can eat more fruits and vegetables even when you are very hungry, feeling depressed, are on vacation, or need a quick meal? How about when tasty but less healthy options are available at a restaurant, at a friend's home, or over the holidays? As you can see, healthy eating is fraught with challenges. Notably, these are just a few of the 30 tempting situations Bandura (2006) identifies in his self-efficacy scale to regulate eating habits. As these examples illustrate, self-efficacy judgments are behavior and situation specific (i.e., it may be strong for some tasks or circumstances but weak for others). For example, earlier I noted that healthy eating involves a variety of different behaviors such as (1) eating fruits and vegetables and fiber, (2) eating whole grains, (3) limiting saturated fats, and (4) avoiding added sugars. Thus, a person may have confidence in their ability to eat more fruits and vegetables but lack confidence in their ability to avoid added sugars. Also, for example, a person may have confidence in their ability to eat more fruits and vegetables when at home but lack confidence in their ability to do so when eating out.

SCT views self-efficacy as the foundation of thought and action (Bandura, 1986). Self-efficacy perceptions impact the behaviors people engage in, the goals they set for themselves, the outcomes people expect their efforts to produce, and how long they persist when confronted with obstacles. Thus, self-efficacy plays a prominent role in public health communication interventions. With this in mind, the next section reviews four ways to influence self-efficacy.

### Sources of Self-Efficacy

Bandura (1977a, 1997) identifies four sources of information or types of learning that impact self-efficacy: (1) mastery experience, (2) vicarious experience, (3) verbal persuasion, and (4) emotional arousal (see Figure 7.3).

The most effective way to develop a strong sense of self-efficacy is through *mastery experience*, which is based on personal knowledge or direct involvement with a behavior. Mastery experience is predicated on the proposition that "practice makes perfect." This is one reason why many public health communication interventions provide an opportunity

**FIGURE 7.3    Sources of Self-Efficacy**

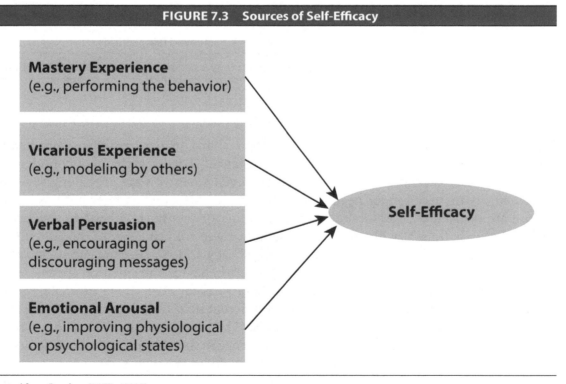

Adapted from Bandura (1977a, 1997).

for participants to learn by doing. For example, as part of an intervention designed to promote gun safety, our team distributed free trigger locks to gun owners so they could try them out and see for themselves how easy they are to use (Roberto et al., 2002). Or, returning to our running example of fruit and vegetable consumption, you might have participants actually plan or prepare one or more healthy meals. However, it is important to keep in mind that while successes can build self-efficacy, failures can undermine it (Bandura, 1997). Thus, it is sometimes best to ask participants to perform a set of attainable but increasingly difficult tasks. For example, you might ask participants to replace one unhealthy meal each week with a healthier one at the start of the intervention, in hopes of getting them to replace most unhealthy meals with healthier ones by the end of the intervention.

Vicarious experience is another important source of self-efficacy. *Vicarious experience* involves observing and learning from other people's behavior. Schunk and Usher (2019) note that observational learning is an efficient alternative to learning by doing as it saves people from the undesirable consequences of acting in potentially dangerous ways. A powerful example of vicarious learning in action is the Mothers Against Drunk Driving (MADD) victim impact panel, where victims and survivors of substance-impaired driving crashes speak about the crash in which they were injured or a loved one was killed or injured (MADD, 2020). Such panels often include live presenters but may also include prerecorded videos. For example, as part of the gun-safety intervention I mentioned earlier, we created a video where five individuals whose lives were impacted by accidental gunshot injuries shared their stories to prevent other gun owners from experiencing a similar fate (Roberto et al., 2000). However, vicarious experiences do not have to be that intense or complex. For example, to encourage healthier eating behaviors, you could simply have someone similar to the individuals you are trying to influence demonstrate a behavior, such planning or preparing some simple healthy meals.

People can also be persuaded to believe that they have the ability to succeed. Generally speaking, *verbal persuasion* involves messages designed to influence how people believe, feel, or behave. For SCT, this entails convincing people they have the capability of performing a behavior (i.e., self-efficacy), and that the behavior will have some desirable consequence (i.e., outcome expectations). The use of verbal persuasion is very common in the realm of public health communication interventions and can take on a variety of different forms (e.g., Ashford et al., 2010; Prestwich et al., 2014). For example, you might encourage or reward people for engaging in a healthy behavior (e.g., a healthy diet) or discourage them from engaging in an unhealthy one (e.g., an unhealthy diet). Also, for example, you might remind people about positive consequences of the healthy behavior (e.g., living a longer and healthier life, looking and feeling their best, etc.), or the negative consequences of the unhealthy behavior (e.g., being overweight or obese, high blood pressure or cholesterol, increased risk of heart disease and stroke, etc.). In short, the goal here is to make people feel they have the ability to engage in the recommended behavior, and to motivate them to do so. However, Bandura (1977a, 1997) notes that the effects of verbal persuasion alone may be limited, and that verbal persuasion works best when combined with the other techniques discussed in this section.

The final source of self-efficacy is *emotional arousal*, which refers to a heightened state of physiological and psychological activity. Bandura (1977a, 1997) notes that our emotional reactions provide us with cues about anticipated success or failure, and that these cues can impact self-efficacy. For example, people usually interpret negative emotional states as a sign of lower self-efficacy (e.g., individuals who find planning or preparing healthier meals to be stressful and frustrating will feel less efficacious). Conversely, positive emotional states are often interpreted as a sign of higher self-efficacy (e.g., individuals who find planning or preparing healthier meals to be relaxing and fun will feel more efficacious). In short, people can improve their sense of self-efficacy by learning how to minimize negative emotions and maximize positive emotions when faced with a difficult task (Prestwich et al., 2014).

## OUTCOME EXPECTATIONS

*Outcome expectations* (sometimes called *behavioral beliefs*; Bandura, 2004; Fishbein & Ajzen, 2010) refers to the perceived consequences of engaging in a behavior. For example, do you believe that eating more fruits and vegetables will improve your health, impact your relationships with friends and family, or make you feel better about yourself? Outcome expectations typically take the form of a conditional statement such as "if I eat more fruits and vegetables, then I will feel more energetic throughout the day." Further, outcome expectations generally vary along three different dimensions: (1) area of consequence, (2) temporal proximity, and (3) valence (Fasbender, 2019; Schwarzer & Luszczynska, 2016).

*Area of consequence* focuses on the form of the outcome (i.e., physical, social, and self-evaluative). *Physical outcome expectations* relate to how a behavior impacts your body. For example, does eating more fruits and vegetables make you feel more energetic (or hungrier) throughout the day? *Social outcome expectations* refer to the impact of a behavior on one's relationships. For example, how does your decision to eat more fruits and vegetables impact your ability to interact with others (i.e., does it make eating out with friends and family easier or more difficult)? *Self-evaluative outcome expectations* deal with how a behavior makes you feel mentally or emotionally. For example, many people feel good when they think about how eating more fruits and vegetables will improve their health, minimizes cruelty to animals, or reduces their impact on climate change.

*Temporal proximity* focuses on when the consequences occur (i.e., in the short-term vs. long-term). *Short-term outcome expectations* are those you expect a behavior to lead to right away. For example, you might expect eating more fruits and vegetables will help you feel better physically and mentally fairly quickly. *Long-term outcome expectations* are those that take an extended period of time to achieve. For example, the long-term benefits of eating more fruits and vegetables include reducing your risk of heart disease, stroke, some cancers, and so forth. Unfortunately, and as noted in Chapter 4, the long-term benefits of many health behaviors can be difficult to observe (Rogers, 2003). Thus, it can be difficult to motivate someone to engage in a healthier behavior now to prevent a health problem that may or may not occur in the future. This highlights the importance of also identifying and addressing shorter-term and easily observable outcome expectations whenever possible.

*Valence* relates to how the consequences are evaluated (i.e., positively vs. negatively). Put differently, while outcome expectations focus on the perceived consequences of engaging in a behavior, *outcome expectancies* (sometimes called *outcome evaluation*; Bandura, 2004; Fishbein & Ajzen, 2010) focuses on the positive or negative assessment of each consequence. For example, a person might believe that eating more fruits and vegetables will help them lose weight (outcome expectations) and evaluate losing weight positively (outcome expectancies). Conversely, they may believe that eating fruits and vegetables is more costly (outcome expectations) but evaluate the additional cost negatively (outcome expectancies). In short, public health communication interventions must find ways to emphasize the pros or advantages and to minimize the cons or disadvantages of the recommended behavior.

## SOCIOSTRUCTURAL FACTORS

*Sociostructural factors* are environmental factors that make it easier or harder to engage in a behavior, but that are largely beyond an individual's control. I reviewed a wide variety of sociostructural factors when discussing ecological models in Chapter 4. Examples include relationship factors (e.g., do important others approve of or eat healthy foods?), community factors (e.g., are healthy foods available where you live and shop?), and societal factors (e.g., do public policies encourage healthy eating?).

Sociostructural factors may facilitate or impede behavior. *Facilitators* are environmental factors that help or enable a person to engage in a behavior. Conversely, *impediments* are environmental factors that hinder or prevent a person from engaging in a behavior. For example, other's approval should help facilitate—and other's disapproval would likely impede—a person's motivation to make healthy food choices. Similarly, the availability of low-cost fruits and vegetables available where you shop would make it easier to eat healthy, while a lack of availability would make it harder to do so. Finally, public policies designed to discourage unhealthy eating (e.g., a tax on sweetened beverages) and encourage healthy eating (e.g., using this tax revenue to make healthier options more readily available) would encourage healthier eating, while the lack of such policies might discourage it.

## GOALS

*Goals* (sometimes called *intention*; Bandura, 2004; Fishbein & Ajzen, 2010) represent a person's readiness or plans to perform (or not perform) a behavior in the future. Goals can be proximal or distal. *Distal goals* are long-term goals that take an extended period of time to achieve, whereas *proximal goals* are short-term goals that can be achieved fairly quickly. Bandura (2004) notes that while "long-term goals set the course of personal change . . . short-term attainable goals help people to succeed by enlisting effort and guiding action in the here and now" (pp. 144–145).

To illustrate, a long-term goal of a healthy diet is to reduce the risk of serious diseases such as heart disease, diabetes, and some cancers. However, given that a "healthy diet" encompasses a variety of different behaviors, coupled with the fact the "the risk of serious diseases" is far off and difficult to observe, means this goal may not be very helpful when it comes to predicting specific daily behaviors. Instead, ask people to set and monitor their progress toward short-term subgoals that will be easier to monitor and maintain, such as how many servings of fruit, vegetables, grain (especially whole grains), dairy (especially non-fat or low-fat dairy), and protein they eat each day. Ultimately, these short-term subgoals should lead to the long-term goal, but be more motivating since they happen daily and are easy to observe.

## SUMMARY

In sum, SCT predicts behavior (i.e., whether or not you eat the recommended number of fruits and vegetables each day) is a function of four factors:

1.  Self-efficacy (i.e., whether or not you believe you have the ability to eat the recommended number of fruits and vegetables each day);

2.  Outcome expectations (i.e., your assessment of the pros and cons of eating the recommended number of fruits and vegetables each day);

3.  Goals (i.e., whether or not you intend to eat the recommended number of fruits and vegetables each day); and

4.  Sociostructural factors (i.e., whether the environment facilitates or impedes your ability to eat the recommended number of fruits and vegetables each day).

Further, self-efficacy represents the core construct of SCT in that it not only influences behavior directly, but also impacts it indirectly by informing the outcomes people expect their behavior to have, the goals they set for themselves, and how they view and respond to the environmental factors that might impact the behavior.

## OPERATIONAL DEFINITIONS

As noted in Chapter 5, an operational definition defines a concept by specifying the procedures used to measure it. Numerous studies have assessed the validity and reliability of SCT measures for a wide variety of topics and intended audiences. Measures of self-efficacy, goals, and behavior tend to be consistent across studies. However, as will be illustrated in more detail below, measures for outcome expectations and sociostructural factors tend to vary depending on the purpose of the study. With this in mind, sample survey items for key SCT constructs are presented in Table 7.2. The next section reviews several guidelines for constructing self-efficacy scales, and the sections after that examine the measurement validity and reliability of the five core SCT constructs.

| TABLE 7.2 | Sample Operational Definitions for Social Cognitive Theory Constructs |
|---|---|
| **Construct** | **Operational Definition** |
| Self-Efficacy [1,3] | How confident are you that you can: <br> ▶ Eat five servings of fruits and vegetables every day? <br> ▶ Eat fruits and vegetables for a snack instead of chips or candy? <br> ▶ Eat fruits and vegetables when eating out at a restaurant? <br> ▶ Eat fruits and vegetables when I am at a social event? |
| Outcome Expectations | **Outcome Expectations** [2,4] <br> ▶ Eating fruits and vegetables can reduce my risk of some illnesses and diseases (e.g., heart disease, diabetes, some cancers, etc.). <br> ▶ Eating fruits and vegetables helps me feel better physically. <br> ▶ Eating fruits and vegetables helps me manage my weight. <br> ▶ Eating fruits and vegetables helps me to feel more energetic throughout the day. <br><br> **Outcome Expectancies** [2,5] <br> ▶ How important is reducing your risk of illness and disease to you? <br> ▶ How important is feeling better physically to you? <br> ▶ How important is managing your weight to you? <br> ▶ How important is feeling more energetic to you? <br><br> **Outcome Expectations (Pros)** [1,5] <br> Please rate how important each statement is to your decision to eat five fruits and vegetables a day. <br> ▶ I would have more energy if I ate fruits and vegetables. <br> ▶ I would be doing something good for my body if I ate more fruits and vegetables. <br> ▶ Eating more fruits and vegetables helps me manage my weight. <br><br> **Outcome Expectations (Cons)** [1,5] <br> Please rate how important each statement is to your decision to eat five fruits and vegetables a day. <br> ▶ It takes too much time to prepare fruits and vegetables. <br> ▶ Fruits and vegetables do not satisfy my hunger for very long. <br> ▶ Fresh fruits and vegetables are too expensive. |

| TABLE 7.2    Continued | |
|---|---|
| **Construct** | **Operational Definition** |
| Sociostructural Factors | **Social Support / Injunctive Norms** [1,6] <br> How often in the PAST three months have your family or friends done the following? <br> ▸ Encouraged you to eat fruits and vegetables. <br> ▸ Discussed the benefits of eating fruits and vegetables. <br> ▸ Reminded you to choose fruits and vegetables. <br> ▸ Eat healthy meals with you. |
| | **Situation / Environment** [1,4] <br> ▸ There is at least one option at school where I can select fruits and vegetables for snacks or meals. <br> ▸ There is a wide variety of fresh fruits and vegetables where I shop. <br> ▸ The fruits and vegetables where I shop are at good prices. |
| Goals [2,7] | In the NEXT three months, do you ... <br> ▸ Intend to eat at least five servings of fruit and vegetables each day? <br> ▸ Intend to choose low-fat foods and drinks whenever you have a choice. <br> ▸ Intend to choose food and drinks that are low in added sugar whenever you have a choice? <br> ▸ Intend to eat healthier portion sizes during meals? |
| Behavior [2,6] | In the PAST three months, how often did you ... <br> ▸ Eat at least five servings of fruit and vegetables each day? <br> ▸ Did you choose low-fat food and drinks when they were available? <br> ▸ Did you choose food and drinks that are low in added sugar when available? <br> ▸ Did you leave food on your plate once you felt full during a meal? |

[1] Sample items taken or adapted from Norman et al. (2010).
[2] Sample items taken or adapted from Dewar et al. (2012).
[3] Response categories ranged from "not at all confident" to "extremely confident."
[4] Response categories ranged from "strongly disagree" to "strongly agree."
[5] Response categories ranged from "not important" to "extremely important."
[6] Response categories ranged from "never" or "almost never" to "always" or "almost always."
[7] Response categories ranged from "not at all true of me" to "very true of me."

## GUIDELINES FOR CONSTRUCTING SELF-EFFICACY SCALES

Bandura (1997, 2006) provides several recommendations for constructing self-efficacy scales. Much of this advice is applicable to the measurement of all the theoretical constructs discussed elsewhere in this book, including the importance of assessing measurement reliability and validity (see Chapter 5) and minimizing survey response bias (see Chapter 12). Thus, these and related issues will not be reviewed again here. Instead, I will draw your attention to three important guidelines for constructing self-efficacy scales in particular.

First, self-efficacy scales should accurately reflect the construct. Bandura (2006) notes that self-efficacy items "should be phrased in terms of *can do* rather than *will do*. *Can* is a judgment of capability; *will* is a statement of intention" (p. 308). Thus, the general wording for self-efficacy items should look something like this: "I am confident I can [insert recommended behavior] even when [insert barrier here]" (e.g., "I am confident I can eat a healthy diet even when visiting family and friends during the holidays"). Second, self-efficacy scales should be behavior specific, as general self-efficacy scales are weaker predictors of behavior than self-efficacy scales tailored to a particular behavior. For example, people may feel differently about their ability to eat fruits and vegetables, fiber and whole grains, or fat-free or low-fat dairy, so you will want to include separate items for each behavior under investigation. Third, self-efficacy scales should focus on behavior, not outcomes. For example, instead of focusing on outcomes such as losing weight, self-efficacy scales should focus on the specific behavior(s) over which people have some control, such as diet and exercise.

## MEASUREMENT VALIDITY

As a reminder, measurement validity refers to the extent to which an instrument fully and accurately measures the construct it is designed to measure. As noted in Chapter 5, measurement validity is typically assessed in three ways: (1) content validity—which focuses on the match between the conceptual and operational definition, (2) factor analysis—to determine how well a set of survey items measures the construct(s) they were designed to measure, and (3) criterion-related validity—which involves comparing the measure to some external standard or criteria. In this section I review two studies that assessed the validity of scales developed to measure SCT constructs in the realm of dietary behavior (Dewar et al., 2012; Norman et al., 2010). These two studies were chosen because they complement each other in a number of important ways. To illustrate:

▸ Norman et al. studied college students and overweight and obese adults while Dewar et al. studied adolescents.

▸ Norman et al. measured outcome expectations as pros and cons while Dewar et al. measured outcome expectations and outcome expectancies.

▸ Norman et al. did not conduct confirmatory factor analysis (CFA) while Dewar et al. did.

▸ Norman et al. provided evidence for criterion-related validity while Dewar et al. did not.

Thus, when considered together these studies assess the three key types of measurement validity introduced in Chapter 5.

That said, Norman et al. (2010) developed and tested measures for self-efficacy, outcome expectations (both pros and cons), and social support for three dietary behaviors (i.e., fat, fiber and whole grains, and fruits and vegetables). Here, I will focus on just the fruits and vegetables measures. To ensure content validity of their measures, Norman et al. generated a pool of potential items for each construct from previously published measures, had three judges evaluate each pool of items, and retained only the highest rated items for each scale. To assess criterion-related validity, Norman et al. looked at the relationship between dietary behavior (e.g., fruit and vegetable consumption) and the scores on their self-efficacy, pros, cons, and social support scales. As expected, cons were negatively related to fruit and vegetable consumption, and self-efficacy and social support were positively related to fruit and vegetable consumption. However, contrary to expectations, pros were unrelated to fruit and vegetable consumption. In sum, they interpret their results as providing evidence of criterion-related validity for only some of their measures.

Dewar et al. (2012) set out to develop measures for self-efficacy, outcome expectations, outcome expectancies, social support, goals, and behavior. The authors undertook an especially rigorous four-step process to assess content validity of each scale. First, they reviewed the literature and examined the content and psychometric properties of existing measures of SCT constructs. Second, they had four judges with expertise in nutrition, SCT, or scale development review and provided feedback on the items in each scale. Third, they conducted focus groups with members of the intended audience to examine the thought processes used to interpret and respond to each item. Finally, after all necessary changes were made, they returned the scales to the expert judges for final review.

Once content validity was established, Dewar et al. (2012) conducted CFA to test the assumption that items from each scale measured the same construct. In some cases (i.e., for self-efficacy, outcome expectations, social support, intention) preliminary results indicated that further refinement was necessary, in which case an iterative process was employed to progressively remove problematic items until acceptable results were obtained. Results for the final versions of the self-efficacy (7 items), outcome expectations (5 items), outcome expectancies (5 items), social support (5 items), intentions (5 items), and behavior (6 items) scales were consistent with the prediction that each set of items measured the same construct.

## MEASUREMENT RELIABILITY

Also, as a reminder, measurement reliability refers to the extent to which the items in a scale consistently measure the intended target. Further, Cronbach's alpha (α) is commonly used to assess measurement reliability, with an alpha of .70 or higher indicating strong reliability. With this in mind, and as you can see from the sample reliability estimates presented in Table 7.3, Cronbach's alphas for each of the SCT scales typically (but not always) meet or exceed the .70 threshold. This holds true regardless of how the variables are conceptualized (see footnotes 1 through 6 in Table 7.3), and for a wide variety of topics and intended audiences.

| Study (Year) | Topic | Self-Efficacy | Outcome Expectations | Sociostructural Factors | Goal |
|---|---|---|---|---|---|
| Nagy & Watts (2003) [1] | Sexual Abstinence | .69 | .78 | .75 | .74 |
| Wójcicki et al. (2009) [2] | Exercise | .99 | .82 .84 .81 | – | – |
| Norman et al. (2010) [3] | Diet | .76 | .61 .73 | .91 .82 | – |
| Dewar et al. (2012) [4] | Diet | .70 | .72 .65 | .71 .79 | .71 |
| Yang et al. (2016) [5] | Condom Use | .89 | .82 | .60 .66 | – |
| Sheu et al. (2017) [6] | Academic Well-Being | .90 | .94 | .82 | .87 |
| Knowlden et al. (2018) [7] | Diet Physical Activity Sleep | .86 .88 .93 | .81 .85 .87 | .79 .90 .99 | .93 .94 .94 |

TABLE 7.3    Sample Alpha (α) Coefficients for Social Cognitive Theory Constructs

[1] Sociostructural factors represented by injunctive norms.
[2] Alphas reported separately for physical, self-evaluative, and social dimensions of outcome expectations.
[3] Alphas reported for fruit and vegetable consumption at baseline. Alphas reported separately for pros and cons dimensions of outcome expectations. Sociostructural factors represented by (and alphas reported separately for) social support and environment.
[4] Alphas reported separately for outcome expectations and outcome expectancies. Sociostructural factors represented by (and alphas reported separately for) social support and situation.
[5] Alphas reported separately for facilitators and impediments dimensions of sociostructural factors.
[6] Sociostructural factors represented by social support.
[7] Alphas reported separately for fruit and vegetable consumption, physical activity, and sleep behaviors.

## SOCIAL COGNITIVE THEORY: ADVANCES THROUGH META-ANALYSIS

In this section I review eight meta-analyses focusing on three key aspects of SCT research. The first set assessed the relationship between self-efficacy and other SCT constructs, as well as some of the factors that moderate the strength of the self-efficacy-behavior relationship (Chen et al., 2017; Holden, 1992; Kim et al., 2019; Robbins et al., 2014). The second set assessed how well SCT as a whole predicts behavior (Young et al., 2014; Zimmerman & Vernberg, 1994). The third set focused on the most (and least) effective strategies for increasing self-efficacy (Ashford et al., 2010; Prestwich et al., 2014).

## RELATIONSHIPS BETWEEN SELF-EFFICACY AND OTHER SOCIAL COGNITIVE THEORY VARIABLES

### Main Effects

Table 7.4 provides a detailed description and breakdown from the four meta-analyses reviewed for this section, including number of subjects ($N$), number of studies ($k$), and the effect sizes between self-efficacy and other SCT constructs (i.e., outcome expectations, sociostructural factors, goals, and behavior). As a reminder, when reporting effect sizes using correlations, or $r$, as is done in Table 7.4, values of .10, .30, .50 are considered small, medium, and large effects, respectively (Cohen, 1988). Thus, the relationships between self-efficacy and other SCT variables tend to fall in the medium to large range.

| TABLE 7.4    Effect Sizes (r) Between Self-Efficacy and Other Social Cognitive Theory Constructs | | | | | |
|---|---|---|---|---|---|
| **Study** | **N** **(k)**[1] | **Outcome Expectations** | **Sociostructural Factors** | **Goals** | **Behavior** |
| Holden (1992)— Various Health Behaviors[2] | 3,527 (49) | – | – | – | .26[*] |
| Robbins et al. (2004)— Academic Performance and Persistence[3] | 26,263 (109) | – | .43[*] | .49[*] | .50[*] .36[*] |
| Chen et al. (2017)— Cyberbullying[4] | 99,741 (81) | – | .27[*] | – | .21[*] −.04[*] |
| Kim et al. (2019)— Job Search Behavior[5] | 31,586 (74) | .37[*] | .33[*] −.04 | .33[*] | .26[*] |

[*] $p < .05$.

[1] $N$ = total number of participants included in the meta-analysis. $k$ = total number of studies included in the meta-analysis.

[2] $N$, $k$, and $r$ reported for adjusted results.

[3] $N$ was not reported in this meta-analysis, so $N$ from the largest individual analyses is reported here. Sociostructural factors represented by social support. Results for behavior reported separately for academic performance (grade point average) and academic persistence (retention).

[4] Sociostructural factors represented by social norms. Results for behavior reported separately for perpetration (i.e., self-efficacy) and victimization (i.e., self-efficacy in defending).

[5] Sociostructural factor represented by and results reported separately for social support and barriers.

## Moderator Effects

Also, as a reminder, a moderator variable changes the strength of the relationship between two other variables. So, this section looks at some key factors that strengthened or weakened the relationships between self-efficacy and behavior. More specifically, results indicate that the self-efficacy-behavior relationship is moderated by:

1. Time interval—as the time interval between the measurement of self-efficacy and the measurement of behavior increased, the strength of the self-efficacy-behavior relationship decreased (Holden, 1992).

2. Research design—the self-efficacy-behavior relationship is stronger for cross-sectional than for longitudinal designs (Kim et al., 2019).

3. Health outcomes—the self-efficacy-behavior relationship is stronger for some health outcomes (e.g., pain) than for other health outcomes (e.g., weight loss) (Holden).

4. Type of culture—the self-efficacy-behavior relationship appears to be stronger for collectivist than for individualistic cultures (Kim et al.).

## PREDICTING BEHAVIOR

The meta-analyses discussed so far focused on the relationship between self-efficacy and the four core SCT constructs. Here, I will briefly review the results from two meta-analyses that assessed how well SCT as a whole predicted behavior (Young et al., 2014; Zimmerman & Vernberg, 1994). The SCT portion of the Zimmerman and Vernberg meta-analysis included 15 studies that assessed the impact of behavioral (i.e., skills), environmental (i.e., social support), and personal (i.e., perceived self-efficacy) factors on various health behaviors. Results indicate that these SCT variables explained 34% of the variance in behavior. The Young et al. meta-analysis examined how well the full SCT model (see Figure 7.2) explained physical activity. Their meta-analysis included 44 studies, containing 55 SCT models, and a total of 13,358 participants. Results indicated that self-efficacy, outcome expectations, sociostructural factors, and goals explained 31% of the variance in physical activity behavior.

## EFFECTIVE STRATEGIES FOR INCREASING SELF-EFFICACY

As noted previously, SCT remains one of the most influential theories of public health communication, and the concept of self-efficacy has since been added to most major public health communication theories, including all of those discussed in this book. Given the prominent role self-efficacy plays in public health communication interventions, it seems only natural to ask: What are the best ways to increase self-efficacy? Several meta-analyses sought to answer this question, and this section will review two of them. As a reminder, when reporting effect sizes using $d$ or $g$, as is done by the meta-analyses discussed in this section, values of .20, .50, .80 are considered small, medium, and large effects, respectively (Cohen, 1988).

The Ashford et al. (2010) meta-analysis examined the impact of physical activity interventions in general, and 23 specific behavioral change strategies in particular, on physical activity self-efficacy. This meta-analysis included 27 studies with a total of 5,501 participants. Their general finding was that physical activity interventions had a small but significant impact on physical activity self-efficacy ($d = .16$). However, their moderator analyses suggest that some strategies were more or less effective than others. Specifically, interventions that included (1) vicarious experience, (2) feedback compared to others, (3) feedback compared to past performance, or (4) feedback delivered via email or online were three to four times more effective at increasing physical activity self-efficacy than those that did not. Conversely, interventions that included (1) guided mastery, (2) verbal persuasion, (3) persuasion via other means, (4) feedback given verbally, or (5) barrier identification were less effective at increasing self-efficacy than those that did not.

The Prestwich et al. (2014) meta-analysis examined the impact of diet interventions in general (and 26 specific behavioral change strategies in particular) on dietary self-efficacy. Their meta-analysis included 54 studies with a total of 13,446 participants. Their general finding was that diet interventions had a small but significant impact on dietary self-efficacy ($g = .24$). But, again, they found that some intervention strategies were more effective than others. Their most robust finding was that interventions that included stress management techniques (e.g., stretching, breathing, tips for managing stress, relaxation techniques, etc.) were consistently more effective at increasing self-efficacy than those that did not. Other results suggest that some strategies were more effective at least under certain circumstances (e.g., when interventions were longer, included more sessions, or were delivered face-to-face). These strategies included (1) reviewing of behavioral goals—e.g., reviewing previous goals and setting new goals; (2) self-monitoring of behavior—e.g., tracking diet through food logs; (3) providing feedback on performance—e.g., comparing what the participant ate to nutrition goals for a heart-healthy diet; and (4) providing contingent rewards—e.g., small reinforcements for attendance and behavior change.

## CONCLUSION

The goal of this chapter was to introduce key elements of SCT from a public health communication perspective. In doing so, this chapter introduced the notion of triadic reciprocal causation, reviewed the four key elements of SCT for health promotion, provided sample operational definitions for major SCT constructs, and summarized results from numerous SCT-related meta-analyses. I will conclude this chapter by reiterating two important points. First, SCT takes a comprehensive approach by highlighting the importance of moving beyond the individual level and also considering one's social and physical environment when developing public health communication interventions. Second, SCT views self-efficacy as the foundation of human thought and action (Bandura, 1986, 1997). People must believe they are capable of performing the recommended behavior before they will be inclined to adopt it. With this in mind, and "as you venture forth to promote your own health and that of others, may the efficacy force be with you" (Bandura, 2004, p. 162).

## REFERENCES

Ashford, S., Edmunds, J., & French, D. P. (2010). What is the best way to change self-efficacy to promote lifestyle and recreational physical activity? A systematic review with meta-analysis. *British Journal of Health Psychology, 15*, 265–288. https://doi.org/10.1348/135910709X461752

Bandura, A. (1977a). Self-efficacy: Toward a unifying theory of behavioral change. *Psychological Review, 84*(2), 191–215. https://doi.org/10.1037/0033-295X.84.2.191

Bandura, A. (1977b). *Social learning theory.* Prentice-Hall.

Bandura, A. (1978). The self system in reciprocal determinism. *American Psychologist, 33*(4), 344–358. https://doi.org/10.1037/0003-066X.33.4.344

Bandura, A. (1986). *Social foundations of thought and action: A social cognitive theory.* Prentice Hall.

Bandura, A. (1997). *Self-efficacy: The exercise of control.* W.H. Freeman and Company.

Bandura, A. (1999). A social cognitive theory of personality. In L. Pervin & O. John (Eds.), *Handbook of personality: Theory and research* (2nd ed., pp. 154–196). Guilford Publications.

Bandura, A. (2001). Social cognitive theory of mass communication. *Media Psychology, 3*, 265–299. https://doi.org/10.1207/S1532785XMEP0303_03

Bandura, A. (2004). Health promotion by social cognitive means. *Health Education and Behavior, 31*, 143–164. https://doi.org/10.1177/1090198104263660

Bandura, A. (2006). Guide for constructing self-efficacy scales. In F. Pajares & T. Urdan (Eds.) *Self-efficacy beliefs of adolescents* (pp. 307–337). Information Age Publishing.

Breastcancer.org. (2020). *What does healthy eating mean?* https://www.breastcancer.org/tips/nutrition/healthy_eat

Chen, L., Ho, S. S., & Lwin, M. O. (2017). A meta-analysis of factors predicting cyberbullying perpetration and victimization: From the social cognitive and media effects approach. *New Media and Society, 19*(8), 1194–1213. https://doi.org/10.1177/1461444816634037

Cohen, J. (1988). *Statistical power analysis for the behavioral sciences* (2nd ed.). Laurence Erlbaum Associates.

Dewar, D. L., Lubans, D. R., Plotnikoff, R. C., & Morgan, P. J. (2012). Development and evaluation of social cognitive measures related to adolescent dietary behaviors. *International Journal of Behavioral Nutrition and Physical Activity, 9*(36), 1–10. https://doi.org/10.1186/1479-5868-9-36

Fasbender, U. (2019). Outcome expectations. In V. Zeigler-Hill & T. K. Schckelford (Eds.), *Encyclopedia of personality and individual differences*. Springer. https://doi.org/10.1007/978-3-319-28099-8_1802-1

Firth, J., Marx., W., Dash, S., Carney, R., Teasdale, S. B, Solmi, M., Stubbs, B., Schuch, F. B., Carvalho, A., Jacka, F., & Sarris, J. (2019). The effects of dietary improvement on symptoms of depression and anxiety: A meta-analysis of randomized control trials. *Psychosomatic Medicine, 81*(3), 165–280. https://doi.org/10.1097/PSY.0000000000000673

Fishbein, M., & Ajzen, I., (2010). *Predicting and changing behavior: The reasoned action approach*. Psychology Press.

Holden, G. (1992). The relationship of self-efficacy appraisals to subsequent health related outcomes: A meta-analysis. *Social Work in Health Care, 16*(1), 53–93. https://doi.org/10.1080/J010v16n01_05

Kelder, S. H., Hoelscher, D., & Perry, C. L. (2015). How individuals, environments, and health behaviors interact: Social cognitive theory. In K. Glanz, B. K. Rimer, & K. Viswanath (Eds.), *Health behavior: Theory, research, and practice* (5th ed.) (pp. 159–181). Jossey-Bass.

Kim, J. G., Kim, H. J., & Lee, K. H. (2019). Understanding behavioral job search self-efficacy through the social cognitive lens: A meta-analytic review. *Journal of Vocational Behavior, 112*, 17–34. https://doi.org/10.1016/j.jvb.2019.01.004

Knowlden, A. P., Robbins, R., & Grandner, M. (2018). Social cognitive models of fruit and vegetable consumption, moderate physical activity, and sleep behavior in overweight and obese men. *Health Behavior Research, 1(2)*, 1–21. https://doi.org/10.4148/2572-1836.1011

Lassale, C., Batty, G. D., Baghdadli, A., Jacka, F., Sánchez-Villegas, A., Kivimäki, M., & Akbaraly, T. (2019). Healthy dietary indices and risk of depressive outcomes: A systematic review and meta-analysis of observational studies. *Molecular Psychiatry, 24*(7), 965–986. https://doi.org/10.1038/s41380-018-0237-8

Loughrey, D. G., Lavecchia, S., Brennan, S., Lawlor, B. A., & Kelly, M. E. (2017). The impact of the Mediterranean diet on the cognitive functioning of healthy older adults: A systematic review and meta-analysis. *Advances in Nutrition, 8*(4), 571–586. https://doi.org/10.3945/an.117.015495

Luszczynska, A., & Schwarzer, R. (2005). Social cognitive theory. In M. Conner & P. Norman (Eds.), *Predicting health behaviour: Research and practice with social cognition models* (2nd ed., pp. 127–186). Open University Press.

Mothers Against Drunk Driving. (2020). *Victim impact panels*. https://maddvip.org/

Nagy, S., Watts, G. F., & Nagy, M. C. (2003). Scales measuring psychosocial antecedents of coital initiation among adolescents in a rural southern state. *Psychological Reports, 92*(3), 981–990. https://doi.org/10.2466/pr0.2003.92.3.981

Norman, G. J., Carlson, J. A., Sallis, J. F., Wagner, N., Calfas, K. J., & Patrick, K. (2010). Reliability and validity of brief psychosocial measures related to dietary behaviors. *International Journal of Behavioral Nutrition and Physical Activity, 7*, 1–10. https://doi.org/10.1186/1479-5868-7-56

Prestwich, A., Kellar, I., Parker, R., MacRae, S., Learmonth, M., Sykes-Muskett, B., Taylor, N. J., & Castle, H. (2014). How can self-efficacy be increased? Meta-analysis of dietary interventions. *Health Psychology Review*, 8(3), 270–285. https://doi.org/10.1080/17437199.2013.813729

Robbins, S. B., Lauver, K., Le, H., Davis, D., Langley, R., & Carlstrom, A. (2004). Do psychosocial and study skill factors predict college outcomes? A meta-analysis. *Psychological Bulletin*, 130, 261–288. https://doi.org/10.1037/0033-2909.130.2.261

Roberto, A. J., Meyer, G., Johnson, A. J., & Atkin, C. K. (2000). Using the extended parallel process model to prevent firearm injury and death: Field experiment results of a video-based intervention. *Journal of Communication*, 50(4), 157–175. https://doi.org/10.1111/j.1460-2466.2000.tb02867.x

Roberto, A. J., Meyer, G., Johnson, A. J., Atkin, C. K., & Smith, P. K. (2002). Promoting gun trigger-lock use: Insights and implications from a radio-based health communication intervention. *Journal of Applied Communication Research*, 30(3), 210–230. https://doi.org/10.1080/00909880216584

Rogers, E. M. (2003). *Diffusions of innovation* (5th ed.). Free Press.

Schunk, D. H., & Usher, E. L. (2019). Social cognitive theory of motivation. In R. M. Ryan (Ed.), *The Oxford handbook of human motivation* (2nd ed., pp. 11–26). Oxford University Press.

Schwarzer, R. & Knoll, N. (2010). Social support. In D. French, K. Vedhara, A. A. Kaptein, & J. Weinman (Eds.), *Health psychology* (2nd ed., pp. 283–293). Blackwell.

Schwarzer, R., & Luszczynska, A. (2016). Self-efficacy and outcome expectancies. In Y. Benyamini, M. Johnston, & E. C. Karademas (Eds.), *Assessment in health psychology* (pp. 31–44). Hogrefe.

Sheu, H. B., Liu, Y., & Li, Y. (2017). Well-being of college students in China: Testing a modified social cognitive model. *Journal of Career Assessment*, 25(1), 144–158. https://doi.org/10.1177/1069072716658240

Sofi, F., Cesari, F., Abbate, R., Gensini, G. F., & Casini, A. (2008). Adherence to Mediterranean diet and health status: Meta-analysis. *BMG*, 337, 673–680. https://doi.org/10.1136/bmj.a1344

U.S. Department of Health and Human Services and U.S. Department of Agriculture. (2015). *2015–2020 dietary guidelines for Americans* (8th ed.). https://health.gov/dietaryguidelines/2015/guidelines/

Wójcicki, T. R., White, S. M., & McAuley, E. (2009). Assessing outcome expectations in older adults: The multidimensional outcome expectations for exercise scale. *Journals of Gerontology: Psychological Sciences*, 64(1), 33–40. https://doi.org/10.1093/geronb/gbn032

Wood, R., & Bandura, A. (1989). Social cognitive theory of organizational management. *The Academy of Management Review*, 14(3), 361–384. https://doi.org/10.2307/258173

Yang, Y., Yang, C., Latkin, C. A., Luan, R., & Nelson, K. E. (2016). Condom use during commercial sex among male clients of female sex workers in Sichuan China: A social cognitive theory analysis. *AIDS and Behavior*, 20(10), 2309–2317. https://doi.org/10.1007/s10461-015-1239-z

Young, M. D., Plotnikoff, R. C., Collins, C. E., Callister, R., & Morgan, P. J. (2014). Social cognitive theory and physical activity: A systematic review and meta-analysis. *Obesity Reviews*, 15(12), 983–995. https://doi.org/10.1111/obr.12225

Zimmerman, R. S., & Vernberg, D. (1994). Models of preventive health behavior: Comparison, critique, and meta-analysis. In G. Albrecht (Ed.), *Advances in medical sociology, health behavior models: A reformulation* (pp. 45–67). JAI Press.

## CHAPTER 8

# Fear Appeals: The Extended Parallel Process Model

## CHAPTER OUTLINE

## INTRODUCTION

A *fear appeal* is "a persuasive message designed to both create and alleviate the emotion of fear in audience members" (Roberto et al., 2018, p. 144). Introductions to most fear appeal literature reviews invariably begin with a statement similar to the following: Although the effects of fear appeals have been studied for over six decades, the empirical evidence is disappointingly contradictory, conflicting, inconsistent, uncertain, or unclear (Peters et al., 2013; Sheeran et al., 2014; Tannenbaum et al., 2015; Witte, 1992; Witte & Allen, 2000). The premise of this chapter is that fear appeals can be an effective way to change attitudes, intentions, and behavior *if they are implemented and studied correctly*. Thus, the main goal of this chapter is to provide a set of best practices for developing and evaluating fear appeal messages. Toward this end, this chapter will (1) provide a brief history of fear appeals; (2) describe the extended parallel process model—and provide conceptual definitions for all key constructs; (3) provide sample operational definitions for all key constructs; (4) review results of several recent fear appeal meta-analyses; and (5) identify the practical implications for designing theory- and research-based fear appeal messages.

## A VERY BRIEF HISTORY OF FEAR APPEALS

The extended parallel process model (EPPM; Witte, 1992) integrates and extends three earlier efforts to explain the effects of fear appeal messages: (1) drive theories, (2) the parallel process model, and (3) protection motivation theory. While a detailed review of these three earlier approaches is beyond the scope of this chapter (i.e., existing evidence suggests they are either inaccurate or incomplete; Dillard, 1994; Mongeau, 2013; Witte, 1992), each approach incrementally added important elements to current fear appeal science and practice. To illustrate, drive theories (Hovland et al., 1953; Janis, 1967) introduced the idea that fear appeal messages should have two components: one that instills fear and another that reduces it (Dillard, 1994). The parallel process model (Leventhal, 1971) made the distinction between the cognitive danger control and emotional fear control reactions to fear appeal messages, but did not clearly specify when one process should dominate over another (Witte, 1992). Finally, protection motivation theory (PMT; Rogers, 1975, 1983) clearly explicated the role of perceived severity, susceptibility, self-efficacy, and response efficacy in the danger control process, but did not address the fear control portion of the parallel process model (Witte, 1992).

Thus, "the EPPM picks up where the original PMT left off. Specifically, the EPPM adopts the original PMT's explanation of danger control processes that lead to message acceptance (one side of the parallel process model) and defines and expands the fear control process which lead to message rejection (the other side of the parallel process model)"

(Witte, 1992, p. 337). More specifically, the EPPM (1) stresses the importance of focusing on both threat and efficacy in fear appeal messages as first suggested by drive theories; (2) extends the original parallel process model's cognitive (danger control) and emotional (fear control) reactions to fear appeals; and (3) keeps protection motivation theory's explanation for the cognitive danger control processes that lead to message acceptance. The key difference between the EPPM and previous fear appeal theories, then, is that earlier approaches focused largely on individuals who adopted the recommended response (i.e., danger control) after being exposed to a fear appeal message, placing everyone else into the no-response category. However, the EPPM proposes that the no-response category was made up of two groups: (1) those who truly had no response to the campaign and (2) those who engaged in fear control. The EPPM specifies how interactions between perceived threat and efficacy lead to danger control or fear control and explains when one process would be expected to dominate over the other. With this general overview of fear appeals in mind, I now turn to a more detailed discussion of the EPPM. For your convenience, Table 8.1 on the following page contains conceptual definitions for all EPPM constructs, and each of these constructs is discussed in more detail in the sections that follow.

## PUTTING THE FEAR BACK INTO FEAR APPEALS: THE EXTENDED PARALLEL PROCESS MODEL

The EPPM (Witte, 1992) is concerned with the effects of four variables on behavior change: perceived susceptibility, perceived severity, response-efficacy, and self-efficacy. Since there is strong evidence that regular physical activity helps prevent heart disease, the most common types of cancer, stroke, and diabetes—which represent the first, second, fifth, and seventh leading causes of death in the US respectively (U.S. Department of Health and Human Services, 2008), it will serve as the running example throughout this section. This example was also selected since recent meta-analysis results indicate that fear appeals messages have small to moderate effects on exercise intentions and behavior (Sheeran et al., 2014). Throughout this example, please keep in mind that when I say, "regular physical activity," I am referring to the physical activity guidelines for adults issued by the federal government (U.S. Department of Health and Human Services, 2008). According to these guidelines, adults should engage in:

1. At least 150 minutes (2 hours and 30 minutes) a week of *moderate-intensity* aerobic physical activity.  Examples include walking briskly (at least 3 miles per hour), bicycling (less than 10 miles per hour), tennis (doubles), golfing (carrying clubs), weight training, general gardening, ballroom dancing, heavy cleaning, mowing the lawn, etc.

2.  At least 75 minutes (1 hour and 15 minutes) a week of *vigorous-intensity* aerobic physical activity. Examples include jogging, bicycling (over 10 miles per hour), tennis (singles), heavy gardening, aerobics classes, swimming laps, hiking uphill, many competitive sports (basketball, soccer, football, rugby, hockey, lacrosse), etc.
3.  An equivalent combination of moderate- and vigorous-intensity aerobic activity.

| TABLE 8.1 | Conceptual Definitions for Key Extended Parallel Process Model Constructs |
| --- | --- |
| **Construct** | **Conceptual Definition** |
| Fear | A negative emotion accompanied by a high level of arousal that is caused by the belief that a serious and personally relevant threat exists. |
| Perceived Threat | Thoughts a person has about a danger that exists in the environment. |
| Severity | Beliefs about the significance, magnitude, or seriousness of a health threat. |
| Susceptibility | Beliefs about the likelihood or chances that one will experience a health threat. |
| Perceived Efficacy | Thoughts a person has about the effectiveness and ease with which a recommended response can prevent the threat. |
| Response-Efficacy | Beliefs about the safety or effectiveness of effectiveness of the recommended behavior. |
| Self-Efficacy | Beliefs about one's ability to perform a behavior under various challenging circumstances. |
| Fear Control | An emotional coping process or psychological defense tactic where listeners strive to reduce the fear—but not the actual threat—generated by a message. |
| Defensive Avoidance | Conscious efforts to ignore or not think about an issue or message. |
| Issue Derogation | Criticizing the message or the source of the message. |
| Danger Control | A cognitive, problem-solving process where listeners strive to reduce the danger—or threat—presented in a message. |
| Behavior | What a person does or the way a person acts in a particular situation. |
| Intention | A person's readiness, motivation, or plans to perform a behavior in the future. |
| Attitude | How favorably or unfavorably a person feels toward a behavior. |

## PERCEIVED THREAT

*Perceived threat* refers to the thoughts a person has about a danger that exists in the environment. Perceived threat is comprised of two components: perceived susceptibility and perceived severity. *Perceived susceptibility* concerns the likelihood or chances that one will experience a health threat. For example, perceptions of susceptibility would be high if a person feels a threat (i.e., heart disease) is likely to happen to them. *Perceived severity* concerns the magnitude or seriousness of the threat. For example, those who perceive heart disease as less dangerous would score lower in severity, whereas those who view heart disease as more dangerous would score higher in severity. Taken together, an individual's level of perceived susceptibility combined with their level of perceived severity comprises their overall level of perceived threat. Notably, both perceived susceptibility and perceived severity must be high for one's overall perception of threat to be high. That is, unless a person believes both that the threat is likely and that the threat has serious consequences, they will not be motivated to engage in the recommended behavior.

## PERCEIVED EFFICACY

*Perceived efficacy* focuses on the effectiveness and ease with which a recommended response can prevent the threat. Perceived efficacy is also comprised of two components: response-efficacy and self-efficacy. *Response-efficacy* refers to one's beliefs about the safety or effectiveness of the recommended response (i.e., regular physical activity). For example, if one believes that physical activity is an effective way to prevent heart disease, then response-efficacy would be high (and vice versa). *Self-efficacy* concerns the extent to which an individual believes they are capable of performing the recommend behaviors under various challenging circumstances. For example, if an individual feels they do not have the time for regular physically activity, or if they are worried about getting injured while exercising, then self-efficacy would be low. On the other hand, if a person felt they could make time for regular physical activity and if they were confident that they could do so without getting injured, then perceived self-efficacy would be high. Notably, both perceived response-efficacy and perceived self-efficacy must be high for one's overall perception of efficacy to be high. That is, unless a person believes both that they can perform the recommended behavior and that the recommended behavior works, they will be unlikely to engage in the recommended behavior.

## THREE RESPONSES TO FEAR APPEAL MESSAGES

Three outcomes are possible depending on one's levels of perceived threat and efficacy: (1) no response, (2) a response that controls or limits perceived fear (i.e., fear control), and (3) a response that controls or limits the actual danger (i.e., danger control). Figure 8.1 provides a visual representation of the EPPM.

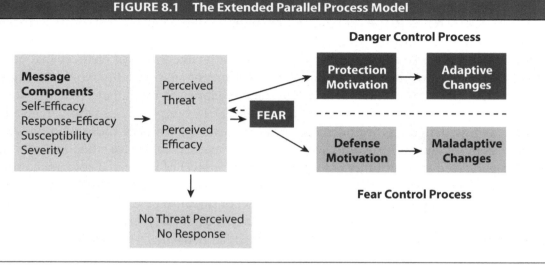

FIGURE 8.1    The Extended Parallel Process Model

Adapted from Witte (1992).

When utilizing the EPPM to develop public health communication messages, it is important to first identify a goal (i.e., the recommended response) and the threat (i.e., what motivates the recommended response). To illustrate the three possible outcomes mentioned previously, suppose you wanted to evaluate the effect of a hypothetical fear-appeal intervention designed to get people to engage in regular physical activity. The goal (or recommended response) of the intervention is to get adults to engage in regular physical activity each week to reduce their risk of heart disease (which is the threat). The following section illustrates the three paths an individual might take depending on their levels of perceived threat and efficacy.

### Low-Threat Path (No Response)

According to the EPPM, no response will occur when perceived threat is low (see Figure 8.2). Thus, if a person does not believe that they are susceptible to the threat (e.g., "Heart disease does not run in my family"), or if they do not believe that the threat has severe consequences (e.g., "Many people with heart disease lead a normal life"), the person will not be motivated to pay attention to the message and, therefore, will not respond to it. In other words, the hypothetical intervention has failed to promote a perception of threat, and since perceived threat is low the person will not be motivated to process the rest of the message or change their behavior.

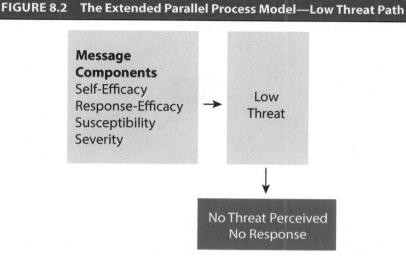

**FIGURE 8.2 The Extended Parallel Process Model—Low Threat Path**

### High-Threat/Low-Efficacy Path (Fear Control Response)

According to the EPPM, an individual will engage in fear control when perceived threat is high and perceived efficacy is low (see Figure 8.3). That is, if an individual believes that they are susceptible to a threat (e.g., "Heart disease runs in my family") and believes that the threat has severe consequences (e.g., "Heart disease is the leading cause of death in the US"), their level of perceived threat will be high. Since perceived threat is high, the person will be motivated to process the message and engage in the second appraisal of efficacy. If, during the appraisal of efficacy, the person does not believe the recommended response is effective (low response-efficacy—"Regular physical activity alone is not enough to prevent heart disease") or does not believe that they can engage in the recommended response (low self-efficacy—"I do not have the time for regular physical activity"), the person's level of perceived efficacy will be low. In this case, the intervention has promoted high perceptions of threat but not high perceptions of efficacy (i.e., although the person perceives a threat, they do not perceive a realistic option to reduce it). Since being afraid (high threat) is an uncomfortable state, the person will take steps to reduce the fear that do not necessarily decrease the actual danger. Two common strategies for reducing fear are defensive avoidance and issue derogation (Witte, 1992; Witte et al., 1994). *Defensive avoidance* refers to conscious efforts to ignore or not think about an issue or message. Examples of defensive avoidance might include looking away, closing a webpage, ignoring a conversation, refusing to read, or changing the channel to prevent exposure to information about heart disease. *Issue derogation* involves criticizing the message or the source of the message. For

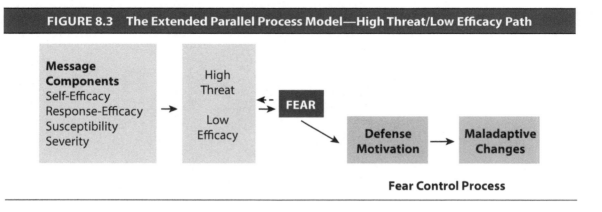

FIGURE 8.3    The Extended Parallel Process Model—High Threat/Low Efficacy Path

example, an individual might believe the message is exaggerated or that the source is deliberately trying to manipulate their feelings. In short, *fear control* is an emotional coping process or psychological defense tactic where listeners strive to reduce the fear—but not the actual threat—generated by a message.

### High-Threat/High-Efficacy Path (Danger Control Response)

An individual will engage in danger control when both perceived threat and perceived efficacy are high (see Figure 8.4). In this instance, the hypothetical intervention has accomplished all its goals by convincing the person that both a personally relevant and serious threat exists (i.e., high susceptibility and high severity) and, by providing an effective means to reduce the threat (high response efficacy—"Regular physical activity helps prevent heart disease"), that they are able to perform (high self-efficacy—"I can make the time for regular physical activity"). Put differently, *danger control* is a cognitive, problem-solving process where listeners strive to reduce the danger—or threat—presented in the message. That is, they will think carefully about the recommended response and change their behavior to reduce the danger.

In sum, the EPPM predicts that perceived threat is necessary to motivate action, and that perceived efficacy determines the nature of that action (i.e., whether people attempt to control the danger or control their fear). Thus, it is important to fully consider both perceived threat and perceived efficacy when developing fear appeal messages for public health communication interventions. I will also point out that the exercise example used in this section, which is adapted from Witte and Roberto (2009), is just one of the many examples that my colleagues and I have created. For those who may be interested in other topics, similar examples have been developed for disaster preparedness (Roberto et al.,

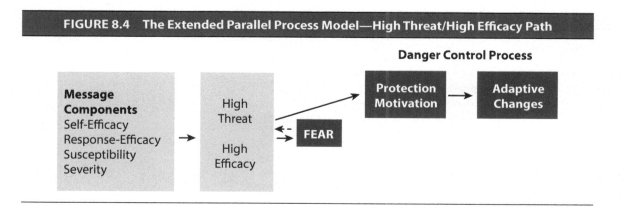

**FIGURE 8.4    The Extended Parallel Process Model—High Threat/High Efficacy Path**

2009), breast cancer screening (Ferrara et al., 2012), concussion reporting (Roberto et al., 2017), and bicycle safety (Lederman et al., 2017).

## OPERATIONAL DEFINITIONS: THE RISK BEHAVIOR DIAGNOSTIC SCALE (RBDS)

The primary tool used to measure EPPM constructs is the risk behavior diagnostic scale (RBDS, Witte et al., 1996). The RBDS includes 12 items, or three each, for severity, susceptibility, self-efficacy, and response efficacy. However, some researchers include one or two additional items per construct to increase the scales' reliability for their topic or intended audience. The RBDS is reported in such a way that it is possible for researchers to develop topic-specific items to increase accuracy and precision (Fishbein & Ajzen, 2010; Witte et al., 1996). To illustrate, consider these sample items for severity, susceptibility, self-efficacy, and response efficacy:

> I believe that [health threat] is serious.
> I am at risk for getting [health threat].
> I can [perform recommended response] to prevent [health threat].
> [Performing recommended response] prevents [health threat].

To further illustrate, Table 8.2 contains sample items for all EPPM variables using our running example of regular physical activity (the recommended response) to reduce the risk of heart disease (the health threat).

**TABLE 8.2    Sample Operational Definitions for Key Extended Parallel Process Model Constructs[1]**

| Construct | Operational Definition [2] |
|---|---|
| Severity | ► I believe that heart disease is serious.<br>► Heart disease is harmful to my health.<br>► Heart disease is dangerous.<br>► Heart disease has severe health consequences. |
| Susceptibility | ► I am at risk for getting heart disease.<br>► I am vulnerable to getting heart disease.<br>► It is likely that I will get heart disease.<br>► I am susceptible to getting heart disease. |

| Fear | Overall, how did the message make you feel about heart disease? |
|---|---|

|  | None of this feeling |  |  |  | A great deal of this feeling |
|---|---|---|---|---|---|
| Fearful | ❏ | ❏ | ❏ | ❏ | ❏ |
| Afraid | ❏ | ❏ | ❏ | ❏ | ❏ |
| Scared | ❏ | ❏ | ❏ | ❏ | ❏ |
| Worried | ❏ | ❏ | ❏ | ❏ | ❏ |
| Anxious | ❏ | ❏ | ❏ | ❏ | ❏ |
| Concerned | ❏ | ❏ | ❏ | ❏ | ❏ |

| Construct | Operational Definition |
|---|---|
| Self-Efficacy | ► I can engage in regular physical activity.<br>► I am able to engage in physical activity.<br>► It is simple for me to engage in regular physical activity.<br>► It is easy for me to engage in regular physical activity. |
| Response-Efficacy | ► Regular physical activity prevents heart disease.<br>► Engaging in regular physical activity reduces my chances of getting heart disease.<br>► Regular physical activity is an effective way to prevent heart disease.<br>► If I regularly engage in physical activity, I am less likely to get heart disease. |
| Fear Control | **Defensive Avoidance**<br>► When I was learning about the negative effects of heart disease, my first instinct was to avoid thinking about these effects.<br>► When I was learning about the negative effects of heart disease, my first instinct was to ignore what was being said.<br>► When I was learning about the negative effects of heart disease, my first instinct was to <u>NOT</u> think about my chance of experiencing these effects.<br><br>**Issue Derogation/Message Minimization**<br>► The information provided about heart disease was overblown.<br>► The information provided about heart disease was exaggerated.<br>► The information provided about heart disease was overstated.<br>► The information provided about heart disease was distorted. |

| TABLE 8.2   Continued | |
|---|---|
| **Construct** | **Operational Definition** |
| Danger Control | **Behavior**<br>I engaged in regular physical activity for at least 25 minutes over the past 30 days.<br>☐ No    ☐ Yes |
| | **Intention**<br>▸ I intend to engage in regular physical activity over the next 30 days.<br>▸ I will engage in regular physical activity for the next 30 days.<br>▸ I plan to engage in regular physical activity for the next 30 days. |
| | **Attitude**<br>My engaging in regularly physical activity for the next 30 days would be: |

| | | | | | | | |
|---|---|---|---|---|---|---|---|
| Bad | ☐ | ☐ | ☐ | ☐ | ☐ | ☐ | ☐ | Good |
| Unimportant | ☐ | ☐ | ☐ | ☐ | ☐ | ☐ | ☐ | Important |
| Useless | ☐ | ☐ | ☐ | ☐ | ☐ | ☐ | ☐ | Useful |
| Harmful | ☐ | ☐ | ☐ | ☐ | ☐ | ☐ | ☐ | Beneficial |
| Undesirable | ☐ | ☐ | ☐ | ☐ | ☐ | ☐ | ☐ | Desirable |

[1] See U.S. Department of Health and Human Services (2008) definition of "regular physical activity" provided earlier in this chapter. Such instructions are often included in the survey, so a researcher does not have to be continually provide such detailed information in each survey item.

[2] Measures adapted from Dillard and Anderson (2004); Hatchell et al. (2013); Fishbein & Ajzen (2010); Witte (1994); and Witte et al. (1996). Unless otherwise noted, all variables are typically measured using four- to seven-point Likert items ranging from strongly agree to strongly disagree.

## VALIDITY

Witte et al. (1996) assessed three types of validity for the RBDS. First, content validity was assessed to see how well the RBDS items accurately reflected the conceptual definitions of the four constructs it was designed to measure. To do this, trained raters classified each of the 12 RBDS items as measuring severity, susceptibility, self-efficacy, or response-efficacy. Items were correctly classified 88% of the time, which the authors interpreted as evidence of content validity. Second, construct validity, or the extent to which each of the RBDS subscales measures the variable it was designed to measure, was assessed using confirmatory factor analysis. Results were generally consistent with the prediction that severity, susceptibility, self-efficacy, and response efficacy items measured unique constructs (see also Kim & Nan, 2015; Maguire et al., 2010). Third, predictive validity was assessed by looking at how well each of the RBDS sub-scales predicted various danger control and fear control outcomes. The RBDS scores accurately predicted all three danger control outcomes under investigation (i.e., attitude, intention, and behavior), and one of the three fear control outcomes under investigation (i.e., defensive avoidance).

## RELIABILITY

As you can see in Table 8.3, Cronbach's alphas (α) for each of the RBDS subscales typically (but not always) fall above the .70 threshold for a wide variety of topics and intended

**TABLE 8.3   Sample Alpha (α) Coefficients for Extended Parallel Process Model Constructs**

| Study (Year) | Topic | Severity | Susceptibility | Self-Efficacy | Response Efficacy | Fear | Attitude | Intention | Defensive Avoidance | Issue Derogation |
|---|---|---|---|---|---|---|---|---|---|---|
| Witte et al. (1993) | Use safety Measures to Prevent Farm Equipment Injuries | .87 | .68 | .53 | .92 | .87 | .86 | .91 | .81 | .95 |
| Witte et al. (1996)[1] | Condom Use to Prevent Genital Warts | .90 | .85 | – | – | – | .89 | .98 | .81 | .95 |
| Ordoñana et al. (2009)[2] | Get Vaccinated to Prevent Tetanus | .89 | .82 | – | – | .87 | – | .95 | .88 | .80 |
| Meczkowski et al. (2016)[3] | Floss to Prevent Periodontal Disease | .87 | .81 | .84 | .85 | .91 | – | .95 | – | – |
| Roberto et al. (2019) | Annual Influenza Vaccine | .82 | .78 | .80 | .92 | .94 | .95 | .97 | – | – |
| Roberto et al. (2021) | Social Distancing During COVID-19 | .81 | .86 | .65 | .76 | .88 | – | .79 | .75 | .89 |

[1] Witte et al. (1996) did not report individual alphas for self-efficacy and response efficacy. Instead, they combined their three self-efficacy and three response efficacy items into a single efficacy measure with an alpha of .71.

[2] Ordoñana et al. (2009) did not report individual alphas for self-efficacy and response efficacy. Instead, they combined their three self-efficacy and four response efficacy items into a single efficacy measure with an alpha of .75.

[3] Meczkowski et al. (2016) measured fear at three points in time. Only the lowest alpha for the fear measures is reported here.

– = Variable not measured or alpha not reported.

audience, indicating strong measurement reliability. Further, Cronbach's alphas for all danger control and fear control variables typically fall in the very strong range (i.e., .86–.89 for attitude, .91–.98 for intention, .81–.88 for defensive avoidance, and .80–.95 for issue derogation).

While most EPPM studies focus on a single recommended response or health threat, some studies have successfully used slight variations of these RBDS items to study multiple related health threats. For example, Witte et al. (1993) combined response efficacy items that assessed the effectiveness of farm equipment safety measures at preventing (1) injuries, (2) deaths, and (3) disfigurement ($\alpha$ = .92). Also, for example, Hatchell et al.'s (2013) severity, susceptibility, and response-efficacy items each focused on four different health threats associated with low physical activity. That is, instead of changing the root question and keeping the threat the same, they kept the same root question and changed the threat. For example, their severity questions read, "I believe that [obesity/erectile dysfunction/chronic disease] is a severe condition" ($\alpha$ = .81). Their susceptibility questions read, "I am at risk for [becoming obese/developing erectile dysfunction/developing chronic disease]" ($\alpha$ = .97). Further, their response efficacy items read, "If I engage in the recommended amount of physical activity, I will decrease my risk of [becoming obese/developing erectile dysfunction/developing chronic disease] ($\alpha$ = .92). Alternatively, researchers sometimes define important key terms in instructions so large amounts of text do not have to be repeated in each item. For example, in the instructions for their tractor-safety study, Witte et al. (1993) defined safety measures as "seatbelts, roll bars, PTO covers, auger covers, etc.," and then just used the phrase "safety measures" in the items (e.g., "farm equipment safety measures are effective in preventing injuries," p. 321).

## FEAR APPEALS: ADVANCES THROUGH META-ANALYSIS

To date, at least a dozen meta-analyses have been conducted to assess the effects of fear appeal messages on attitude, intention, and behavior (Boster & Mongeau, 1984; de Hoog et al., 2007; Earl & Alberracín, 2007a, 2007b; Floyd et al., 2000; Good & Abraham, 2007; Milne et al., 2000; Mongeau, 1998; Peters et al., 2013; Sheeran et al., 2014; Sutton, 1982; Tannenbaum et al., 2015; Witte & Allen, 2000). In this section, four meta-analyses are reviewed, including the first one to explicitly test several key propositions from the EPPM (Witte & Allen, 2000), plus the three most recent fear appeal meta-analyses (Peters et al., 2013; Sheeran et al., 2014; Tannenbaum et al., 2015). Table 8.4 summarizes some of the key information from these four meta-analyses, including the number of subjects ($N$), number of studies ($k$), and the effect sizes for threat (broken down by severity and susceptibility when possible) and efficacy (broken down by self-efficacy and response-efficacy when possible) on attitude, intention, and behavior. The following section will focus on: (1) main

| TABLE 8.4 | Effect Sizes (Cohen's *d*) for Fear Appeal Message Features on Attitudes, Intentions, and Behaviors | | | | | |
|---|---|---|---|---|---|---|
| Study | N (k)[1] | Dependent Variable(s) | Threat[2] | | Efficacy[3] | |
| | | | Severity | Susceptibility | Self- | Response- |
| Witte & Allen (2000)[4]—Various Health Behaviors | 12,735 (98) | Attitude | .30* | .24 | .28* | .24* |
| | | Intention | .28* | .35* | .35* | .35* |
| | | Behavior | .26* | .28* | .26 | .26 |
| Peters et al. (2013)—Various Health Behaviors | 459 (6) | Behavior | .11 | | .49* | |
| Sheeran et al. (2014) —Various Health Behaviors | 52,976 (239) | Intention | .32* | .36* | – | |
| | | Behavior | .34* | .25* | – | |
| Tannenbaum et al. (2015)[5]—Various Health Behaviors | 27,372 (127) | Attitude | .23* | | – | |
| | | Intention | .31* | | – | |
| | | Behavior | .27* | | – | |

* *p* < .05.
[1] *N* = total number of participants included in the meta-analysis. *k* = total number of studies included in the meta-analysis.
[2] Effect sizes are reported separately for severity and susceptibility when available. Otherwise, they are reported for overall threat (which may include severity, susceptibility, or both).
[3] Effect sizes are reported separately for self-efficacy and response-efficacy when available. Otherwise, they are reported for overall efficacy (which may include self-efficacy, response-efficacy, or both).
[4] Originally reported effect sizes using *r*, which were converted to Cohen's *d* throughout this chapter using Ellis' (2009) Effect Size Calculator. *N* was not reported in this meta-analysis, so *n* from the largest individual analyses is reported here.
[5] Individual effect sizes reported in Tannenbaum et al. (2015) Appendix B.

effects for threat; (2) main effects for efficacy; (3) the combined effects of threat and efficacy; (4) moderator variables that do and do not appear to impact the effectiveness of fear appeal messages; and (5) fear control outcomes. Finally, as a reminder, when reporting effect sizes using Cohen's *d* (as is done in Table 8.4 and throughout this chapter) values of .20, .50, .80 are considered small, medium, and large effects, respectively (Cohen, 1988).

## MAIN EFFECTS OF THREAT ON DANGER CONTROL OUTCOMES

All four meta-analyses assessed the effects of threat on one or more danger control outcomes (i.e., attitudes, intentions, and/or behavior). These meta-analyses differ, however, in whether they present separate effect sizes for both severity and susceptibility or whether they present a single effect size for threat (which may include severity, susceptibility, or both; see Table 8.4). These meta-analyses indicated that severity has small to medium main effects on attitudes, intention, and behavior. In addition, susceptibility has a small but insignificant effect on attitudes, and small to medium significant effects on intention and behavior. Finally, global threat (which may include severity, susceptibility, or both) had small to medium main effects on attitudes, intention, and behavior, though the effect of threat on behavior was not significant in the Peters et al. (2013) meta-analysis.

Sheeran et al. (2014) reported the separate effects of increasing severity and susceptibility on intentions and behavior which sheds additional light on the findings reported in the previous paragraph and in Table 8.4. Specifically, each threat component moderated the effect of the other threat component. That is, severity increased the impact of susceptibility on intentions by $d = .11$ (from .29 to .40) and behavior by $d = .20$ (from .16 to .36). Moreover, susceptibility increased the impact of severity on intentions by $d = .18$ (from .22 to .40). In short, these results indicate that increasing both severity and susceptibility leads to greater changes in intentions and behavior than does increasing only one component. Not only are these results consistent with EPPM predictions, they also suggest the influence of threat in many studies and meta-analyses may be attenuated given that the threat component often includes either just susceptibility or just severity.

Tannenbaum et al. (2015), on the other hand, report that fear appeals were similarly effective regardless of whether they depicted high severity, high susceptibility, or both. Differential inclusion criteria may explain the apparent contradiction between findings. That is, the Sheeran et al. (2014) analyses only included studies that generated significant differences in both perceived susceptibility and severity, whereas Tannenbaum et al. (2015) had no such requirement (i.e., the studies included in their meta-analyses only had to attempt to manipulate severity or susceptibility, but they did not have to do so successfully). It is possible that the manipulations of severity or susceptibility in some studies included in this meta-analysis were ineffective, and therefore may have attenuated individual study and meta-analytic results. In sum, based on the Sheeran et al. (2014) meta-analyses, it seems reasonable to conclude that to be maximally effective, fear appeals must consider both perceived severity and perceived susceptibility.

## MAIN EFFECTS OF EFFICACY ON DANGER CONTROL OUTCOMES

As Table 8.4 indicates, two of the reviewed meta-analyses also assessed the main effects of self-efficacy, response-efficacy, or efficacy in general (which may include self-efficacy, response-efficacy, or both) on danger control outcomes. With this in mind, self-efficacy had small to medium main effects on attitudes and intentions, and a small but insignificant effect on behavior. In addition, response-efficacy had small to medium main effects on attitudes and intentions, and a small but insignificant effect on behavior. Finally, global efficacy (which may include self-efficacy, response efficacy, or both) had a medium main effect on behavior.

## COMBINED EFFECTS OF THREAT AND EFFICACY ON DANGER CONTROL OUTCOMES

Working from the protection motivation explanation (Rogers, 1975, 1983), the EPPM predicted that fear appeal messages will be persuasive only if they include both threat components (i.e., severity and susceptibility) and both efficacy components (i.e., self-efficacy and/or response-efficacy). Moreover, messages that lack strong threat and/or efficacy components will be unpersuasive (though for different reasons). In short, the EPPM predicts that threat and efficacy should interact to influence persuasive outcomes. This is typically referred to as the *strong hypothesis* (a.k.a., the *EPPM hypothesis*).

Tannenbaum et al. (2015) note that research suggests a second, competing, hypothesis regarding the importance of threat and efficacy in fear appeal messages: The *weak hypothesis* (a.k.a., the *additive hypothesis*) suggests that threat and efficacy will not interact, but will have separate main effects on attitude, intention, and behavior. In other words, although having both high threat and high efficacy messages will be optimal, messages with one strong component (either threat or efficacy) will be more persuasive than low-threat/low-efficacy message.

It is worth noting that the strong and weak models are very similar and, therefore, highly correlated (Mongeau, 2013; Roberto & Goodall, 2009). For example, both models predict larger effects when both threat and efficacy are high, and smaller (or no) effects when both threat and efficacy are low. Thus, data consistent with one model will likely be consistent with the other model as well. With this in mind, all four of the reviewed meta-analyses analyzed the effects of both threat and efficacy on danger control outcomes (i.e., attitude, intention, or behavior).

Witte and Allen (2000) tested both the strong and weak hypotheses by creating four groups—high threat/high efficacy (HTHE), high threat/low efficacy (HTLE), low threat/high efficacy (LTHE), and low threat/low efficacy (LTLE)—and using those groups to compare two effects-coded models. First, they tested the strong hypothesis, which predicts a specific threat × efficacy interaction, expressed as: HTHE > HTLE = LTHE = LTLE. Put differently, the EPPM predicts that only the high threat/high efficacy group will generate danger control outcomes. The other three groups should generate no danger control outcomes. Second, they tested the weak hypothesis, expressed as: HTHE > HTLE = LTHE > LTLE. Witte and Allen (2000) conclude that while the data were consistent with both the strong EPPM hypothesis ($\eta^2 = .21$; $p < .05$) and the weak additive hypothesis ($\eta^2 = .29$; $p < .05$), the cell means favored the weak additive hypothesis over the strong EPPM hypothesis.

The Peters et al. (2013) meta-analysis sought to provide the most rigorous test of fear appeal studies to date. To be included in their meta-analysis a study had to: (1) manipulate threat—i.e., severity, susceptibility, or both; (2) manipulate efficacy—i.e., self-efficacy, response-efficacy, or both; (3) perform those manipulations in such a way as to create a

2 × 2 full factorial design; and (4) include behavior as a dependent variable. Given the straightforward nature of the selection criteria, it is surprising that only six studies met all four criteria. Results were consistent with the strong EPPM hypothesis. That is, the threat × efficacy interaction was significant, and the high-treat/high-efficacy messages had the greatest impact on behavior.

Sheeran et al. (2014) investigated the effects of both threat and efficacy on intentions and behavior. A significant change in self-efficacy increased the impact of threat on intentions by $d = .31$ (from .28 to .59) and on behavior by $d = .13$ (from .16 to .29). Further, a significant change in response-efficacy increased the impact of threat on intentions by $d = .30$ (from .23 to .53), and on behavior by $d = .19$ (from .24 to .43). Perhaps most notable, however, is that increasing both response-efficacy and self-efficacy had the greatest impact. That is, significant changes in both self-efficacy and response-efficacy increased the impact of threat on intentions by $d = .75$ (from .23 to .98), and on behavior by $d = .32$ (from .12 to .45). In sum, the authors concluded that the pattern of results from this meta-analysis are largely consistent with predictions of the strong EPPM hypothesis.

Tannenbaum et al. (2015) examined the effect of including efficacy statements (i.e., self-efficacy, response-efficacy, or both) in fear appeal messages. Results indicate that fear appeals are twice as effective when they include efficacy statements ($d = .43$) than when they do not ($d = .21$). Given that fear appeals were effective with or without efficacy statements, the authors concluded that their meta-analytic data were consistent with the weak additive hypothesis and not the strong EPPM hypothesis.

In sum, the preponderance of the meta-analytic evidence indicates that fear appeals that include both a threat component and an efficacy component are generally more effective at changing attitudes, intentions, and behavior than fear appeals that focus only on threat. Further, messages that contain both threat (i.e., severity and susceptibility) components appear to be the most effective of all. In short, and at a minimum, there appears to be an additive effect for threat and efficacy, and at a maximum, threat and efficacy interact in such a way that the effects of one depend on the value of the other.

## MODERATOR EFFECTS

As a reminder, moderator analysis is used to determine if the strength or direction of a relationship between two variables depends on (i.e., is moderated by) a third variable. Together, the four meta-analyses reviewed here assessed the effects of dozens of descriptive (e.g., topic, gender, education, age, culture, stage of change), theoretical (e.g., efficacy, trait anxiety), and methodological (e.g., study setting, media of message) moderators on fear appeal effectiveness. Results indicate that fear appeals tend to be more effective for women than for men, when they focus on one-time rather than repeated behaviors, and for some topics over others (Sheeran et al., 2014; Tannenbaum et al., 2015). None of the other moderators included in these meta-analyses appear to impact the effects of fear appeal messages. These include, but are not limited to, (1) type of change (i.e., response encouragement vs. response discouragement vs. response maintenance; Sheeran et al. 2014); (2) target behavior type (i.e., detection behaviors vs. promotion/prevention behaviors; Sheeran et al., 2014; Tannenbaum et al., 2014); (3) message media (i.e., text vs. pictures/videos; Tannenbaum et al., 2015); (4) participant age (Sheeran et al., 2014; Tannenbaum et al., 2015); and (5) study source (i.e., published vs. thesis/other; Sheeran et al., 2014; Tannenbaum et al.. 2015). The fact that so few moderators are consistently associated with fear appeal effectiveness provides important information about their robustness.

## FEAR CONTROL

One of the EPPM's major contributions is that it distinguished between individuals who had no response to a fear appeal message and those who had a fear control response. Recall that no response is predicted when perceived threat is low, and a fear control response is predicted when perceived threat is high and perceived efficacy is low. Under such circumstances, individuals will focus on managing their emotional reaction rather than reducing the threat.

Notably, only one of the reviewed meta-analyses explicitly assessed fear control outcomes (Witte & Allen, 2000). This is likely because fewer fear appeal studies focused on fear control (Popova, 2012). To illustrate, only 13 of the 93 studies included in the Witte and Allen (2000) meta-analysis included fear control outcomes. That said, the authors report that perceived threat was positively related to fear control outcomes ($d = .41$) and perceived efficacy was negatively related to fear control outcomes ($d = -.22$). Finally, although the Peters et al. (2013) meta-analysis did not explicitly test the EPPM's fear-control prediction, they do note that their findings are consistent with the EPPM's fear control predictions.

In sum, existing evidence, while admittedly minimal, appears to be consistent with EPPM fear-control predictions. As Peters et al. (2013) and Kok et al. (2018) note, fear control responses provide an element of risk to using threatening communication "if the intervention developer is not very certain that either the population is high in response *and* self-efficacy, or that a given relevant intervention will manage to considerably increase response *and* self-efficacy" (Peters et al., 2013, p. S24, emphasis original).

## PRACTICAL IMPLICATIONS

Meta-analytic results suggest that threatening communication alone (i.e., severity or susceptibility) can have small effects on attitude, intention, and behavior. Moreover, these effects are substantially increased when such messages focus on (1) both components of threat—susceptibility and severity, (2) both components of efficacy—response-efficacy and self-efficacy, and (3) both threat and efficacy. The implications of these findings are discussed next.

## THE IMPORTANCE OF FOCUSING ON BOTH THREAT AND EFFICACY

Based on the definition of fear appeals advanced at the beginning of this chapter, efficacy is more than a moderator variable, it is an integral component of fear appeal messages (Dillard, 1994; Roberto et al., 2018; Witte, 1994; Witte & Allen, 2000). Consistent with this notion, the most important finding from the reviewed meta-analyses is that to be optimally persuasive, fear appeals must include both threat and efficacy components. These concepts have long been important in fear appeal explanations (Hovland et al., 1953; Rogers, 1975, 1983; Witte, 1992). It is curious, then, that so few studies include both threat and efficacy components (e.g., 24% in Witte & Allen, 2000; 33% in Tannenbaum et al., 2015).

Put differently, it appears that researchers and practitioners are spending considerable amount of time focusing on the creation of fear, but an insufficient time focusing on alleviating fear. The reviewed meta-analyses generally report that increasing perceptions of threat alone can have small positive effects on attitude, intention, and behavior. However, the reviewed meta-analyses clearly indicate that efficacy enhances the effectiveness of fear appeal messages. At a minimum, efficacy has an additive effect, and at a maximum threat and efficacy interact (e.g., Peters et al., 2013; Sheeran et al., 2014; Tannenbaum et al., 2015; Witte & Allen, 2000). Thus, failure to include an efficacy component with fear appeal messages will, in most cases, lead to suboptimal results (e.g., unless the intended audience is already known to be high in response- and self-efficacy; Peters et al., 2013; Popova, 2012; Rimal & Real, 2003; Roberto et al., 2018).

## THE IMPORTANCE OF FOCUSING ON BOTH SEVERITY AND SUSCEPTIBILITY

Even when focusing on the creating fear portion of the definition of fear appeals, research often comes up short. According to the EPPM, perceived susceptibility and perceived severity do not work independently; they should interact (Peters et al., 2013; Rogers, 1975, 1983; Witte, 1992). That is, "no matter how severe an outcome might be, it would be irrational to expend effort to prevent the outcome if it has no chance of occurring. Similarly, it would be irrational to take precautions if the outcome is not undesirable, regardless of its likelihood" (Weinstein, 2000, p. 65). Results from the Sheeran et al. (2014) meta-analysis indicate that each threat component moderates the effect of the other threat component is consistent with this supposition. Unfortunately, only a small minority of studies included both severity and susceptibility components (e.g., 33% in Tannenbaum et al., 2015). Again, failure to focus on both the severity and susceptibility components of threat will, in most cases, lead to suboptimal results.

## THE IMPORTANCE OF FOCUSING ON BOTH
## SELF-EFFICACY AND RESPONSE-EFFICACY

The largest effect sizes in the Sheeran et al. (2014) meta-analysis came from messages that simultaneously increased threat, response-efficacy, and self-efficacy. Both self-efficacy and response-efficacy are critical to the success of fear appeals. That is, no matter how easy it might be to perform a behavior (self-efficacy), why expend effort if it is ineffective (low response-efficacy) and vice versa? These findings, when combined with the finding that efficacy alone often has an equally large, or larger, effect than threat alone (see Table 8.4), highlight the importance of focusing on both components of efficacy if one wants to obtain optimal results from fear appeal messages. As was true with threat, the number of studies that include both efficacy components is small (e.g., only 3% in the Sheeran et al., 2014 meta-analysis). This is curious as efficacy components have been important parts of fear appeal explanations for over four decades (e.g., Rogers, 1975, 1983; Witte, 1992).

## BEHAVIOR AS A DEPENDENT VARIABLE

Table 8.4 reveals that threatening communication tends to have a smaller influence on behavior when compared with attitudes or intentions. Unfortunately, while most fear appeal studies include attitudes or intentions as a dependent variable, far fewer studies include actual behavior. The two most recent meta-analyses (Sheeran et al., 2014, Tannenbaum et al., 2015) included far more tests for intentions than for behavior (218 vs. 92 and 166 vs. 68, respectively). Notably, Sheeran et al. (2014) explicitly identified small cell sizes when behavior was the dependent variable as a potential meta-analytic limitation.

The most striking example of the paucity of behavioral measures in fear appeal studies comes from Peters et al. (2013). Using the most stringent (but quite reasonable) inclusion criteria, the authors identified just six studies that: (1) manipulated at least one component of threat, (2) manipulated at least one component of efficacy, and (3) included behavior as a dependent variable. A review of Tannenbaum et al. (2015) indicates that only 24 (19%) of the 127 articles included in their meta-analysis manipulated both threat and efficacy and measured behavior. The discrepancies between these two meta-analyses are that (1) Peters et al. (2013) included only published studies, whereas 9% of the studies in Tannenbaum et al. (2015) were unpublished; (2) Peters et al. (2013) searched through January 2012, whereas Tannenbaum et al. (2015) searched through February 2015; and perhaps most importantly, (3) Peters et al. (2013) required full-factorial, orthogonal, manipulations of threat and efficacy where Tannenbaum et al. (2015) did not.

## CONCLUSION

As noted at the outset of this chapter, there has been considerable confusion regarding the effectiveness of fear appeal messages over the past six decades. A large part of that confusion stems from differences in terminology and methodology. For example, terms like threatening communication and fear appeals are often used interchangeably even though the former is just one important component of the latter. Moreover, as the reviewed meta-analyses demonstrate, threatening communication is qualitatively very different, and quantitatively has very different effects, than theory- and research-based fear appeal messages. For example, and as was demonstrated throughout this chapter, (1) messages that focus on just one threat component are not as effective as those that focus on both threat components; (2) messages that focus on efficacy component are not as effective as those that focus on both efficacy components; and (3) messages that focus on just threat are not as effective as those that focus on both threat and efficacy. Thus, it makes little sense to treat all of these messages the same or to expect them all to have similar effects. Nonetheless, this is exactly what has and continues to happen (see Kok et al., 2018).

In summary, fear appeals can be effective; especially if they are designed, implemented, and studied correctly. However, this does not mean that fear appeals will always be the best or most appropriate choice. For example, if formative research suggests that one or more of the key components of fear appeals cannot be successfully manipulated, fear appeals will be less effective, or even risky (Peters et al., 2013; Witte, 1992). Nor is it reasonable to expect any type of message to be equally effective across all topics, contexts, and audiences. But, all things considered, theory- and researched-based fear appeal messages represent one viable option for public health communication researchers and practitioners interested in changing attitude, intention, and behavior under the appropriate circumstances.

## REFERENCES

Boster, F. J., & Mongeau, P. (1984). Fear-arousing persuasive messages. In R. N. Bostrom (Ed.), *Communication Yearbook 8* (pp. 330–375). SAGE.

Cohen, J. (1988). *Statistical power analysis for the behavioral sciences* (2nd ed.). Laurence Erlbaum Associates.

de Hoog, N., Stroebe, W., & de Wit, J. B. F. (2007). The impact of vulnerability to and severity of a health risk on processing and acceptance of fear-arousing communications: A meta-analysis. *Review of General Psychology, 11*(3), 258–285. https://doi.org/ 10.1037/1089-2680.11.3.258

Dillard, J. P. (1994). Rethinking the study of fear appeals: An emotional perspective. *Communication Theory, 4*, 295–323. https://doi.org/10.1111/j.1468-2885.1994.tb00094.x

Dillard, J. P., & Anderson, J. W. (2004). The role of fear in persuasion. *Psychology & Marketing, 21*(11), 909–926. https://doi.org/10.1002/mar.20041

Earl, A., & Albarracín, D. (2007a). Nature, decay, and spiraling of the effects of fear-inducing arguments and HIV counseling and testing: A meta-analysis of the short- and long-term outcomes of HIV-prevention interventions. *Health Psychology, 26*(4), 496–506. https://doi.org/10.1037/0278-6133.26.4.496

Earl, A., & Albarracín, D. (2007b). Correction to Earl and Albarracin (2007). *Health Psychology, 26*(6), 815–816.

Ellis, P. D. (2009). *Effect size calculators.* https://www.polyu.edu.hk/mm/effectsizefaqs/calculator/calculator.html

Ferrara, M. H., Roberto, A. J., & Witte, K. (2012). Managing fear to promote healthy change. In R. Obregon & S. Waisbord (Eds.), *The handbook of global health communication* (pp. 274–287). Wiley and Blackwell.

Fishbein, M., & Ajzen, I. (2010). *Predicting and changing behavior: The reasoned action approach.* Psychology Press.

Floyd, D. L., Prentice-Dunn, S., & Rogers, R. W. (2000). A meta-analysis of research on protection motivation theory. *Journal of Applied Social Psychology, 30*(2), 407–429. https://doi.org/10.1111/j.1559-1816.2000.tb02323.x

Good, A., & Abraham, C. (2007). Measuring defensive responses to threatening messages: A meta-analysis of measures. *Health Psychology Review, 1*(2), 208–229. https://doi.org/10.1080/17437190802280889

Hatchell, A. C., Bassett-Gunter, R. L., Clarke, M., Kimura, S., & Latimer-Cheung, A. E. (2013). Messages for men: The efficacy of EPPM-based messages targeting men's physical health. *Health Psychology, 32*(1), 24–32. https://doi.org/10.1037/a0030108

Hovland, C. I., Janis, I. L., & Kelley, H. H. (1953). *Communication and persuasion: Psychological studies of opinion change.* Yale University Press.

Janis, I. L. (1967). Effects of fear arousal on attitude change: Recent developments in theory and experimental research. *Advances in Experimental Social Psychology, 3*, 166–224. https://doi.org/10.1016/S0065-2601(08)60344-5

Kim, J., & Nan, X. (2015). Consideration of future consequences and HPV vaccine uptake among young adults. *Journal of Health Communication, 20*(9), 1033–1040. https://doi.org/10.1080/10810730.2015.1018583

Kok, G., Peters, G.-J. Y., Kessels, L. T. E., ten Hoor, G., & Ruiter, R. A. C. (2018). Ignoring theory and misinterpreting evidence: The false belief in fear appeals. *Health Psychology Review, 12*(2), 111–125. https://doi.org/10.1080/17437199.2017.1415767

Lederman, L. C., Kreps, G. L., & Roberto, A. J. (2018). *Health communication and everyday life.* Kendall-Hunt Publishing.

Leventhal, H. (1971). Fear appeals and persuasion: The differentiation of a motivational construct. *American Journal of Public Health, 61*(6), 1208–1224. https://doi.org/10.2105/AJPH.61.6.1208

Maguire, K. C., Gardner, J., Sopory, P., Jian, G., Roach, M., Amschlinger, J., Moreno, M., Pettey, G., & Piccone, G. (2010). Formative research regarding kidney disease health information in a Latino American sample: Associations among message frame, threat, efficacy, message effectiveness, and behavioral intention. *Communication Education, 59*(3), 344–359. https://doi.org/10.1080/03634521003628271

Meczkowski, E. J., Dillard, J. P., & Shen, L. (2016). Threat appeals and persuasion: Seeking and finding the elusive curvilinear effect. *Communication Monographs, 83*(3), 373–395. https://doi.org/10.1080/036377 51.2016.1158412

Milne, S., Sheeran, P., & Orbell, S. (2000). Prediction and intervention in health-related behavior: A meta-analytic review of protection motivation theory. *Journal of Applied Social Psychology, 30*(1), 106–143. https://doi.org/10.1111/j.1559-1816.2000.tb02308.x

Mongeau, P. A. (1998). Another look at fear-arousing persuasive appeals. In M. Allen & R. W. Preiss (Eds.), *Persuasion: Advances through meta-analysis* (pp. 53–68). Hampton Press.

Mongeau, P. A. (2013). Fear appeals. In J. P. Dillard & L. Shen (Eds.), *The SAGE handbook of persuasion* (2nd ed., pp. 184–199). SAGE.

Ordoñana, J. R., González-Javier, F., Espín-López, L., Gómez-Amor, J. (2009). Self-report and psychophysiological responses to fear appeals. *Human Communication Research, 35*(2), 195–220. https://doi.org/10.1111/j.1468-2958.2009.01344.x

Peters, G. J. Y., Ruiter, R. A., & Kok, G. (2013). Threatening communication: Acritical re-analysis and a revised meta-analytic test of fear appeal theory. *Health Psychology Review, 7*(1), S8–S31. https://doi.org/10.1080/17437199.2012.703527

Popova, L. (2012). The extended parallel process model: Illuminating the gaps in research. *Health Education and Behavior, 39*(4), 455–473. https://doi.org/10.1177/1090198111418108

Rimal, R. N., & Real, K. (2003). Perceived risk and efficacy beliefs as motivators of change: Use of the risk perception attitude (RPA) framework to understand health behaviors. *Human Communication Research, 29*(3), 370–399. https://doi.org/10.1111/j.1468-2958.2003.tb00844.x

Roberto, A. J., & Goodall, C. E. (2009). Using the extended parallel process model to explain physicians' decisions to test their patients for kidney disease. *Journal of Health Communication, 14*(4), 400–412. https://doi.org/10.1080/10810730902873935

Roberto, A. J., Goodall, C. E., & Witte, K. (2009). Raising the alarm and calming fears: Perceived threat and efficacy during risk and crisis. In R. Heath and D. O'Hair (Eds.), *Handbook of risk and crisis communication* (pp. 287–303). Routledge.

Roberto, A. J., Mongeau, P. A., & Liu, Y. (2018). A (re)defining moment for fear appeals: A comment on Kok et al. (2018). *Health Psychology Review, 12*(2), 144–146. https://doi.org/10.1080/17437199.2018.1445546

Roberto, A. J., Mongeau, P. A., Liu, Y., & Hashi, E. C. (2019). "Fear the flu, not the flu shot": A test of the extended parallel process model. *Journal of Health Communication, 24*(11), 829–836. https://doi.org/10.1080/10810730.2019.1673520

Roberto, A. J., Zhou, X., & Lu, A. H. (2021). The effects of perceived threat and efficacy on college students' social distancing behavior during the COVID-19 pandemic. *Journal of Health Communication, 26*, 264–271.

Roberto, A. J., van Raalte, L. J., Liu, Y., & Posteher, K. (in press). The role of perceived threat and efficacy in motivating behavior change in sport and exercise communication contexts. In B. Jackson, J. A. Dimmock, & J. Compton (Eds.), *Persuasion and communication in sport, exercise, and physical activity*. Taylor & Francis.

Rogers, R. W. (1975). A protection motivation theory of fear appeals and attitude change. *The Journal of Psychology, 91*(1), 93–114. https://doi.org/10.1080/00223980.1975.9915803

Rogers, R. W. (1983). Cognitive and physiological processes in fear appeals and attitude change: A revised theory of protection motivation. In J. Cacioppo & R. Petty (Eds.), *Social psychophysiology* (pp. 153–176). Guilford.

Sheeran, P., Harris, P. R., & Epton, T. (2014). Does heightening risk appraisals change people's intentions and behavior? A meta-analysis of experimental studies. *Psychological Bulletin, 140*(2), 511–543. https://doi.org/10.1037/a0033065

Sutton, S. R. (1982). Fear-arousing communications: A critical examination of theory and research. In J. R. Eiser (Ed.), *Social psychology and behavioral medicine* (pp. 303–337). Wiley.

Tannenbaum, M. B., Hepler, J., Zimmerman, R. S., Saul, L., Jacobs, S., Wilson, K., & Albarracín, D. (2015). Appealing to fear: A meta-analysis of fear appeal effectiveness and theories. *Psychological Bulletin, 141*(6), 1178–1204. https://doi.org/10.1037/a0039729

U.S. Department of Health and Human Services. (2008). *2008 physical activity guidelines for Americans.* https://health.gov/paguidelines/pdf/paguide.pdf

Weinstein, N. D. (2000). Perceived probability, perceived severity, and health-protective behavior. *Health Psychology, 19*(1), 65–74. https://doi.org/10.1037/0278-6133.19.1.65

Witte, K. (1992). Putting the fear back into fear appeals: The extended parallel process model. *Communication Monographs, 59*(4), 329–349. https://doi.org/10.1080/03637759209376276

Witte, K. (1994). Fear control and danger control: A test of the extended parallel process model (EPPM). *Communication Monographs, 61*(2), 113–134. https://doi.org/10.1080/03637759409376328

Witte, K., & Allen, M. (2000). A meta-analysis of fear appeals: Implications for effective health campaigns. *Health Education & Behavior, 27*(5), 591–615. https://doi.org/10.1177/109019810002700506

Witte, K., Cameron, K. A., McKeon, J. K., & Berkowitz, J. M. (1996). Predicting risk behaviors: Development and validation of a diagnostic scale. *Journal of Health Communication, 1*(4), 317–341. https://doi.org/10.1080/108107396127988

Witte, K., Peterson, T. R., Vallabhan, S., Stephenson, M. T., Plugge, C. D., Givens, V. K., Todd, J. D., Becktold, M. G., Hyde, M. K., & Jarrett, R. (1993). Preventing tractor-related injuries and deaths in rural populations: Using a persuasive health message framework in formative evaluation research. *International Quarterly of Community Health Education, 13*, 219–251. https://doi.org/10.2190/UHU7-W9DM-0LGM-0GV3

Witte, K., & Roberto, A. J. (2009). Fear appeals and public health: Managing fear and creating hope. In L. R. Frey & K. N. Cissna (Eds.), *Handbook of applied communication research* (pp. 584–610). Routledge.

## CHAPTER 9

# The Reasoned Action Approach

## CHAPTER OUTLINE

## INTRODUCTION

The theories reviewed in the previous chapters in this section identified a wide variety of variables that potentially impact behavior. The list includes severity and susceptibility, self-efficacy and response-efficacy, benefits and barriers, facilitators and impediments, attitude and norms, and intention. While there are some differences between the theories discussed so far, there are also many similarities. Further, the reasoned action approach is billed as "unifying conceptual framework" (Fishbein & Ajzen, 2010, p. 2), or meta-theory, that integrates a limited set of variables from multiple theoretical perspectives to predict, explain, and influence behavior. While the reasoned action approach has undergone several modifications over the years, intention remains the central construct as it represents the most important and immediate determinant of behavior. For example, getting an individual to adopt a healthy behavior (or to abandon an unhealthy one) involves first getting them to intend to adopt (or abandon) the behavior.

In this chapter I discuss the evolution of the reasoned action approach. Toward this end, I will describe the theory of reasoned action, the theory of planned behavior, and the integrative model of behavioral prediction—and provide conceptual definitions for all key variables (see Table 9.1). Next, I will provide sample survey items—or operational definitions—for all key variables, and review results of several meta-analyses on the reasoned action approach. Finally, I will identify several practical implications for planning and evaluating public health communication interventions guided by the reasoned action approach. Before I do, however, I will provide some background information about distracted driving, which continues to be a problem among college students (Hill et al., 2015), and will serve as the running example for this chapter.

| TABLE 9.1 | Conceptual Definitions for Reasoned Action Approach Constructs |
|---|---|
| **Construct** | **Conceptual Definition** |
| Behavior | What a person does or the way a person acts in a particular situation. |
| Intention | A person's readiness, motivation, or plans to perform a behavior in the future. |
| Attitude | How favorably or unfavorably a person feels toward a behavior. |
| Instrumental Attitude | One's assessment of the value of performing a behavior (e.g., unimportant-important). |
| Experiential Attitude | One's feelings about or emotional reactions to the idea of performing the behavior (i.e., boring-interesting). |
| Behavioral Beliefs | The perceived consequences of engaging in a behavior. |
| Outcome Evaluation | The positive or negative assessment of each consequence. |
| Perceived Norm | Perceived social pressure to perform a behavior. |
| Injunctive Norm | A person's perception of the behavior expected by important others *as a whole*. |
| Injunctive Normative Beliefs | A person's perceptions of what each important individual or subgroup expects them to do. |
| Motivation to Comply | How motivated an individual is to comply with *each* important individual or subgroup. |
| Descriptive Norm | Perceptions regarding whether or not important others *as a whole* are performing (or will perform) a behavior. |
| Descriptive Normative Beliefs | Beliefs regarding whether or not *each* important individual or subgroup is performing (or will perform) a behavior. |
| Identification with Referent | One's desire to be like *each* important individual or subgroup. |
| Perceived Control | The extent to which a person believes that they are capable of or have control over performing a behavior. |
| Capacity (a.k.a., Self-Efficacy) | Beliefs about one's ability to perform the recommended behavior in various challenging circumstances. |
| Autonomy | The extent to which performing a behavior is up to the individual; that it does not depend on something outside their control. |
| Control Beliefs | The perceived presence of factors that influence one's ability to perform (or have control over) a behavior. |
| Power of Each Control Belief | Beliefs about how each control belief might facilitate or impede one's ability to perform (or have control over) a behavior. |

Distracted driving "is any activity that could divert a person's attention away from the primary task of driving" (U.S. Department of Transportation, n.d.). While this definition potentially includes many different types of behavior ranging from talking to another passenger, eating, or texting while driving, Lantz and Loeb (2013) note that distracted driving is most commonly used to refer to "driving while distracted by any electronic means (texting, games, internet browsing, and so on)" (p. 40). A recent meta-analysis of 28 studies that compared reading or typing text messages while driving to a control or baseline condition found that texting while driving negatively impacted stimulus detection, reaction time, collisions, lane positioning, and speed (Caird et al., 2014). Research from the Transport Research Laboratory (Basacik et al., 2011) suggests that both texting and talking on the phone while driving had a greater negative impact on drivers' reaction times than either alcohol or cannabis (see Figure 9.1).

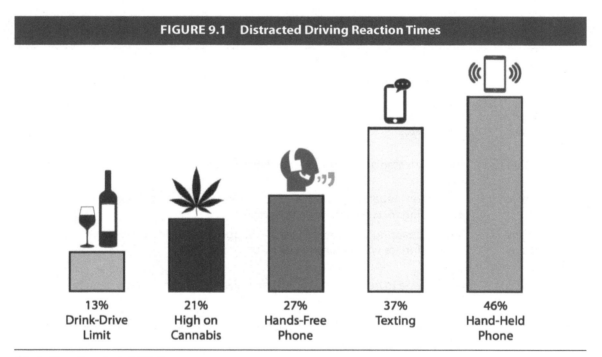

**FIGURE 9.1    Distracted Driving Reaction Times**

| 13% Drink-Drive Limit | 21% High on Cannabis | 27% Hands-Free Phone | 37% Texting | 46% Hand-Held Phone |

Adapted from Basacik et al. (2011).

In the US, 10% of all fatal crashes involve distracted drivers, and every day more than eight people are killed and over 1,100 people are injured in crashes linked to distracted driving (National Highway Traffic Safety Administration, 2015). Research suggests that between 80% and 90% of college students text while driving, even though a majority of them know that doing so is dangerous (Hill et al., 2015; Lantz & Loeb, 2013). These researchers suggest that college students have more confidence in their own driving skills and ability to multitask than they have in other drivers' abilities. Or, as Lantz and Loeb (2013) put it, there seems to be a mentality among college students that use of electronic devices while driving "is dangerous for everyone but me" (p. 40). Please keep this example in mind as I review the reasoned action approach, which begins with a discussion of theory of reasoned action.

## THEORY OF REASONED ACTION

### BEHAVIOR AND INTENTIONS

The theory of reasoned action (TRA) (Ajzen & Fishbein, 1980; Fishbein & Ajzen, 1975) states that the main determinant of *behavior* (i.e., the way a person acts in a particular situation) is *behavioral intention* (i.e., their readiness—or motivation—to perform the behavior in the future; Fishbein & Ajzen, 2010). Obviously, people do not always do what they intend to do. Nonetheless, research indicates that intentions are a strong—though imperfect—predictor of behavior. With this in mind, I will review some of the factors that moderate the intention-behavior relationship later in this chapter.

### ATTITUDE AND SUBJECTIVE NORMS

Behavioral intention, in turn, is determined by a person's *attitude* toward the behavior (i.e., how favorable or unfavorable a person feels about performing the behavior; Fishbein & Ajzen, 2010) and *subjective norms* (sometimes called *injunctive norms*; i.e., the person's perception of the behavior expected by important others as a whole). As was the case for intention, attitude and subjective norms tend to be strong though imperfect predictors of intention. I will review an additional predictor of intention later in this chapter.

Finally, according to the TRA, both attitude and subjective norms each also have two predictors. Attitude is determined by both *behavioral beliefs* (i.e., the perceived consequences of engaging in the behavior) and *outcome evaluation* (i.e., the positive or negative assessment of each consequence).[1] Further, subjective norms are based on both *normative beliefs* (i.e., a person's perceptions of what each important individual or subgroup expects them to do) and *motivation to comply* (i.e., how motivated an individual is to comply with each important individual or subgroup). Given that an individual's beliefs—right or wrong—impact attitude and norms (and ultimately intention and behavior), they represent ripe targets for public health communication interventions.

### BACKGROUND VARIABLES

Finally, *background variables* represent some of the other factors that might affect an individual's beliefs. Examples include a wide variety of individual, social, or informational considerations, such as personality, demographics, and media exposure respectively. Ajzen and Fishbein (1980) note that such factors are not an integral part of the TRA; instead they influence intentions and behavior indirectly via their effect on other variables in the theory. For example, background variables might influence behavioral and normative beliefs, which, in turn, affect attitudes and subjective norms, and ultimately intentions and behavior.

Figure 9.2 contains a simplified model of the TRA. That is, for simplicity's sake this model omits (1) the feedback loop between behavior and beliefs, (2) the feedback loops between attitudes and behavioral beliefs and between subjective norms and normative beliefs, (3) an indication that attitudes and subjective norms may correlate with each other, and (4) an indication that the relative importance of attitudes and subjective norms may vary for each behavior or population being investigated (Ajzen & Fishbein, 2005). Also, for simplicity's sake, I will not focus on these missing features in the example that follows, but they are worth considering during the intervention planning process.

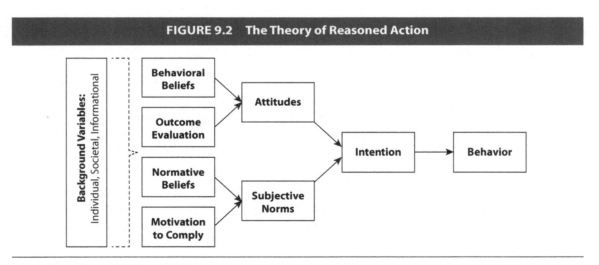

FIGURE 9.2   The Theory of Reasoned Action

Adapted from Ajzen and Fishbein (1980).

Next, I will provide a sample application of the TRA using sending text messages while driving as the referent behavior. As a reminder, this represents an instance of response extinguishing, which means we want to reduce or eliminate any positive beliefs that college students hold about texting while driving, decrease their intentions to text while driving, and *discourage* them from engaging in this unhealthy behavior. With this in mind, according to the TRA, the best determinant of *behavior* (i.e., whether or not I send text messages while driving in the next 7 days) is *behavioral intention* (i.e., whether or not I plan to send text messages while driving in the next 7 days).

Behavioral intention, in turn, is a joint function of a person's *attitude* toward performing the behavior (i.e., how positively or negatively I feel about sending text messages while driving in the next 7 days) and *subjective norms* (i.e., what I think relevant significant others, as a whole, think about my sending text messages while driving in the next 7 days). For example, relevant significant others might include your best friend, other friends, romantic partner, each parent, each sibling, other drivers, and so forth. Notably, for subjective norms we are interested in your overall perceptions of the group as a whole, not each individual or subgroup that makes up this group (your specific assessment of each individual or subgroup comes later). And again, it is worth noting that while attitudes and subjective norms are moderate to strong predictors of intentions, they are not perfect predictors of intention. For example, research indicates that most college students have relatively negative attitudes toward texting while driving and perceive that relevant significant others would disapprove of their texting while driving (Nemme & White, 2010; Prat et al., 2015). Nonetheless, some college students still intend to, and ultimately do, send text messages while driving.

Next, attitude is a joint function of *behavioral beliefs* (i.e., my assessment of the consequences of send text messages while driving in the next 7 days) and *outcome evaluation* (i.e., whether I evaluate each of these consequences as positive or negative). Example behavioral beliefs include saving time or relieving boredom—two outcomes that most people would evaluate positively; as well as loss of concentration, being dangerous to yourself and others, and the fact that it could be illegal in your state—examples of outcomes that most people would view negatively (Benson et al., 2015). Ultimately, when each belief is weighted (or multiplied) by the evaluation of the belief, and these scores are added together, they should predict an individual's overall attitude toward sending text messages while driving.

Finally, subjective norms are based on *normative beliefs* (i.e., _____ thinks I should send text messages while driving in the next 7 days) and *motivation to comply* (i.e., when it comes to sending text messages while driving in the next 7 days, I want to do what _____ thinks I should do). In both cases, each question would be asked multiple times and the blank would be filled in with one specific relevant individual (e.g., mother, father, best friend) or subgroup (e.g., family, friends, other drivers, etc.). Of course, sometimes the individuals you include in your normative component will disagree with each other. For instance, research indicates that students often view young people and some of their friends as approving of texting while driving, and family or relatives, police, the general population, and other friends as disapproving of texting while driving (Benson et al., 2015). The question then becomes, how much are we motivated to comply with each of these individuals? As was the case for attitude, each normative belief is weighted by your motivation to comply with each referent. When these scores are added together, they should predict your overall subjective norms toward texting while driving.

Finally, I wanted to make an explicit distinction between subjective norms and normative beliefs since it is easy to confuse the two given their close relationship to each other. Specifically, subjective norms are more global and deals with your assessment of people who are important to you as a whole, while normative beliefs are more specific and focus on your assessment of each individual or subgroup of individuals. Again, individuals might include your parents, romantic partner, best friend, boss, and example subgroups might include your family, friends, or coworkers, other drivers, or other students at your university. The TRA simply states that your global assessment (i.e., subjective norms) will be based on your individual assessments (i.e., normative beliefs and motivation to comply).

## THEORY OF PLANNED BEHAVIOR

As you can see from the simplified model presented in Figure 9.3, the theory of planned behavior (TPB) (Ajzen, 1985, 1991) shares many things in common with the TRA (i.e., only the shaded components in Figure 9.3 are unique to the TPB). There are three important differences between the TRA and the TPB. First, the TPB predicts that actual control moderates the intention-behavior relationship. However, since actual control is difficult to measure, the TPB uses perceived control (defined below) as a proxy for actual control

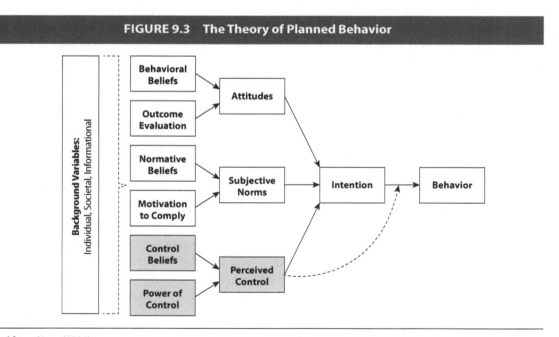

**FIGURE 9.3　The Theory of Planned Behavior**

Adapted from Ajzen (1991).
Note: Unshaded components are the theory of reasoned action, and shaded components are additions for the theory of planned behavior.

(thus, the reason for the dashed rather than solid line between perceived control and the intention-behavior relationship). Second, the TPB predicts that intentions are determined by three factors (instead of just two): attitude and subjective norms (defined above), plus perceived control (defined below). Third, the TPB posits that perceived control is influenced by both control beliefs and power of each control belief (also defined below).

## PERCEIVED CONTROL

*Perceived control* (a.k.a., *perceived behavioral control*) is the extent to which a person believes that they are capable or have control over performing a behavior (Fishbein & Ajzen, 2010). To provide a familiar point of reference, Fishbein and Ajzen also note that "self-efficacy and perceived behavioral control are virtually identical" (p. 161). Furthermore, as a reminder, the concept of self-efficacy is also an important part of the health belief model (from Chapter 6), social cognitive theory (from Chapter 7), and the extended parallel process model (from Chapter 8).

Also, as was the case for attitude and subjective norms, TPB posits that perceived control is influenced by two factors. The first factor is *control beliefs*, which refers to the perceived presence of factors that will influence one's ability to perform—or have control over—a behavior. The second factor focuses on the *power of each control belief*, or beliefs about how each control belief might facilitate or impede one's ability to perform—or have control over—a behavior. In sum, the TPB adds perceived control as a direct predictor of both behavior and intentions and adds two determinants for perceived control.

To continue with the texting while driving example that we started earlier, according to the TPB, whether or not I send text messages while driving in the next 7 days (i.e., behavior) is a function of my intention to send text messages while driving in the next 7 days. And, the intention-behavior relationship will be moderated by *perceived behavioral control*—which serves as a proxy for actual control in this theory (i.e., whether or not I send text messages while driving in the next 7 days is entirely up to me). Intention, in turn, is determined by my attitude, subjective norms, and perceived control regarding texting while driving in the next 7 days. Finally, perceived control is a joint function of both *control beliefs* (i.e., I will get an important text message while driving in the next 7 days) and *power of each control factor* (i.e., getting an important text would make it more likely that I will send text messages while driving in the next 7 days). Here is a list of some of the reasons (i.e., control beliefs) related to sending text messages while driving: stopped at traffic lights, urgent or emergency circumstances, needing to read or reply to an important message, traveling in fast-moving traffic, needing to concentrate on driving, presence of police while driving (Benson et al., 2015). The first three factors are the types of things that might encourage someone to send text messages while driving, while the last three factors are things that might discourage someone from sending text messages while driving. And, as was the case for attitude and subjective norms, each control belief is weighted by the power of that belief, and when these scores are added together, they should predict your overall perceived control regarding sending text messages while driving in the next 7 days.

## THE INTEGRATIVE MODEL OF BEHAVIORAL PREDICTION

The integrative model of behavioral prediction (hereafter the integrative model) (Fishbein, 2000, 2008; Fishbein & Ajzen, 2010; Institute of Medicine, 2002) represents the most recent iteration of the reasoned action approach. As you can see from the simplified model presented in Figure 9.4, while the TPB and the integrative model share many things in common, the integrative model extends the TPB in at least two important ways. First, the integrative model adds two explicit factors that influence actual control over a behavior: (1) knowledge and skills and (2) environmental constraints. Further, as was the case in the TPB, these variables moderate the intention-behavior relationship (that is, they influence the strength of the relationship between intention and behavior). Second, the integrative model subdivides attitude, perceived norm, and perceived control into two distinct, but related, subcomponents. In this section of the chapter, I will review these additions to the reasoned action approach.

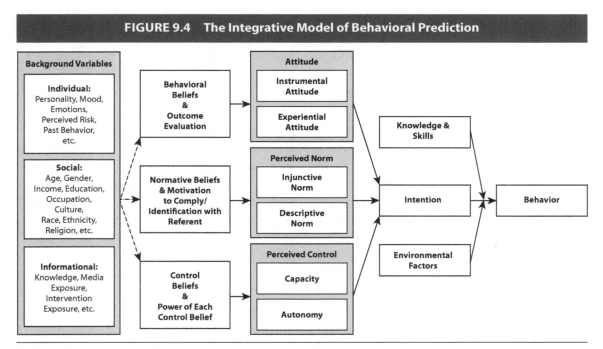

**FIGURE 9.4    The Integrative Model of Behavioral Prediction**

Adapted from Fishbein (2000), Fishbein and Ajzen (2010), Institute of Medicine (2002), and Montano and Kasprzyk (2015).

## FACTORS THAT MODERATE THE INTENTION-BEHAVIOR RELATIONSHIP

In Chapter 4, I noted that the ecological model views behavior as a product of individual and environmental factors. One of the ways the integrative model incorporates these factors is by adding knowledge and skills and environmental constraints as moderators of the intention-behavior relationship. *Knowledge and skills* are additional internal or individual factors that affect an individual's ability to perform the behavior. Examples include understanding how or having the expertise to perform the behavior. *Environmental factors* are external issues that may facilitate or limit behavior. Examples include the many relationships (e.g., social ties), community (e.g., the physical environment), and societal factors (e.g., public policy) that influence behavior.

In short, the integrative model posits intention will best predict behavior (1) when an individual has the necessary knowledge and skills necessary to engage in the behavior, and (2) when there are no significant environmental constraints preventing them from performing the behavior. Again, Ajzen and Fishbein (2010) make an important distinction between *perceived control* which predicts intentions and *actual control* which moderates the intention-behavior relationship. In short, people are most likely to engage in a behavior when they have both the motivation (e.g., intention) and ability (e.g., the knowledge, skills, and environment) to do so. Practically this means that different interventions will be required for people who are not motivated to engage in the recommended behavior versus people who are motivated but unable to do so.

## ADDITIONAL PREDICTORS OF INTENTION

In addition to explicitly noting that knowledge, skills, and environmental constraints moderate the intention-behavior relationship, the integrative model reconceptualizes the attitude, perceived norm, and perceived control components of the reasoned action approach. This section concludes by reviewing the differences between experiential and instrumental attitudes, injunctive and descriptive norms, and capacity and autonomy. This discussion will continue into the following section where I will discuss measurement issues regarding these variables.

### Instrumental Attitude vs. Experiential Attitude

Take a moment to consider how strongly you disagree or agree with each of the following statements: "Sending text messages while driving is *important*" versus "Sending text messages while driving is *interesting*." The distinction between "important" and "interesting" also represents the essential difference between instrumental and experiential attitudes. On the one hand, *instrumental attitude* represents one's assessment of the value of performing a behavior. For example, is texting while driving unimportant or important, unhealthy or unhealthy, bad or good, unwise or wise, and so forth. On the other hand, *experiential attitude* represents one's feelings about or emotional reactions to the idea of performing the behavior. For example, is texting while driving boring or interesting, dull or exciting, unpleasant or pleasant, aggravating or satisfying, and so forth.

### Injunctive Norms vs. Descriptive Norms

I already defined injunctive norms (sometimes called *subjective norms*; Fishbein & Ajzen, 2010) above. But as a reminder, *injunctive norms* refer to a person's perception of the behavior expected by important others as a whole. For example, a sample injunctive norms item might ask how strongly you disagree or agree that, "most people who are important to me approve of my sending text messages while driving in the next 7 days." *Descriptive norms*, on the other hand, refer to a person's perception about whether or not important others as a whole are performing a behavior. A sample descriptive norms item might ask how strongly you disagree or agree that, "most people who are important to me will send text messages while driving in the next 7 days." In short, injunctive norms focus on what others think you should do, while descriptive norms focus on what others are doing.

Most of the predictors of perceived norms will also look familiar. For example, perceived injunctive norms (a.k.a., subjective norms) are still based on both *injunctive normative beliefs* (i.e., a person's perceptions of what each important individual or subgroup expects them to do) and *motivation to comply* (i.e., how motivated an individual is to comply with each important individual or subgroup). However, in the integrative model, *(descriptive) normative beliefs* take on a second meaning, and a new variable called "identification with referent" has been added. In tandem, these two variables inform an individual's perceived descriptive norms. More specifically, *descriptive normative beliefs* represent one's view regarding whether or not each individual or subgroup is performing a behavior (i.e., _____ will send text messages while driving in the next 7 days), while *identification with referent* refers to one's desire to be like each individual or subgroup (i.e., when it comes to sending text messages while driving in the next 7 days, I want to be like _____). Also, as a reminder, injunctive and descriptive norms are more global and deal with your assessment of the group as a whole, while injunctive and descriptive normative beliefs, motivation to comply, and identification with referent are more specific and focus on your assessment of each individual in the group.

### Capacity vs. Autonomy

Finally, perceived control also taps into two separate but related constructs: capacity and autonomy. *Capacity* (sometimes called *self-efficacy*) focuses on one's ability to perform the recommended behavior. For example, does the individual view the behavior as easy to do, or feel confident in their ability to do it? *Autonomy*, on the other hand, focuses on the extent to which an individual believes performing a behavior is up to them. For example, that it does not depend on something outside of their control. Hence, if we want to discourage texting while driving among colleges students, one objective might be to reduce their perceived capacity regarding texting while driving (i.e., we do not want college students to be confident in their ability to do it), while another objective might be to increase perceived autonomy regarding texting and driving (i.e., we want college students to know that whether or not they text while driving is completely up to them rather than something outside of their control).

## OPERATIONAL DEFINITIONS

### GUIDELINES FOR CONSTRUCTING A REASONED ACTION SURVEY

Ajzen and Fishbein (1980) and Fishbein and Ajzen (2010) provide specific guidelines for constructing a reasoned action survey. These guidelines include two general steps: (1) defining the behavior and formulating items for direct measures, and (2) eliciting salient beliefs and formulating items to assess the strength and evaluation of each belief. This section will review these steps and provide sample survey items for each variable. As a reminder, all variables (with the possible exception of behavior) should be measured with a minimum of three items, and preferably four or more items. Formative evaluation should be used to pilot test potential items and to select reliable and valid items for the final survey.

### *Defining the Behavior*

The first step in developing a reasoned action questionnaire is to define the behavior of interest and develop direct measures for behavior, intention, attitude, perceived norms, and perceived control. Many decisions must be made during this process. For example, an intervention might focus on specific activity such as "sending text messages," or it might focus on general categories or sets of activities such as "texting" (which includes sending or reading text messages). Or, intervention planners must decide if they are interested in the intended audience performing the behavior at a particular time (e.g., "during rush hour"), during a general time frame (e.g., "in the next 7 days"), or "always." In short, when defining a behavior one must clearly identify the action, target, context, and time elements of the behavior.

To illustrate, consider the following behavior: *Send text messages while driving in the next 7 days*. In this example, (1) "Send" is the *action*, or the specific behavior we are interested in; (2) "text messages" is the *target*, or the focus of the behavior; (3) "while driving" is the *context*, in this case where we *do not* want the behavior to occur; and (4) "during the next 7 days" is the *time* frame, or when we want the intended audience to refrain from engaging in the behavior. Table 9.2 includes additional examples for action, target, context, and time for a variety of different topics

| TABLE 9.2 | Example Action, Target, Context, and Time of a Behavior | | |
|---|---|---|---|
| **Action** | **Target** | **Context** | **Time** |
| Attend | A Walking Event | On Campus | During the Fall Semester |
| Send | Text Messages | While Driving | In the Next 7 Days |
| Attend [1] | Aerobics Class | At Sun Devil Fitness Complex | Thursday Night |
| Order [2] | A Salad | When Eating Out | Always |
| Recycle [3] | Paper | At Work | During "Recycle-Mania" |

[1] Adapted from Ajzen & Fishbein (2010).
[2] From DiClemente et al. (2013).
[3] Adapted from Frymier & Nadler (2017).

## The Principle of Compatibility

Fishbein (2008) notes that "irrespective of how one chooses to define a behavior, once that behavior has been defined, a reasoned action approach suggests that a change in any one of these elements changes the behavior under consideration" (p. 836). Thus, the *principle of compatibility* states that all reasoned action variables must be measured at the same level of specificity or generality by focusing on the same action, target, context and time. For example, measures should not mix and match "attending a walking event" with "exercise," "on campus" with "anywhere," or "Saturday afternoon" with "during the fall semester." Altering one or more of these elements not only changes the behavior being explained but will weaken the relationships between the reasoned action variables. Table 9.3 contains compatible items for all reasoned action variables. In some cases, I have included more sample items than you may need to include in your survey, in which case you should select or modify those items that make the most sense for your topic or intended audience. Next, I will review how to elicit salient beliefs for other topics and intended audiences.

| TABLE 9.3 | Sample Operational Definitions for Reasoned Approach Constructs |
|---|---|
| **Construct** | **Operational Definition** |
| Behavior * | Did you send any text messages while driving in the past 7 days?  ❑ No    ❑ Yes |
|  | In the past 7 days, how often have you sent text messages while driving?  Never  ❑  ❑  ❑  ❑  ❑  ❑  ❑  Very Frequently |
|  | In the past 7 days, how many text messages did you send while driving?  ❑ 0  ❑ 1  ❑ 2  ❑ 3  ❑ 4  ❑ 5  ❑ 6  ❑ 7  ❑ 8 or more |
|  | In the past 7 days, how many text messages did you send while driving?  _____ (open-ended) |

| TABLE 9.3    Continued | |
|---|---|
| **Construct** | **Operational Definition** |

| | |
|---|---|
| Intention [1] | ▶ I intend to send text messages while driving in the next 7 days. |
| | ▶ I will send text messages while driving in the next 7 days. |
| | ▶ I plan to send text messages while driving in the next 7 days. |
| | ▶ I expect to send text messages while driving in the next 7 days. |
| | ▶ I will try to send text messages while driving in the next 7 days. |

Attitude

**Instrumental Attitude** [2]

For me, sending text messages while driving in the next 7 days would be:

| | | | | | | | | |
|---|---|---|---|---|---|---|---|---|
| Unimportant | ❑ | ❑ | ❑ | ❑ | ❑ | ❑ | ❑ | Important |
| Bad | ❑ | ❑ | ❑ | ❑ | ❑ | ❑ | ❑ | Good |
| Unwise | ❑ | ❑ | ❑ | ❑ | ❑ | ❑ | ❑ | Wise |
| Negative | ❑ | ❑ | ❑ | ❑ | ❑ | ❑ | ❑ | Positive |
| Dangerous | ❑ | ❑ | ❑ | ❑ | ❑ | ❑ | ❑ | Safe |
| Unhealthy | ❑ | ❑ | ❑ | ❑ | ❑ | ❑ | ❑ | Health |
| Harmful | ❑ | ❑ | ❑ | ❑ | ❑ | ❑ | ❑ | Beneficial |
| Useless | ❑ | ❑ | ❑ | ❑ | ❑ | ❑ | ❑ | Useful |
| Worthless | ❑ | ❑ | ❑ | ❑ | ❑ | ❑ | ❑ | Valuable |

**Experiential Attitude** [2]

For me, sending text messages while driving in the next 7 days would be:

| | | | | | | | | |
|---|---|---|---|---|---|---|---|---|
| Boring | ❑ | ❑ | ❑ | ❑ | ❑ | ❑ | ❑ | Interesting |
| Dull | ❑ | ❑ | ❑ | ❑ | ❑ | ❑ | ❑ | Exciting |
| Unpleasant | ❑ | ❑ | ❑ | ❑ | ❑ | ❑ | ❑ | Pleasant |
| Painful | ❑ | ❑ | ❑ | ❑ | ❑ | ❑ | ❑ | Enjoyable |
| Aggravating | ❑ | ❑ | ❑ | ❑ | ❑ | ❑ | ❑ | Satisfying |
| Stressful | ❑ | ❑ | ❑ | ❑ | ❑ | ❑ | ❑ | Stress free |

**Behavioral Beliefs** [3]

▶ My sending text messages while driving in the next 7 days will result in my losing concentration on driving.

▶ My sending text messages while driving in the next 7 days will result in my causing a crash or accident.

▶ My sending text messages while driving in the next 7 days will result in my injuring myself or someone else.

▶ My sending text messages while driving in the next 7 days will result in my receiving a fine or penalty points on my license.

▶ My sending text messages while driving in the next 7 days will stop me from getting bored.

▶ My sending text messages while driving in the next 7 days will save me time.

**Outcome Evaluation** [4]

▶ Losing my concentration while driving is:

▶ Causing a crash or accident is:

▶ Injuring myself or someone else is:

▶ Receiving a fine or penalty points on my license is:

▶ Not getting bored is:

▶ Saving time is:

| | TABLE 9.3    Continued |
|---|---|
| **Construct** | **Operational Definition** |
| Perceived Norm | **Injunctive Norm** [3]<br>▸ Most people who are important to me would approve of my sending text messages while driving in the next 7 days.<br>▸ Most people whose opinions I value want me to send text messages while driving in the next 7 days.<br>▸ Most people I respect and admire think I should send text messages while driving in the next 7 days. |
| | **Injunctive Normative Beliefs** [3]<br>▸ My spouse or partner would approve of my sending text messages while driving in the next 7 days.<br>▸ My close friends think that I should send text messages while driving in the next 7 days.<br>▸ My parents would approve of my sending text messages while driving in the next 7 days.<br>▸ Other drivers think that I should send text messages while driving in the next 7 days.<br>▸ Most _____ State University students would approve of my text messages while driving in the next 7 days. |
| | **Motivation to Comply With Injunctive Normative Beliefs** [1]<br>▸ When it comes to sending text messages while driving in the next 7 days, I want to do what my spouse or partner thinks I should do.<br>▸ When it comes to sending text messages while driving in the next 7 days, I want to do what my close friends think I should do.<br>▸ When it comes to sending text messages while driving in the next 7 days, I want to do what my parents think I should do.<br>▸ When it comes to sending text messages while driving in the next 7 days, I want to do what other drivers think I should do.<br>▸ When it comes to sending text messages while driving in the next 7 days, I want to do what other _____ State University students think I should do. |
| | **Descriptive Norm** [3,**]<br>▸ Most people who are important to me will send text messages while driving in the next 7 days.<br>▸ Most people whose opinions I value will send text messages while driving in the next 7 days.<br>▸ Most people I respect and admire will send text messages while driving in the next 7 days. |
| | **Descriptive Normative Beliefs** [3,**]<br>▸ My spouse or partner will send text messages while driving in the next 7 days.<br>▸ My close friends will send text messages while driving in the next 7 days.<br>▸ My parents will send text messages while driving in the next 7 days.<br>▸ Other drivers will send text messages while driving in the next 7 days.<br>▸ Most _____ State University students will send text messages while driving in the next 7 days. |

| TABLE 9.3    Continued | |
|---|---|
| **Construct** | **Operational Definition** |
| Perceived Norm (Continued) | **Identification With Referent**[5]<br>▸ When it comes to sending text messages while driving in the next 7 days, how much do you want to be like your spouse or partner?<br>▸ When it comes to sending text messages while driving in the next 7 days, how much do you want to be like your close friends?<br>▸ When it comes to sending text messages while driving in the next 7 days, how much do you want to be like your parents?<br>▸ When it comes to sending text messages while driving in the next 7 days, how much do you want to be like other drivers?<br>▸ When it comes to sending text messages while driving in the next 7 days, how much do you want to be like _____ State University students? |
| Perceived Control (a.k.a., Self-efficacy) | **Capacity**[1]<br>▸ I am confident I can send text messages while driving in the next 7 days.<br>▸ I believe I have the ability to send text messages while driving in the next 7 days.<br>▸ I am capable of sending text messages while driving in the next 7 days.<br>▸ It is easy for me to send text messages while driving in the next 7 days. |
| | **Autonomy**[1]<br>▸ I have complete control over whether or not I send text messages while driving in the next 7 days.<br>▸ Whether or not I send text messages while driving in the next 7 days is entirely up to me.<br>▸ I am in complete control of whether or not I send text messages while driving in the next 7 days.<br>▸ The decision to text while driving is beyond my control. (Reverse Code) |
| | **Control Beliefs**[3]<br>▸ I will get an important text message while driving in the next 7 days.<br>▸ I will be under pressure or running late while driving in the next 7 days.<br>▸ I will run into urgent circumstances while driving in the next 7 days.<br>▸ I will have to pay attention or concentrate on driving in the next 7 days.<br>▸ I will see or encounter police while driving in the next 7 days.<br>▸ I will be in fast-moving traffic in the next 7 days.<br>▸ I will be stopped or stuck in slow traffic in the next 7 days.<br>▸ I will be stopped at a traffic light in the next 7 days. |

| TABLE 9.3 Continued | |
|---|---|
| **Construct** | **Operational Definition** |
| Perceived Control (a.k.a., Self-efficacy) (Continued) | **Power of Each Control Belief** [6] <br> ► Having to reply to an important text message makes sending a text message while driving in the next 7 days: <br> ► Being under pressure or running late makes sending a text message while driving in the next 7 days: <br> ► Urgent circumstances make sending a text message while driving in the next 7 days: <br> ► Paying attention or concentrating on driving makes sending a text message while driving in the next 7 days: <br> ► Seeing or encountering police while driving makes sending a text message while driving in the next 7 days: <br> ► Being in fast-moving traffic makes sending a text message while driving in the next 7 days: <br> ► Being stopped or stuck in slow traffic makes sending a text message while driving in the next 7 days: <br> ► Being stopped at a traffic light makes sending a text message while driving in the next 7 days: |

Adapted from Ajzen and Fishbein (1980); Bazargan-Hejazi et al. (2017); Benson et al. (2015); Fishbein and Ajzen (2010); and Nemme and White (2010).

* The number and type of behavior items may vary for one-time or infrequent behaviors (e.g., in the past year, did you get a flu shot?) versus repeated or frequent behaviors (e.g., in the past 7 days, how many text messages did you send while driving?). A variety of potential behavior measures are provided here for your convenience.

** Fishbein and Ajzen (2010) recommend that descriptive norms and descriptive normative beliefs be measured in one of two ways depending on the nature of the problem under investigation. For example, you might ask (emphasis added): (1) "Most people who are important to me *will send* text messages while driving in the *next* 7 days," or (2) "Most people who are important to me *sent* text messages while driving in the *past* 7 days."

[1] Measured using seven-point scales ranging from "strongly disagree" to "strongly agree."
[2] Measured using seven-point scales using semantic differential items similar to those shown.
[3] Measured using a seven-point scale ranging from "very unlikely" to "very likely."
[4] Measured using a seven-point scale ranging from "very bad" to "very good."
[5] Measured using a seven-point scale ranging from "not at all" to "very much."
[6] Measured using a seven-point scale ranging from "more difficult" to "easier."

## Soliciting Salient Beliefs

According to the reasoned action approach, behavior is guided by *salient beliefs* (a.k.a., *accessible beliefs*), or the thoughts that come readily to mind when you think about a behavior. Information about the intended audience's salient behavioral, normative, and control beliefs is typically gathered during pre-production formative evaluation. Fishbein and Ajzen (2010) argue that at any given time only a small number of readily accessible beliefs inform a person's attitude, perceived norms, and perceived control about the behavior.

Understanding these salient beliefs serves at least two important functions when it comes to planning and evaluating a public health communicating intervention.

For intervention planning, salient beliefs supply vital information for developing objectives (i.e., the cognitive and behavioral changes you want your public health communication intervention to produce) and strategies (i.e., the specific communication activities you will use to accomplish your objectives). In other words, if we want to explain, predict, and ultimately influence behavior, we must also understand the behavioral, normative, and control beliefs that come to mind when the intended audience thinks about that behavior. Only then can we make informed decisions about how to best add or shape new beliefs, change or replace unsupportive beliefs, or strengthen or reinforce supportive beliefs.

For intervention evaluation, salient beliefs help identify what evidence must be collected and analyzed to inform, improve, or assess the effectiveness of an intervention. Understanding salient beliefs plays a key role during both formative and outcome evaluation. For example, one purpose of pre-production formative evaluation is to learn as much as possible about the topic and intended audience (including their salient beliefs), and one purpose of post-production formative research is to test one or more components of your public health communication intervention on a smaller scale to determine if your messages are having the anticipated effects on these beliefs. Also, for example, the aim of outcome evaluation is to test the cause-effect relationship between an intervention and changes in the intended audience on key variables of interest (including their salient beliefs).

With this in mind, eliciting and measuring salient beliefs is a three-step process that consists of (1) administering a pilot survey that includes a series of open-ended items designed to elicit readily accessible beliefs, (2) content analyzing responses to identify the salient beliefs held with the greatest frequency by the intended audience, and (3) using the most frequent salient beliefs to construct the final survey (Fishbein & Ajzen, 2010). For example, to elicit salient beliefs regarding texting while driving, Benson et al. (2015) asked about the advantages and disadvantages of sending text messages while driving, the individuals or groups that would approve or disapprove of sending text messages while driving, and the factors or circumstances that would make it easier or more difficult to send text messages while driving (see Table 9.4). They then content analyzed responses and used the most frequently occurring salient beliefs for each construct to create items for the final survey.

## MEASUREMENT RELIABILITY AND VALIDITY

As noted above, Fishbein and Ajzen (2010) provide detailed instructions for developing a reasoned action survey. They also provide considerable evidence regarding the reliability and validity of these measures. Given that the integrative model of behavioral prediction was advanced relatively recently, I was unfortunately unable to find an exemplar that

| TABLE 9.4    Open-Ended Items for Eliciting Salient Beliefs |
| --- |

**To Elicit Behavioral Beliefs:**
1.  Please list what you see as the advantages of sending text messages while driving in the next 7 days.
2.  Please list what you see as the disadvantages of sending text messages while driving in the next 7 days.

**To Elicit Injunctive Normative Beliefs:**
1.  Please list the individuals or groups that would approve of or support your sending text messages while driving in the next 7 days.
2.  Please list the individuals or groups that would disapprove of or be against your sending text messages while driving in the next 7 days.

**To Elicit Descriptive Normative Beliefs:**
1.  Please list the individuals or groups who are most likely to send text messages while driving in the next 7 days.
2.  Please list the individuals or groups who are least likely to send text messages while driving in the next 7 days.

**To Elicit Control Beliefs:**
1.  Please list any factors or circumstances that would make it easy or enable you to send text messages while driving in the next 7 days.
2.  Please list any factors or circumstances that would make it difficult to or prevent you from sending text messages while driving in the next 7 days.

Note: Respondents should be asked to list the thoughts that come immediately to mind, and five or six lines should be provided to answer each item.
Adapted from Benson et al. (2015) and Fishbein and Ajzen (2010).

included direct measures for the eight key variables in this theory (i.e., instrumental and experiential attitudes, injunctive and descriptive norms, capacity and autonomy, intention, and behavior). Instead, I will review two studies that were explicitly conducted to test the validity and reliability of scales used to measure key variables in the TPB (i.e., attitude, perceived norms, perceived control, and intention). These exemplars were specifically selected because they deal with health issues discussed elsewhere in this book (i.e., the HPV vaccine and physical activity). I will also review results from some texting while driving studies (though these studies were designed to test the theory, they also include some useful information regarding measurement validity and reliability). Finally, I will review some general recommendations regarding the measurement of instrumental and experiential aspects of attitudes, the injunctive and descriptive components of perceived norms, and capacity and autonomy elements of perceived control.

## Measurement Validity

Gonzalez et al. (2012) developed a 21-item TPB survey to measure attitudes (eight items), perceived norms (four items), perceived control (five items), and intentions (four items) regarding physical activity. Content validity was assessed by asking seven professionals with extensive knowledge in the TPB or survey construction to assess how adequately the items appeared to measure the intended TPB construct (and making minor changes to the survey based on their feedback). To assess construct validity, exploratory and confirmatory factor analysis were used to organize items into constructs (also known as variables or factors) and to ensure that the expected items measured the same underlying constructs. After deleting two problematic attitude items, results were consistent with the prediction that the attitude, perceived norm, perceived control, and intention items measured unique constructs. Finally, convergent validity was assessed comparing the final TPB scales to scales measuring internal and external motivations and general self-efficacy. As expected, internal motivations were positively related to attitude and negatively related to norms, external motivations were negatively related to attitude and positively related to norms, and self-efficacy was most strongly related to perceived control.

Similarly, Priest (2015) designed a 20-item survey to measure male undergraduate students' attitudes (seven items), perceived norms (four items), perceived control (six items), and intentions (three items) regarding obtaining the human papillomavirus (HPV) vaccine. Content validity was assessed by asking seven researchers and practitioners with expertise in measurement development, the HPV vaccine, the TPB, or college populations to assess how adequately the items appeared to measure the intended TPB construct (again, minor changes to the survey were made based on the obtained feedback). To test construct validity, confirmatory factor analysis was conducted to ensure that the expected items measured the same underlying constructs, or factors. Results were consistent with the prediction that the attitude, perceived norm, perceived control, and intention items measured unique constructs. Finally, predictive validity was assessed to see if the attitude, perceived norm, and perceived control predicted intention. The model had adequate fit and explained 58% of the variance in intention.

## Measurement Reliability

As you can see from the sample reliability estimates presented in Table 9.5, Cronbach's alphas ($\alpha$) for all reasoned action scales typically fall at or well above the .70 threshold. This remains true when instrumental and experiential attitudes, injunctive and descriptive norms, or capacity and autonomy are each measured separately (e.g., Elliot & Ainsworth, 2012; Elliot & Thomson, 2010), when they are combined into a single scale (e.g., Gonzalez et al., 2012; Priest, 2015), or when only one component of these variables is measured (e.g., Bazargan-Hejazi et al., 2017). It also holds true for a wide variety of

| TABLE 9.5 | Sample Alpha (α) Coefficients for Direct Measures of Reasoned Action Approach Constructs | | | | | | | |
| Study (Year) | Topic | Attitude [1] | | Norms [1] | | Control [1] | | Intention |
| | | Inst. | Exp. | Inj. | Desc. | Cap. | Auto. | |
| Elliott & Thomson (2010) | Driver's Speeding | .95 | .93 | .96 | .94 | .90 | .89 | .89 |
| Elliott & Ainsworth (2012) | Binge-Drinking | – | .91 | .89 | .84 | .84 | .73 | .93 |
| Gonzalez et al. (2012) | Physical Activity | .88 [2] | | .85 | – | .87 [3] | | .89 |
| Priest (2015) | HPV Vaccine | .92 [2] | | .96 | – | .92 [3] | | .97 |
| Bazargan-Hejazi et al. (2017) | Send Text Messages While Driving | .75 | – | .72 | – | – | | .90 |
| | Read Text Messages While Driving | .79 | – | .79 | – | – | | .89 |

[1] When available, effect sizes are reported separately from instrumental and experiential attitudes, injunctive and descriptive norms, and autonomy and capacity.
[2] General attitude scale containing both instrumental and experiential items.
[3] General control scale containing both capacity and autonomy items.
– = Variable not measured or measured using only two items so alpha not reported.

behaviors, ranging from fairly general behavior categories such as physical activity which may include many different types of activities (e.g., Gonzalez et al., 2012) to very specific behaviors such as sending *or* reading text messages while driving (e.g., Bazargan-Hejazi et al., 2017).

## CONCLUSION

I will conclude this section by noting that to date, few studies have fully tested the integrative model of behavioral prediction. For example, I was able to find only one meta-analysis that examined this model (McEachan et al., 2016), and only 14 of the 86 studies included in that meta-analysis included direct measures for all eight variables in the model. Based on existing evidence, Fishbein and Ajzen (2010) acknowledge that instrumental and experiential attitudes, injunctive and descriptive norms, and autonomy and capacity sometimes emerge as distinct concepts. However, sometimes the variables within each pair are highly correlated with each other, and scales containing both types of items will also have high internal consistency. This suggests that experiential and instrumental attitudes may be indicators of the same underlying concept (i.e., a person's overall attitude), that injunctive and descriptive norms may be indicators of a person's overall norm, and that autonomy and capacity may be indicators of a person's overall control. Fishbein and Ajzen (2010) suggest that in all instances both types of items should be included on a reasoned action survey, and that formative research should be conducted to determine which items and variables work best for a particular topic or target audience.

## THE REASONED ACTION APPROACH: ADVANCES THROUGH META-ANALYSIS

This section summarizes six meta-analyses conducted to assess how well the reasoned action approach predicts and explains intentions and behavior (Armitage & Conner, 2001; Downs & Hausenblas, 2005; McEachan et al., 2011; McEachan et al., 2016; Rich et al., 2015; Topa & Moriano, 2010). These meta-analyses were selected from the many available for three reasons. First, they included all the necessary information to complete Table 9.6, which summarizes some of the key points made in this section. The provided information includes number of subjects ($N$), number of studies ($k$), effect sizes (i.e., weighted mean correlations), and the proportion of variance explained for both intention and behavior. Second, these meta-analyses focus on a variety of different topics. For example, some focus on more specific topics like smoking and exercise, while others combine anywhere from a few related topics to many different topics. Third, together these meta-analyses test a variety of different moderators that provide important information for those interested in planning and evaluating public health communication interventions guided by the reasoned action approach. Thus, the following section will examine (1) the main effects between key reasoned action variables—i.e., attitude, perceived norms, perceived control, intention, and behavior, (2) how well the reasoned action approach predicts intention and behavior, and (3) factors that moderate the strength of the relationships between reasoned action variables.

### MAIN EFFECTS: RELATIONSHIPS BETWEEN REASONED ACTION VARIABLES

As a reminder, a main effect refers to the impact of one independent variable on a dependent variable, ignoring the effects of all other variables. For example, the reasoned action approach posits that attitude, perceived norms, and perceived control should each correlate with intention, and that intention should correlate with behavior. Also, as a reminder, when reporting effect sizes using correlations, or $r$, as is done in Table 9.6, values of .10, .30, and .50 are considered small, medium, and large effects respectively (Cohen, 1988). As you can see in Table 9.6, the main effects for the attitude-intention, control-intention, and intention-behavior correlations tended to be large in size, while the main effects for the norms-intention and control-behavior tended to be medium in size. The primary exception was the Topa and Moriano (2010) meta-analysis on smoking, where the relationships between all reasoned action variables were small to medium in size.

| Study & Topic | N (k)[1] | A-I[2] Inst. | A-I[2] Exp. | PN-I[2] Inj. | PN-I[2] Desc. | PC-I[2] Auto. | PC-I[2] Cap. | PC-B[2] Auto. | PC-B[2] Cap. | I-B | Variance Explained (Intention) | Variance Explained (Behavior) |
|---|---|---|---|---|---|---|---|---|---|---|---|---|
| Armitage & Conner (2001) —Various Behaviors | NA (185) | .49 | | .34 | | .43 | | .37 | | .47 | 39% | 27% |
| Downs & Hausenblas (2005)[3] —Exercise | 35,742 (111) | .47 | | .28 | | .41 | | .25 | | .45 | 34% | 21% |
| Topa & Moriano (2010)[4] —Smoking | 267,977 (27) | .16 | | .20 | | −.24 | | −.20 | | .30 | 13% | 12% |
| McEachan et al. (2011)[5] —Six Health Behaviors | 23,996 (237) | .57 | | .40 | | .54 | | .31 | | .43 | 44% | 19% |
| Rich et al. (2015) —Treatment Adherence | 4,771 (27) | .41 | | .32 | | .51 | | .24 | | .28 | 33% | 9% |
| McEachan et al. (2016)[5] —Various Health Behaviors | 21,245 (86) | .38 | .55 | .39 | .35 | .27 | .60 | .20 | .39 | .48 | 59% | 32% |

**TABLE 9.6    Effect Sizes (r) Between Reasoned Action Variables (and Percentage of Variance Explained)**

[1] N = total number of participants included in the meta-analysis. k = total number of studies (or total number of independent tests when available) included in the meta-analysis.

[2] A = attitude, PN = perceived norms, PC = perceived control, I = intention, and B = behavior. Also, when available, effect sizes are reported separately for instrumental and experiential attitudes, injunctive and descriptive norms, and autonomy and capacity.

[3] Originally reported effect sizes using Hedge's g, which were converted to r using Ellis' (2009) Effect Size Calculator.

[4] As perceived control went up, smoking intentions and behavior went down.

[5] McEachan et al. (2011) and McEachan et al. (2016) did not report a total N. Thus, the largest n provided among the bivariate relationships reported in these meta-analyses is reported here.

## PREDICTING INTENTION AND BEHAVIOR

While the preceding paragraph reviewed the relationships between each pair of variables in the reasoned action approach, it did not tell us about the combined effects of these variables on intention or behavior. Thus, the following paragraph reviews the impact of attitude, perceived norms, and perceived control on intention (and intention and perceived control on behavior) when considered together. The paragraphs after that consider the relative contribution of each of these variables on intention or behavior.

A glance at the last two columns in Table 9.6 reveals that when considered together attitude, perceived norms, and perceived control explain between 13% and 59% of the variance for intention. With the exception of smoking (where the percentage of variance explained translates to a small effect), these percentages of variance explained indicate that these three variables have medium to large effects on intention (Cohen, 1988). Further, when considered together intention and perceived control explain between 9% and 32% of the variance for behavior (which represent small to medium effects).

Thus, as the following summary will illustrate, when all reasoned action variables are considered together, attitude tends to be the strongest predictor of intention, followed by perceived control, and finally perceived norms. Further, while intention always emerges as the strongest predictor of behavior, the impact of perceived control on behavior can fluctuate. In short, while general patterns do exist, they vary for different topics and intended audiences, further highlighting the importunate of conducting formative evaluation to inform your public health communication intervention. The importance of this point will become more obvious as you read the next two paragraphs.

### *Predicting Intention*

When attitude, perceived norms, and perceived control are considered together, attitude emerged as a significant predictor of intention in all six meta-analyses included in Table 9.6; and was among the strongest predictors of intention in four of these meta-analyses (i.e., Armitage & Conner, 2001; Downs & Hausenblas, 2005; McEachan et al., 2011; McEachan et al., 2016). Norms was a significant predictor of intention in five of these meta-analyses (the exception being the Downs & Hausenblas, 2005 meta-analysis); and was among the weakest predictors of intention in four meta-analyses (Armitage & Conner, 2001; Downs & Hausenblas, 2005; McEachan et al., 2011; Rich et al., 2015). Finally, control (or the capacity dimension of control) was a significant predictor of intention in all six meta-analyses; though the autonomy aspect of control was not a significant predictor of intention in the McEachan et al. (2016) meta-analysis. Further, control emerged as among the strongest predictors of intention in three of the six meta-analyses (Armitage & Conner, 2001; McEachan et al., 2016; Rich et al., 2015), and among the second strongest predictors of intention in the remaining three meta-analyses (Downs & Hausenblas, 2005; McEachan et al., 2011; Topa & Moriano, 2010).

### Predicting Behavior

As noted above, intention typically proves to be a stronger predictor of behavior than perceived control. This is not surprising given perceived control both serves as a proxy for actual control, and that it also has an indirect effect on behavior via intention. To provide a few points of reference, control (or the capacity dimension of control) was a significant predictor of behavior in five of the six meta-analyses included in Table 9.6. Control did not emerge as a significant predictor of behavior in the Downs and Hausenblas (2005) meta-analyses, nor did the autonomy dimension of control emerge as a significant predictor of behavior in the McEachan et al. (2016) meta-analysis. Further, even when perceived control does contribute to the prediction of behavior, its impact tends to be small. For example, Armitage and Conner (2001) report that perceived control added a small but significant 2% to the prediction of behavior (also see Albarracin et al., 2001). In short, while perceived control does provide some advantages when it comes to predicting behavior, its primary contribution to the reasoned action approach is via intention.

## MODERATOR EFFECTS

To conclude this section, I will review several variables that have been shown to moderate the relationships between various reasoned action variables, with an emphasis on the intention-behavior relationship. As a reminder, a moderator variable changes the strength of the relationship between two variables. Therefore, this section focuses on factors that strengthen or weaken the relationships between the variables reviewed in the preceding section.

### The Principle of Compatibility

As a reminder, the reasoned action approach stresses the importance of measuring all variables at the same level of specificity or generality (i.e., all measures should include the same action, target, context, and time). Two of the reviewed meta-analyses assessed the principle of compatibility as a moderator variable. Downs and Hausenblas (2005) found a significantly larger intention-behavior relationship when scales corresponded versus when they did not ($rs$ =.60 vs. .41). Similarly, Topa and Moriano (2010) report that scale correspondence positively impacted the attitude-intention ($rs$ = .31 vs. .10), norm-intention ($rs$ = .23 vs. .19), control-intention ($rs$ = -.36 vs. -.20), and intention-behavior ($rs$ = .35 vs. .28) relationships. These results clearly illustrate the advantages of compatible measures. In spite of these advantages, compatible measures are not the norm in reasoned action research as only 15% of studies in the Downs and Hausenblas meta-analysis and only 33% of studies in the Topa and Moriano meta-analysis included compatible measures.

## Time Interval Between the Measures of Intention and Behavior

Four of the reviewed meta-analyses assessed how the time interval between the measurement of intention and the measurement of behavior influenced the strength of the relationship between these variables (Downs & Hausenblas, 2005; McEachan et al., 2011; McEachan et al., 2016; Topa & Moriano, 2010). The specific time intervals investigated in these meta-analyses varied greatly and included anything ranging from "one week or less" to "one year or more." Taken together, results from these meta-analyses consistently indicate that significantly larger intention-behavior associations are observed with *shorter* time frames of 4 weeks or less.

## Prospective Versus Retrospective Studies

Somewhat related to the time interval issue are issues regarding the prospective versus retrospective measurement of behavior. *Prospective studies* look forward and attempt to predict future behavior. For the reasoned action approach this typically involves measure attitudes, perceived norms, perceived control, and intention at one point in time, and measuring behavior at a second, later point in time. Per the principle of compatibility, the time frames for all measures should be the same, and overlap with the behavior measures (e.g., if the intention measure asks about "the next 30 days" at Time 1, the behavior measure should ask about "the past 30 days" 1 month later at Time 2). *Retrospective studies* look back and attempt to "postdict" past behavior after the fact. This typically involves collecting cross-sectional data by measuring all reasoned action variables at a single point in time. Under these circumstances you are measuring intention after the behavior already happened. The Topa and Moriano (2010) meta-analysis indicates that correlations between intention and future behavior are significantly lower than correlations between intention and *past* behavior ($rs = .33$ vs. $.59$). These results corroborate those of an earlier meta-analysis not reviewed in this chapter (Albarracin et al., 2001) which also reports that the intention-behavior relationship was significantly lower in prospective versus retrospective studies ($rs = .45$ vs. $.57$).

## Subjective Versus Objective Behavior Measures

*Subjective measures* of behavior involve asking participants to recall and report on their own actions. Common subjective measures include self-report surveys (i.e., "In the past 7 days, how many times did you hard break while driving?"), or daily diaries where participants log each time they engage in the behavior of interest over a certain time period. *Objective measures* of behavior involve directly observing or tracking a person's actions. For example, you might observe people in a driving simulator or install an in-vehicle monitoring system similar to those many car insurance companies have started to use to track instances of hard breaking. Also, for example, pedometers, cyclometers, or heart rate monitors are often used as objective measures for physical activity.

Three of the reviewed meta-analyses included type of behavior measure (i.e., subjective vs. objective) as a moderator variable (Armitage & Conner, 2001; McEachan et al., 2011; Rich et al., 2015). These meta-analyses reveal that about 80% of reasoned action studies use subjective measures of behavior. Both Armitage and Connor ($rs = .55$ vs. .44) and McEachan et al. ($rs = .50$ vs. .34) report that the intention-behavior relationship was significantly stronger when subjective versus objective measures of behavior were used. McEachan et al. also report that that control-behavior relationship was stronger when subjective versus objective measures of behavior were used ($rs = .36$ vs. .18). However, Rich et al. report that type of behavior measure did not moderate the intention-behavior relationship ($rs = .30$ vs. .28) or the control-behavior ($rs = .25$ vs. .22) relationship. Taken together, it seems reasonable to conclude that the way behavior is measured will moderate the intention-behavior relationship more often than not. That being said, it is encouraging that these effect sizes are typically in the medium to large range regardless of what type of behavior measure is used.

### Topic and Intended Audience

The only clear pattern regarding the effects of topic and intended audience on the relationships between reasoned action variables is that there is no clear pattern. For topic, McEachan et al. (2011) compared six types of health behavior (i.e., risk, detection, physical activity, dietary, safe sex, and abstinence) and report that while the strength intention-behavior relationship was lower for safe sex than for physical activity, no other differences were observed. Rich et al. (2015) compared four types of treatment adherence behaviors (i.e., medication, exercise, diet, and self-care) and report that topic did not moderate the strength of the intention-behavior relationship. Finally, McEachan et al. (2016) compared three types of health behaviors including protection (e.g., physical activity, using condoms, etc.), risk (e.g., alcohol, tobacco, or drug use, etc.), or other (e.g., detection behaviors, breastfeeding, etc.), and report that the strength of the intention-behavior relationship was lower for protective than for risk behaviors (unfortunately, there were not enough studies in the "other" category to compare). Similar inconsistencies arise regarding the impact of topic on the relationships between other reasoned action variables—that is, sometimes some of these relationships are moderated by topic (McEachan et al., 2011; McEachan et al., 2016), and other times they are not (Rich et al., 2015).

For intended audiences, consider the four meta-analyses that looked at age as a potential moderator of the intention-behavior relationship. Two of these meta-analyses report age did moderate intention-behavior relationship—i.e., it was stronger for adult versus children and adolescents (Downs & Hausenblas, 2005; Topa & Moriano, 2010), while the other two report that age did not influence the strength of the intention-behavior (McEachan et al., 2016; Rich et al., 2015). Similar inconsistencies arise regarding the impact of age on the relationships between other reasoned action variables—that is, sometimes these relationships are moderated by age and other times they are not (McEachan et al., 2016; Rich et al., 2015; Topa & Moriano, 2010). It is also worth noting that attempts to assess gender, ethnicity, or socioeconomic status as moderators have been largely unsuccessful, "because of the lack of studies segregating their sample by sex and the small number of studies reporting the subject ethnicity and socioeconomic status" (Downs & Hausenblas, 2005, p. 86—see also Rich et al., 2015).

In short, sometimes the relationships between reasoned action variables are moderated by topic or intended audience. And, sometimes they are not. So, the best way to understand the relationships between the reasoned action variables for a given topic and intended audience is to conduct pre-production and post-production formative evaluation research with this specific purpose in mind.

## PRACTICAL IMPLICATIONS

As I have tried to stress throughout this chapter, the reasoned action approach offers a considerable amount of practical advice for planning and evaluating public health communication interventions. Furthermore, interventions represent a key informational background variable that impact the beliefs that ultimately impact intentions and behavior (see Figure 9.4). In the final section of this chapter I review some key practical implications identified so far (to make sure they are not missed) and add a few new ones to the list.

### BEHAVIOR

The reasoned action approach highlights the importance of clearly defining the behavior(s) of interest in terms of action, target, context, and time. For example, in terms of action, you might focus on a general category of behavior such as physical activity, more specific groups of behavior such as aerobic, strength, flexibility, or balance training, or very specific behaviors such as biking or jogging, lifting weights, stretching, or using a BOSU or balance ball. Similar decisions must also be made for the target, context, and time elements of a behavior. Having a precise definition of the behavior(s) of interest will inform and often simplify many of the other decisions that must be made during other stages or phases of the public health communication process. For example, once a behavior has been clearly defined, the reasoned action approach stresses the importance of conducting formative research to better understand what and how various factors impact that behavior.

### INTENTION

The reasoned action approach makes a number of important distinctions regarding the reasons behind an individual's intentions to perform or not perform a behavior. For example, individuals who do not intend to perform a behavior may do so "because they have given little thought to it or because they have thought long and hard and decided not to" (Fishbein & Ajzen, 2010, p. 355). Further, individuals who intend to perform a behavior may not have acted upon their intentions "because they haven't had an appropriate opportunity, because they didn't act even though they had the opportunity, or because they attempted to act on their intention but failed" (Fishbein & Ajzen, 2010, p. 355). The reasoned action approach suggests that different types of interventions may be required to shape, change, or reinforce intentions.

## ATTITUDE, PERCEIVED NORMS, AND PERCEIVED CONTROL

Formative research can also shed light on the potential effectiveness of targeting the various predictors of intention. To illustrate, gathering mean scores for attitudes, perceived norms, and perceived control can help you identify which factors might be most or least susceptible to change. For example, if the intended audience perceives they have very little control over the behavior, you might spend the additional time and effort to understand why and to figure out how to best influence the perceived control components from the reasoned action approach. Conversely, if the intended audience already holds a very positive attitude (or norm), scarce resources can be directed elsewhere. Further, understanding the relative weight of each factor will help you determine which ones should have strongest and weakest impact on the behavior of interest. For example, if perceived norms prove to be an especially strong predictor of intention for a given topic and target audience, you can create strategies and objectives to influence the normative components from the reasoned action approach.

## BEHAVIORAL, NORMATIVE, AND CONTROL BELIEFS

On a related note, if we want to explain, predict, and ultimately influence behavior, understanding the salient behavioral, normative, and control beliefs that come to mind when the intended audience thinks about that behavior provides a good place to start. For example, information about beliefs will help you develop specific, measurable, achievable, relevant, and time-bound (SMART) objectives during the intervention planning process. It will also provide valuable clues for designing intervention strategies.

To illustrate, Fishbein and Ajzen (2010) suggest that public health communication interventions might attempt to change behavior in any or all of the following ways. First, an intervention might attempt to influence an existing behavioral, normative, or control belief. To return to the sending text messages while driving example (see Table 9.3), this might involve convincing the intended audience (1) that sending text messages while driving is more likely to lead to a crash or accident, (2) that their spouse or partner is less likely to approve of their sending text messages while driving, or (3) that they are more likely to have to pay attention or concentrate on driving than they currently believe. Second, an intervention might attempt to influence the current evaluation of a behavioral, normative, or control belief. This might involve convincing the intended audience (1) that getting into a crash or accident is more serious than they think, (2) to be less motivated to comply with a partner or spouse that approves of their sending text messages while driving—or vice versa, or (3) that sending text messages while driving makes it more difficult to pay attention or concentrate on driving than they currently believe. Third, an intervention can add new behavioral, normative, or control beliefs, and shape the evaluation of these added beliefs. For example, perhaps you notice when eliciting salient beliefs during formative evaluation that the intended audience fails to mention a particularly important fact uncovered during your other primary or secondary research. This gap can be addressed by one or more of your existing strategies or objectives, or perhaps serve as the basis for new ones. In short, because beliefs provide the basis for attitudes, perceived norms, and perceived control, an intervention must attempt to shape, change, or reinforce the beliefs that underlie the factors that are most likely to lead to behavior change.

## EVALUATION RESEARCH

Throughout this chapter I have highlighted how the reasoned action approach can inform formative evaluation efforts and facilitate the planning process. For example, it provides guidance for defining the behavior of interest, eliciting salient behavioral, normative, and control beliefs about the behavior, and using this information to develop strategies and objectives targeting these beliefs. But, as Fishbein and Ajzen (2010) note, the reasoned action approach also provides "a conceptual and methodological framework for evaluating the effectiveness of interventions" (p. 359).

As a reminder, even though outcome evaluation occurs during the latter stages of the Health Communication Program Cycle (Chapter 3) or PRECEDE-PROCEED Model (Chapter 4), the task actually begins much earlier. For example, by now you will know who the intended audience is and have already gained access to them. Your objectives will tell you what variables to measure, previous research will tell you how to measure them (see Table 9.3), and formative research will provide an opportunity to test and refine the messages, measures, and procedures for your topic and intended audience. Also, under the right circumstances (see Chapter 13), these measures will tell you whether or not the intervention was effective at meeting its goal and objectives. Either way, outcome evaluation results will provide important information that will allow us to improve (if effective) or redesign (if not) an intervention. For example, if an intervention did change behavior it may be worth asking if there is even more room for improvement in any or all of the reasoned action variables. Or, if the intervention did not change behavior, the reasoned action approach can provide important clues as to why (e.g., perhaps it did not change one or more of the beliefs or other factors inform behavior).

## CONCLUSION

The goal of this chapter was to provide an overview of the reasoned action approach. It began by reviewing how this approach evolved from the theory of reasoned action, to the theory of planned behavior, and ultimately the integrative model of behavioral prediction. It provided conceptual and operational definitions for all key terms, and presented meta-analytic results supporting the reasoned action approach's ability to predict and explain behavior (as well as several factors that might moderate its ability). Finally, it identified several practical implications for planning and evaluating public health communication interventions guided by the reasoned action approach. In short, the reasoned action approach provides important information regarding *why* people perform (or do not perform) a given behavior. It notes that influencing behavior begins by influencing beliefs, and provides a systematic way to identify the behavioral, normative, and control beliefs that guide behavior and therefore can be targeted by public health communication interventions.

## FOOTNOTE

[1] Note that the reasoned action approach uses the phrase "outcome evaluation" differently than it is used elsewhere in this book. As a reminder, during the later stages or phases of the intervention planning process, "outcome evaluation" refers to the assessment of the specific effects an intervention had on the intended audience (i.e., objective-based evaluation). For example, what effect did the intervention have on an intended audience's beliefs, attitudes, or behavior? However, the reasoned action approach uses the phrase "outcome evaluation" to refer to a specific variable in the theory (i.e., as a predictor of a person's attitude; or, how they feel about performing the behavior).

## REFERENCES

Ajzen, I. (1985). From intentions to actions: A theory of planned behavior. In J. Kuhl & J. Beckman (Eds.), *Action control: From cognition to behavior* (pp. 11–39). Springer-Verlag.

Ajzen, I. (1991). The theory of planned behavior. *Organizational Behavior and Human Decision Processes, 50*(2), 179–211. https://doi.org/10.1016/0749-5978(91)90020-T

Ajzen, I., & Fishbein, M. (1980). *Understanding attitudes and predicting social behavior*. Prentice-Hall.

Ajzen, I., & Fishbein, M. (2005). The influence of attitudes on behavior. In D. Albarracin, B. T. Johnson, & M. P. Zanna (Eds.), *The handbook of attitudes* (pp. 173–221). Lawrence Erlbaum Associates Publishers.

Albarracin, D., Johnson, B. T., Fishbein, M., & Muellerleile, P. A. (2001). Theories of reasoned action and planned behavior as models of condom use: A meta-analysis. *Psychological Bulletin, 127*(1), 142–161. https://doi.org/ 10.1037/0033-2909.127.1.142

Armitage, C. J., & Conner, M. (2001). Efficacy of the theory of planned behaviour: A meta-analytic review. *British Journal of Social Psychology, 40*(4), 471–499. https://doi.org/10.1348/014466601164939

Basacik, D., Reed, N., & Robbins, R. (2011). *Smartphone use while driving: A simulator study*. Transport Research Laboratory.

Bazargan-Hejazi, S., Teruya, S., Pan, D., Lin, J., Gordon, D., Krochalk, P. C., & Bazargan, M. (2017). The theory of planned behavior (TPB) and texting while driving behavior in college students. *Traffic Injury Prevention, 18*(1), 56–62. https://doi.org/10.1080/15389588.2016.1172703

Benson, T., McLaughlin, M., & Giles, M. (2015). Factors underlying texting while driving. *Transportation Research, 35*, 85–100. https://doi.org/10.1016/j.trf.2015.10.013

Caird, J. K., Johnston, K. A., Willness, C. R., Asbridge, M. A., & Steel, P. (2014). A meta-analysis of the effects of texting on driving. *Accident Analysis and Prevention, 71*, 311–318. https://doi.org/ 10.1016/j.aap.2014.06.005

Cohen, J. (1988). *Statistical power analysis for the behavioral sciences* (2nd ed.). Laurence Erlbaum Associates.

DiClemente, R. J., Salazar, L. F., & Crosby, R. A. (2013). *Health behavior theory for public health: Principles, foundations, and applications*. Jones & Bartlett Publishers.

Downs, D. S., & Hausenblas, H. A. (2005). The theories of reasoned action and planned behavior applied to exercise: A meta-analytic update. *Journal of Physical Activity and Health, 2*(1), 76–97. https://doi.org/10.1123/jpah.2.1.76

Elliott, M. A., & Ainsworth, K. (2012). Predicting university undergraduates' binge-drinking behavior: A comparative test of the one- and two-component theories of planned behavior. *Addictive Behaviors, 37*(1), 92–101. https://doi.org/ 10.1016/j.addbeh.2011.09.005

Elliott, M. A., & Thomson, J. A. (2010). The social cognitive determinants of offending drivers' speeding behaviour. *Accident Analysis & Prevention, 42*(6), 1595–1605. https://doi.org/10.1016/j.aap.2010.03.018

Ellis, P. D. (2009). *Effect size calculators*. https://www.polyu.edu.hk/mm/effectsizefaqs/calculator/calculator.html

Fishbein, M. (2000). The role of theory in HIV prevention. *AIDS care, 12*(3), 273–278. https://doi.org/10.1080/09540120050042918

Fishbein, M. (2008). A reasoned action approach to health promotion. *Medical Decision Making, 28*(6), 834–844. https://doi.org/10.1177/0272989X08326092

Fishbein, M., & Ajzen, I. (1975). *Belief, attitude, intention, and behavior: An introduction to the theory of reasoned action*. Addison-Wesley.

Fishbein, M., & Ajzen, I. (2010). *Predicting and changing behavior: The reasoned action approach*. Psychology Press.

Frymier, A. B., & Keeshan, M. (2017). *Persuasion: Integrating theory, research, and practice* (4th ed.). Kendall Hunt.

González, S. T., López, M. C. N., Marcos, Y. Q., & Rodríguez-Marín, J. (2012). Development and validation of the theory of planned behavior questionnaire in physical activity. *The Spanish Journal of Psychology, 15*(2), 801–816. https://doi.org/10.5209/rev_SJOP.2012.v15.n2.38892

Hill, L., Rybar, J., Styer, T., Fram, E., Merchant, G., & Eastman, A. (2015). Prevalence and attitudes about distracted driving in college students. *Traffic Injury Prevention, 16*(4), 362–367. https://doi.org/10.1080/15389588.2014.949340

Institute of Medicine. (2002). *Speaking of health: Assessing health communication strategies for diverse populations*. National Academies Press.

Lantz, G., & Loeb, S. (2013). An exploratory study of the psychological tendencies related to texting while driving. *International Journal of Sustainable Strategic Management, 4*(1), 39–49. https://doi.org/10.1504/IJSSM.2013.056384

McEachan, R. R. C., Conner, M., Taylor, N. J., & Lawton, R. J. (2011). Prospective prediction of health-related behaviours with the theory of planned behaviour: A meta-analysis. *Health Psychology Review, 5*(2), 97–144. https://doi.org/10.1080/17437199.2010.521684

McEachan, R., Taylor, N., Harrison, R., Lawton, R., Gardner, P., & Conner, M. (2016). Meta-analysis of the reasoned action approach (RAA) to understanding health behaviors. *Annals of Behavioral Medicine, 50*(4), 592–612. https://doi.org/10.1007/s12160-016-9798-4

Montano, D. E., & Kasprzyk, D. K. (2015). Theory of reasoned action, theory of planned behavior, and the integrated behavioral model. In K. Glanz, B. K. Rimer, & K. Viswanath (Eds.), *Health behavior: Theory, research, and practice* (5th ed., pp. 95–124). Jossey-Bass.

National Highway Traffic Safety Administration. (2015). Distracted driving 2013. *Traffic Safety Facts: Research Notes.* Author.

Nemme, H. E., & White, K. M. (2010). Texting while driving: Psychosocial influences on young people's texting intentions and behaviour. *Accident Analysis & Prevention, 42*(4), 1257–1265. https://doi.org/10.1016/j.aap.2010.01.019

Prat, F., Gras, M. E., Planes, M., Gonzalez-Iglesias, B., & Sullman, M. J. M. (2015). Psychological predictors of texting while driving among university students. *Transportation Research, 34,* 76–85. https://doi.org/10.1016/j.trf.2015.07.023

Priest, H. M. (2015). *Development and validation of a theory of planned behavior-based instrument to predict human papillomavirus vaccination intentions of college males at a southeastern university* [Unpublished doctoral dissertation]. The University of Alabama.

Rich, A., Brandes, K., Mullan, B., & Hagger, M. S. (2015). Theory of planned behavior and adherence in chronic illness: A meta-analysis. *Journal of Behavioral Medicine, 38*(4), 673–688. https://doi.org/10.1007/s10865-015-9644-3

Topa, G., & Moriano, J. A. (2010). Theory of planned behavior and smoking: Meta-analysis and SEM model. *Substance abuse and rehabilitation, 1,* 23–33. https://doi.org/10.2147/SAR.S15168

U.S. Department of Transportation. (n.d.). *Facts and statistics.* http://www.distraction.gov/stats-research-laws/facts-and-statistics.html

# The Transtheoretical Model

## Chapter Outline

## INTRODUCTION

The transtheoretical model (TTM) was originally proposed by Prochaska and DiClemente to explain an individual's readiness to change their behavior (DiClemente et al., 2013; Prochaska & DiClemente, 1983; Prochaska et al., 2015). The TTM is a stage-based model that views behavior change as a dynamic process that unfolds over time, rather than as a discrete, either-or, event. Its four key elements—(1) stages of change, (2) processes of change, (3) decisional balance, and (4) self-efficacy—"can be used to describe and influence the 'when' (Stage of Change), 'why' (Decisional Balance and Self Efficacy), and 'how' (Processes of Change) of changing a behavior" (Amoyal et al., 2013, p. 1281). The TTM posits that public health communication interventions that customize messages to individuals based on these four elements should be more effective than those that do not.

The TTM was first introduced 40 years ago, and it remains one of the most prominent stage-based models of behavior change to this day. However, it is not the only one. For example, the precaution adoption process model (PAPM) adopts a different approach that emphasizes mental states (i.e., unaware, unengaged, undecided, decided not to act, decided to act, and acting) rather than days or months until action (Weinstein et al., 2008). Nonetheless, the TTM remains the most widely used stage-based approach to intervention design and evaluation and is therefore the primary focus of this chapter.

With this in mind, I begin this chapter defining and discussing the relationships between stages of change, process of change, decisional balance, and self-efficacy. Next, I provide sample operational definitions for all TTM variables, and review information regarding the reliability and validity of these measures. Finally, I review results from six meta-analyses that either assess the effectiveness of TTM-based interventions or test the relationships between the stages of change and other key elements of the TTM. Before continuing, however, I will provide some background information regarding condom use as a means to prevent sexually transmitted disease (STD), which will serve as the running example for this chapter.

*Sexually transmitted diseases (STDs)* are infections "that are passed from one person to another through sexual activity including vaginal, oral, or anal, sex" (Planned Parenthood, 2020). According to Centers for Disease Control and Prevention (CDC) (2019), adolescents and young adults make up one-quarter of the sexually active population, but account for one-half of new STD diagnoses in the United States each year. The most common STDs in the U.S. include the human papillomavirus (HPV), chlamydia, and genital herpes, though gonorrhea and syphilis recently reached unprecedented highs (CDC, 2019). The CDC (2020) recommends a variety of safe sex practices to protect yourself or your partner(s) from STDs, including abstinence, mutual monogamy, or having fewer sex partners, getting vaccinated or tested, or using condoms correctly and consistently. Unfortunately, while condoms have been shown to be highly effective in reducing STD transmission (CDC, 2020), only 47% of college students who had vaginal intercourse and only 27% of college students who had anal intercourse in the past 30 days report using a condom "most of the time" or "always" (American College Health Association, 2019).

The TTM suggests that public health communication interventions designed to change college students' condom use behavior can use this information to develop stage-appropriate interventions that are more likely to be effective. In other words, it is important to develop a different set of strategies to influence individuals who have (1) never, (2) inconsistently, and (3) always used condoms. The TTM also suggests that instead of taking an all-or-nothing approach, it is better to view behavior change as taking place through a series of stages, with any forward momentum through these stages being an indicator of success. In short, the TTM suggest you "begin 'where people are' and move them one step (one stage) closer to lasting behavior change" (DiClemente et al., 2013, p. 106). The remainder of this chapter will take a closer look at the TTM in action.

## STAGES OF CHANGE

The TTM includes five main stages of change: precontemplation (not thinking about changing), contemplation (thinking about changing), preparation (planning for change), action (adopting the change), and maintenance (continuing the change). However, progression through the stages is not always linear, and individuals may move back and forth between the stages of change before maintenance is achieved (DiClemente et al., 2013; Prochaska et al., 2015). A key advantage of viewing behavior change as a dynamic process is that it allows intervention planners to set more realistic objectives. In other words, just because an intervention does not move people into the action stage does not mean it failed. Instead of taking an all-or-nothing approach, it is better to see behavior change as taking place through the stages (i.e., even if you do not move people to the action stage, moving people from precontemplation to contemplation, contemplation to preparation, etc., still has its advantages). In short, asking individuals to move one stage forward will be more effective in the long run (DiClemente et al., 2013), and movement between any two stages should be considered a success (Prochaska et al., 2015). Conceptual definitions for the stages of change are presented in Table 10.1, and each of the stages of change is discussed in more detail below.

Individuals in the *precontemplation stage* have no intention of changing their behavior anytime soon (e.g., not within the next six months). For example, consider the survey item presented in Table 10.2. It asks, "do you consistently use condoms every time you have sex?" Individuals who answer, "No, and I do NOT intend to start doing so in the next six months," would be placed into the precontemplation stage since they do not plan to engage in the recommended behavior in the foreseeable future. Individuals in this stage may be unaware (or deny) that a problem exists or lack the motivation or ability to do something about it.

| TABLE 10.1 | Conceptual Definitions for Transtheoretical Model Constructs |
|---|---|
| **Construct** | **Conceptual Definition** |
| Stages of Change | A person's readiness to act that evolves over time. |
| Precontemplation | Individuals who have no intention of engaging in the recommended behavior in near future (e.g., not within the next six months). |
| Contemplation | Individuals who intend to engage in the recommended behavior in the near future (e.g., within the next six months). |
| Preparation | Individuals who intend to change their behavior in the immediate future (e.g., within the next month), but have not yet done so. |
| Action | Individuals who have recently changed their behavior (e.g., within the past six months). |
| Maintenance | Individuals who have sustained their changed behavior over a significant period of time (e.g., six months or more). |
| Processes of Change | Essential cognitive and behavioral activities that help individuals move through the stages of change. |
| Consciousness Raising | Increasing awareness or getting a better understanding of the (un)healthy behavior |
| Emotional Arousal | Experiencing the positive or negative emotions associated with the (un)healthy behavior. |
| Environmental Reevaluation | Understanding how the (un)healthy behavior impacts one's physical and social environment. |
| Self-Reevaluation | Understanding how the (un)healthy behavior makes a person feel about themself. |
| Social Liberation | Noticing how the physical and social environments are changing in ways that support the healthy behavior. |
| Self-Liberation | Believing that one can change an unhealthy behavior and making a commitment to so. |
| Counterconditioning | Replacing unhealthy thoughts and behaviors with healthier ones. |
| Helping Relationships | Seeking or accepting assistance from others who support the healthy behavior change. |
| Reinforcement Management | Using rewards to help change an unhealthy behavior or maintain a healthy one. |
| Stimulus control | Controlling cues that trigger the (un)healthy behavior. |
| Decisional Balance | The process of comparing the pros and cons of engaging in the recommended behavior. |
| Pros | Any benefits or advantages that help or encourage a person to engage in a behavior. |
| Cons | Any barriers or disadvantages that hinder or discourage a person from engaging in a behavior. |
| Self-Efficacy | Beliefs about one's ability to perform the recommended behavior under various challenging circumstances. |
| Confidence | The primary component of self-efficacy (DiClemente et al., 2013); beliefs about one's ability to perform a behavior under various challenging circumstances. |
| Temptation | The converse of self-efficacy (Prochaska et al., 2015); the intensity of urges to engage in the unhealthy behavior in various challenging situations. |

**TABLE 10.2    Operational Definition for Stages of Change (Simple Staging Algorithm)**

Do you consistently use condoms **every time** you have sex?

a.    YES, I have been doing so for MORE than 6 months.
b.    YES, I have been doing so for LESS than 6 months.
c.    No, but I intend to start doing so in the next 30 days.
d.    No, but I intend to start doing so in the next 6 months.
e.    No, and I do NOT intend to start doing so in the next 6 months.

Note: Answer choice (a) = maintenance stage, (b) = action stage, (c) = preparation stage, (d) = contemplation stage, (e) = precontemplation stage.
Adapted from Grimley et al. (1993).

Individuals in the *contemplation stage* are aware that a problem exists and are considering the possibility of changing their behavior in the foreseeable future (e.g., within the next six months). To continue the previous example, individuals who answer, "No, but I intend to start doing so in the next 6 months," would be placed into the contemplation stage since they plan to engage in the recommended behavior at some point, but not immediately. In short, while individuals in this stage may know what they need to do, they are not yet ready to do it.

Individuals in the *preparation stage* intend to change their behavior in the near future (e.g., within the next month), but have not yet done so. To illustrate, individuals who selected "No, but I intend to start doing so in the next 30 days," would be placed into the preparation stage since they plan to change their behavior sometime soon. Individuals in the preparation stage are ready to engage in the recommended behavior and may have taken some steps to facilitate the process (e.g., purchasing condoms, carrying condoms, setting a start date, etc.).

Individuals in the *action stage* have recently changed their behavior (e.g., within the past six months). Thus, individuals who answered, "Yes, I have been doing so for LESS than 6 months," would be placed into the action stage since they implemented the change in the recent past and are likely still working hard to continue the change. In short, this stage is marked by putting the plan created during the preparation stage into motion.

Finally, individuals in the *maintenance stage* have sustained their changed behavior over a significant period of time (e.g., six months or more). Thus, individuals who answered, "Yes, I have been doing so for MORE than 6 months," would be placed into the maintenance stage of change. Those in the maintenance stage have successfully changed their behavior for a considerable length of time and are committed to continuing the behavior in the future.

## PROCESSES OF CHANGE

*Processes of change* are essential principles that help individuals move through the stages of change (DiClemente et al., 2013). The TTM incorporates 10 common processes of change (five experiential and five behavioral). *Experiential processes* (sometimes referred to as the "thinking" processes; Rosen, 2000) are techniques that influence a person's internal thoughts or feelings about a behavior (e.g., their beliefs and attitude about using condoms). *Behavioral processes* (sometimes referred to as the "doing" processes; Rosen, 2000) are observable steps people take to facilitate behavior change (e.g., purchasing condoms or making a public commitment to use condoms).

As a reminder, an underlying assumption of the TTM is that public health communication interventions will be more effective if they "do the right thing (processes) at the right time (stages)" (Prochaska et al., 2013, p. 13). More specifically, the TTM predicts that the experiential (or "thinking") processes will be most useful during the earlier stages of change (i.e., contemplation and preparation), while the behavioral (or "doing") processes will be most useful during the later stages of change (i.e., action and maintenance). The top portion of Figure 10.1 shows the proposed relationship between the stages and processes of change. With this in mind, next I provide definitions and examples for each of the 10 processes of change.

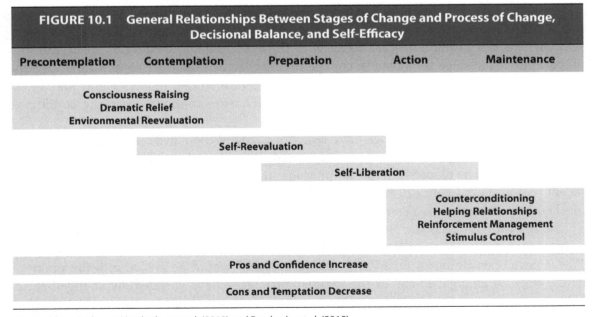

**FIGURE 10.1    General Relationships Between Stages of Change and Process of Change, Decisional Balance, and Self-Efficacy**

| Precontemplation | Contemplation | Preparation | Action | Maintenance |

Consciousness Raising
Dramatic Relief
Environmental Reevaluation

Self-Reevaluation

Self-Liberation

Counterconditioning
Helping Relationships
Reinforcement Management
Stimulus Control

Pros and Confidence Increase

Cons and Temptation Decrease

Adapted from Dishman, Vandenberg et al. (2010) and Prochaska et al. (2015).
Note: Social liberation is omitted due to its unclear relationship to the stages of change.

## EXPERIENTIAL PROCESSES OF CHANGE

*Consciousness raising* refers to any efforts taken to increase awareness or provide a better understanding of the (un)healthy behavior. The objectives here are to get people to look for, think about, or pay attention to information regarding the causes and consequences of a health problem in order to help prevent it.

*Emotional arousal* (sometimes called *dramatic relief*, e.g., Prochaska et al., 2015) concerns the impact of positive or negative emotions on the (un)healthy behavior. For example, someone might feel sad, mad, or scared when they learn that a friend contracted a sexually transmitted disease after engaging in unprotected sex. Emotional appeals designed to create and alleviate the emotion of fear represent a classic strategy for targeting this process of change (see Chapter 8 for more on fear appeals).

*Environmental reevaluation* focuses on how the (un)healthy behavior impacts one's physical and social environment. For example, some colleges students might be persuaded by how their safe-sex practices impact the college environment in general or their sexual partner(s) in particular (e.g., by reducing the spread of sexually transmitted diseases). Whereas others might be persuaded by the fact that using condoms sets a good example that might influence others' behavior.

*Self-reevaluation* focuses on how the (un)healthy behavior makes a person feel about themself. Here, it is important to show people how using condoms is good for them, consistent with their beliefs, and can make them feel more confident and empowered. Alternatively, you might need to convince them that having unprotected sex contradicts their views of themselves as healthy or responsible individuals or might raise concerns about their health and safety.

*Social liberation* entails noticing how the physical and social environments are changing in ways that support the healthy behavior. Social liberation is closely related to environmental factors from the ecological approach to health promotion (see Chapter 4). For example, you might point out that the university started providing easy access to free or reduced-price condoms at various locations around campus. It is also related to the discussion of injunctive norms or descriptive norms from the reasoned action approach (see Chapter 9). Thus, an intervention might point out that others support using condoms (injunctive norms) or are themselves using condoms (descriptive norms).

## BEHAVIORAL PROCESSES OF CHANGE

*Self-liberation* includes both the belief that one can change a behavior and making a commitment to do so. In other words, this process involves making a promise to change and taking steps to keep this promise. For example, some students might make a New Year's resolution to engage in safer sex in the future, and regularly remind themselves that they have the ability to use condoms even in the face of temptation.

*Counterconditioning* involves replacing unhealthy thoughts and behaviors with healthier ones. This might include getting someone to react more positively toward a healthy behavior or more negatively toward an unhealthy one. For example, if someone feels negatively about using condoms, one objective might be to get them to feel more positively about doing so. Alternatively, if someone is comfortable having unprotected sex, an objective might be to get them to feel uncomfortable doing so.

*Helping relationships* includes seeking or accepting assistance from others who support the healthy behavior change. For example, college students might identify existing relationships (or seek out new ones) with people who are engaging in the healthy behavior, that will listen when they need to talk, or who will encourage them when they are having a problem. This way they will have easy access to someone who cares about them, that they can be open with, and that they trust when they need help extinguishing an unhealthy behavior or encouraging a healthy one.

*Reinforcement management* (sometimes called *contingency management*, e.g., DiClemente et al., 2013) entails using rewards to help change an unhealthy behavior or maintain a healthy one. The key objectives here are to increase the rewards associated with a healthy behavior and decrease the rewards associated with an unhealthy behavior. To do this, you might encourage students to set themselves up for success with realistic goals, remind them that STD prevention is a major incentive for using condoms, or reward them in some way for engaging in the healthier behavior.

Finally, *stimulus control* involves controlling cues that trigger the (un)healthy behavior. For example, some students might add prompts to trigger the healthy behavior, such as carrying condoms when they go out. While others might choose to avoid people or situations that trigger the unhealthy behavior, such as partners that do not want to use condoms or being under the influence of alcohol or drugs.

## DECISIONAL BALANCE

*Decisional balance* is the process of comparing the pros and cons of engaging in the recommended behavior. The pros and cons constructs from the TTM are very similar to the benefits and barriers constructs from the health belief model (see Chapter 6). That is, *pros* are any benefits or advantages that encourage or facilitate a person's ability to engage in the recommended behavior, while *cons* are any barriers or disadvantages that discourage or hinder a person's ability to engage in the recommended behavior. For example, the key advantages of using condoms include protecting you and your partner against STDs and unintended pregnancy. Also, for example, some potential disadvantages of using condoms include causing sex to feel less natural, requiring your partner's cooperation, or signaling that you do not trust them.

Unlike the health belief model, however, the TTM makes some fairly specific predictions regarding the relationship between pros and cons and the stages of change. To illustrate, the *strong principle of progress* suggests that the pros of the recommended behavior must increase by about one standard deviation from precontemplation to action, while the *weak principle of progress* proposes that the cons of the recommended behavior must decrease by about one-half standard deviation from precontemplation to action (Hall & Rossi, 2008). Thus, a general objective for many public health communication interventions might be to maximize the pros and minimize the cons of engaging in the recommended behavior. More specifically, and practically speaking, this means that the pros of changing must increase about twice as much as the cons must decrease to move a person from the precontemplation to the action stages of change (Prochaska et al., 2015). The bottom portion of Figure 10.1 shows the proposed relationship between the stages and pros and cons.

## SELF-EFFICACY

In previous chapters I defined *self-efficacy* as a person's beliefs about their ability to perform the recommended behavior (such as using condoms). The TTM conceptualizes self-efficacy as having two related components. *Confidence*, the primary component of self-efficacy (DiClemente et al., 2013), concerns a person's beliefs about their ability to perform the healthy behavior in various challenging situations. For example, how sure are you that you would use a condom (1) when you are sexually aroused, (2) when you are under the influence of alcohol or drugs, (3) when your partner does not want to use a condom, or (4) when the risk seems low? *Temptation*, the converse of self-efficacy (Prochaska et al., 2015), concerns the intensity of urges to engage in the unhealthy behavior in various challenging situations. For example, how tempted would you be to have unprotected sex under each of the aforementioned circumstances?

Generally speaking, "confidence and temptation function inversely across the stages" (Redding & Rossi, 1999, p. 468). More specifically, confidence should increase, and temptation should decrease as individuals move from the precontemplation to the maintenance stage of change. The bottom portion of Figure 10.1 also shows the proposed relationship between the stages of change and confidence and temptation.

## OPERATIONAL DEFINITIONS

As a reminder, an operational definition defines a concept by specifying the procedures used to measure it. A considerable amount of research has focused on the measurement of TTM constructs. In this section (and when available), I will review a series of studies designed to assess the measurement validity and reliability of each construct in the realm of condom use. However, as you will see when you review the various tables in this section, these measures have also been adapted to a wide array of topics and intended audiences.

## STAGES OF CHANGE

The stages of change are typically operationalized using either a categorical staging algorithm or continuous stage of change scales. *Staging algorithms* place individuals into one of the five stages of change based on their responses to a small number of questions regarding their intentions and behavior. For example, Table 10.2 included a simple staging algorithm. This measure consists of a question followed by five response options representing the five main stages of change. Participants are asked to select the option that best describes their current behavioral status and are assigned to a single stage of change based on their response. Also, for example, consider the staging algorithm presented in Figure 10.2,

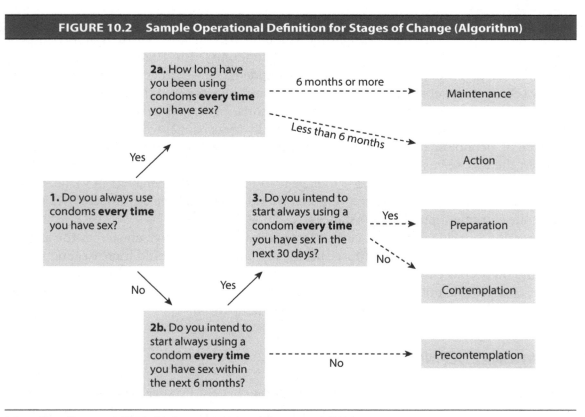

**FIGURE 10.2    Sample Operational Definition for Stages of Change (Algorithm)**

Adapted from Ferrer et al. (2009), Grimley et al. (1997), and Timpson et al. (2001).

Question 1 asks about condom use behavior. Based on the answer to this question, individuals are either asked another question about behavior (i.e., Question 2a) or a question or two about intentions (i.e., Question 2b and Question 3). Ultimately, participants are placed into a single stage of change based on their pattern of answers to these questions.

*Continuous stage of change scales* use multiple items to assess each stage of change. For example, consider McConnaughy and colleagues' (1983) Stages-of-Change Questionnaire (a.k.a., the University of Rhode Island Change Assessment (URICA) Survey), which has been adapted for dozens of topics and intended audiences worldwide. A version of this measure is presented in Table 10.3. While the general procedures for the various iterations of this survey are the same, the number of stages measured, the number of items used to measure them, and the manner in which the items are combined can vary. To illustrate, Rollnick et al. (1992) measured three stages of change using 12 items, while Boswell et al. (2012) measured four stages of change using 32 items; and both assigned participants to stages based on their highest score. Alternatively, these same items have been combined to provide a single, higher order, "readiness to change" score after recoding or subtracting the precontemplation items or scores (e.g., Budd & Rollnick, 1996). Next, I provide information about the measurement reliability and validity of both types of stage of change measures.

| TABLE 10.3 Sample Operational Definitions for Stages of Change (Continuous Measure) | |
| --- | --- |
| **Construct** | **Operational Definition** |
| Precontemplation | ▶ I don't think I engage in risky sex.<br>▶ It's a waste of time to think about my condom use habits.<br>▶ There is no need for me to think about changing my sexual behaviors to be safer. |
| Contemplation | ▶ Sometimes I think I should cut down on my unsafe sexual behavior.<br>▶ Sometimes I have sex without a condom when I would rather not.<br>▶ I am at a stage where I should think about changing my unsafe sexual behavior.<br>▶ My not using a condom during sex is problematic sometimes. |
| Action | ▶ I am trying to use a condom more than I used to.<br>▶ I have just recently begun using condoms more.<br>▶ Anyone can talk about wanting to do something about using condoms more often, but I'm actually trying to do something about it.<br>▶ I'm actually changing my unsafe sexual behaviors right now. |

Source: LaBrie et al. (2005). Stage of change continuous measure typically asks participants to respond using a five-point scale ranging from "strongly disagree" to "strongly agree."

## *Measurement Validity*

As a reminder, content validity focuses on the match between the conceptual definition of a variable and the operational definition used to measure it and is typically assessed via trained judges or expert opinions. For example, to establish the content validity of their stage-of-change algorithm for physical activity, Kosma and Ellis (2010) sought feedback from 14 individuals with expertise in exercise psychology, the TTM, and physical activity promotion. Also, for example, when developing the continuous Stage-of-Change Questionnaire, McConnaughy et al. (1983) had three graduate students in psychology who were familiar with the TTM match 165 potential items with the stages of change. Only items with 100% agreement among all three judges were included in subsequent analysis. Similar procedures are regularly employed when adapting this questionnaire to specific topics and intended audiences (e.g., Hammond et al., 2017; Kheawwan et al., 2016).

Also, as a reminder, confirmatory factor analysis (CFA) is used to test whether or not the expected items measure the same construct. CFA has been used in numerous studies to assess the underlying factor structure of the continuous stage-of-change questionnaire (e.g., Hammond et al., 2017; Kheawwan et al., 2016; McConnaughy et al., 1983; Rollnick et al., 1992). While CFA results are generally consistent with expectations, it is not uncommon for some stages to be omitted, eliminated, or collapsed (e.g., McConnaughy et al., 1983; Kheawwan et al., 2016)—or for some items to be added to or omitted from certain stages (e.g., Hammond et al., 2017; Kheawwan et al., 2016)—when adapting this measure to a specific topic or intended audience. And, again, some research suggests that at least some stages of change (e.g., precontemplation, contemplation, and action) can be combined to provide a single, higher-order, readiness to change score (e.g., Budd & Rollnick, 1996; LaBrie et al., 2005).

Finally, criterion-related validity involves comparing the performance of a measure to some external standard or criteria. Criterion-related validity for both types of stages of change measures has been assessed using a wide variety of criteria. Here are some of the more common ones:

1. The relationship between decisional balance and the stages of change—i.e., pros should increase, and cons should decrease across the stages of change (Kosma & Ellis, 2010; Reed et al., 1997).

2. The relationship between self-efficacy and the stages or change—i.e., self-efficacy should increase across the stages of change (Kosma & Ellis, 2010; Reed et al., 1997).

3.  Subscale-to-subscale correlations—i.e., the correlations between adjacent scales should be higher than the correlations between non-adjacent scales (Kheawwan et al., 2016; Rollnick et al., 1992).

4.  Correspondence between stages of change and reported intentions or behavior—i.e., individuals should demonstrate greater intentions or behavior in later stages of change (Ferrer et al., 2009; Kosma & Ellis, 2010; LaBrie et al., 2005; Reed et al., 1997; Rollnick et al., 1992).

5.  Correspondence between multiple stages of change measures—i.e., different measures should place individuals into the same stage of change (Epler et al., 2005; LaBrie et al., 2005; Reed et al., 1997).

The preponderance of evidence supports the validity of both types of measures. But there are some exceptions. For example, when assessing the fourth criteria, Ferrer et al. (2009) report that "18% of those classified in the maintenance SOC [stage of change] for condom use reported one or more sexual risk behaviors during the matched time period" (p. 13). Similarly, while LaBrie et al. (2005) observed small to medium correlations between their stage of change algorithms and both condom intentions and drinking intentions, the correlations between their continuous stage of change measures and intentions tended to be both small and insignificant. Further, when assessing the fifth criteria, and on average, various stage of change measures place individuals into the same stage between 61% and 69% of the time (Epler et al., 2005; Reed et al., 1997). That said, Reed et al. (1997) conclude that the best stage of change measures (1) select and clearly define a discrete behavior and (2) provide a clear description for each stage of change.

### *Measurement Reliability*

As a reminder, measurement reliability refers to the extent to which the items in a scale consistently measure whatever they measure. Also, as a reminder, Cronbach's alpha ($\alpha$) is commonly used to assess measurement reliability, with an alpha of .70 or higher indicating strong measurement reliability. Table 10.4 on the following page includes sample Cronbach's alphas from a variety of classic and contemporary studies assessing stage of change using a continuous measure. As you can see, these alphas typically (but not always) meet or exceed the .70 threshold. This holds true regardless of the number of stages measured, the language used to measure them, and the topic and intended audience being studied. It also holds true when the stages are measured separately or when they are combined into a single score.

| TABLE 10.4 | Sample Alpha (α) Coefficients for Stages of Change (Continuous Measure) | | | | | | |
|------------|-------|-----|-----|-----|-----|-----|----------|
| Study (Year) | Topic | PC | C | P | A | M | Combined |
| McConnaughy et al. (1983) | Psychotherapy | .88 | .88 | – | .89 | .88 | – |
| Rollnick et al. (1992) | Alcohol Use | .73 | .80 | – | .85 | – | – |
| Budd & Rollnick (1996) | Alcohol Use | – | – | – | – | – | .85 |
| LaBrie et al. (2005) [1] | Alcohol Use | – | – | – | – | – | .72 |
| | Condom Use | – | – | – | – | – | .85 |
| Lerdal et al. (2008) | Exercise | .72 | .72 | .88 | .77 | .92 | – |
| Kheawwan et al. (2016) | Exercise After Cardiac Surgery | .68 | .75 | .72 | .75 | – | – |
| Hammond et al. (2017) [2] | Career Development | .58 | .76 | .76 | .76 | .64 | .75 |

Abbreviations: PC = precontemplation, C = contemplation, P = preparation, A = Action, M = maintenance
[1] Contained separate readiness to change questionnaires for both alcohol use and condom use.
[2] Alpha coefficients for final 15-item measure.

## PROCESS OF CHANGE

Each process of change is typically measured using three or four items. Unfortunately, I was unable to find a published study that included full process of change measures for condom use. Thus, Table 10.5 on the following page includes sample survey items collected from three different studies. Nor was I able to find a published study that assessed the validity of the processes of change scales in the realm of condom use. Thus, below I will review a recent effort to develop and validate processes of change measures for another STD prevention behavior—getting vaccinated against the human papillomavirus (HPV).

### *Measurement Validity*

Fernandez et al. (2013) assessed the validity and reliability of scales applying the process of change to HPV vaccination. Content validity was evaluated via literature and expert reviews, plus 11 focus groups and five in-depth individual interviews with members of the intended audience. Confirmatory factor analysis results were consistent with expectations

**TABLE 10.5   Sample Operational Definitions for Process of Change**

| Construct | Operational Definition |
|---|---|
| Consciousness Raising | ▶ I remember what people have told me about how condoms can help keep me from getting sexually transmitted diseases.<br>▶ I think about how to protect myself from sexual transmitted diseases.<br>▶ I notice condom ads. |
| Emotional Arousal | ▶ I get scared when I hear about people getting sexually transmitted diseases because they did not use condoms.<br>▶ Warnings about the risks of sex without condoms scare me.<br>▶ Warnings about the dangers of having sex without a condom upset me. |
| Environmental Reevaluation | ▶ I stop to think that using a condom protects my partner, as well as myself.<br>▶ I remind myself that I can do my part to help stop the spread of diseases by using condoms.<br>▶ My getting a sexually transmitted disease would have a bad effect on the people around me. |
| Self-Reevaluation | ▶ I feel like a more responsible, caring person when I use condoms regularly.<br>▶ Being content with myself includes always using a condom during sex. |
| Social Liberation | ▶ I notice it is getting easier to find partners who do not mind using condoms.<br>▶ I notice that sex partners are more aware of the need for condom use.<br>▶ I notice that people are more concerned about using condoms. |
| Self-Liberation | ▶ I tell myself that I can choose to have sex with a condom.<br>▶ I make a commitment to avoid risky sexual situations. |
| Counterconditioning | ▶ When I want to have sex but do not have a condom, I find other sexual ways to satisfy myself and my partner.<br>▶ When I am tempted to have sex without condoms, I think about the unhealthy results.<br>▶ Not having sex is a good substitute for having sex without a condom. |
| Helping Relationships | ▶ I have someone I can count on when I'm having a hard time using condoms.<br>▶ I have someone who listens when I need to talk about condom use.<br>▶ People in my life try to make me feel good about using condoms. |
| Reinforcement Management | ▶ I reward myself when I use condoms during sex.<br>▶ I am rewarded by others when I use condoms. |
| Stimulus Control | ▶ I carry condoms when I go out.<br>▶ I check on my supply of condoms to make sure that I do not run out. |

Adapted from Grimley et al. (1997), Noar et al. (2001), and Timpson et al. (2001). Process of change items are typically measured using the following five-point scale: never, seldom, occasionally, frequently, repeatedly (or always).

that the instrument measured 10 related processes of change. Other research indicates these 10 processes can be combined into two, higher-order, factors (i.e., experiential and behavioral) comprised of five processes each (e.g., Prochaska et al., 1988); a technique Fernandez et al. (2013) sometimes employed when testing criterion-related validity (see below).

Finally, to assess the criterion-related validity of their processes of change measure, Fernandez et al. (2013) examined the relationship between each of the processes of change subscales and the stages of change. As expected, individuals in the precontemplation stage used all processes of change less than individuals in all other stages, and the steepest increase in the use of all processes occurred between the precontemplation and contemplation stages of change. Further, Fernandez et al. (2013) assessed the relationship between the five experiential processes of change (combined) and the five behavioral processes (combined) and pros, cons, and self-efficacy/confidence. Results were partially consistent with expectations in that pros and self-efficacy were positively correlated with both experiential and behavioral processes of change, but cons were unrelated to the processes of change.

### Measurement Reliability

Table 10.6 includes sample Cronbach's alphas for the 10 process of change. As you can see, these alphas typically (but not always) meet or exceed the .70 threshold. This holds true for a wide variety of topics and intended audiences.

| TABLE 10.6    Sample Alpha (α) Coefficients for Processes of Change | | | | | |
|---|---|---|---|---|---|
| Study (Year) | Topic | Consciousness Raising | Emotional Arousal | Environmental Reevaluation | Self-Reevaluation |
| Noar et al. (2001)[1] | Condom Use | .72 | .76 | .71 | – |
| de Oliveira et al. (2005) | Fruit & Vegetable Consumption | .83 | .91 | .82 | .81 |
| Dishman, Jackson, & Bray (2010)[2] | Physical Activity | .87 | .85 | .72 | .67 |
| Blaney et al. (2012) | Exercise | .84 | .63 | .73 | .87 |
| Amoyal et al. (2013) | Blood Donation | .79 | .83 | .88 | .91 |
| Fernandez et al. (2013) | HPV Vaccine | .77 | .86 | .92 | .87 |

[1] Self-reevaluation and self-liberation items were combined into a single scale with an alpha of .74.
[2] The self-liberation factor was deleted from the final measure.

## DECISIONAL BALANCE

Sample survey items for pros and cons are included in the top half of Table 10.7 on the following page. I previously discussed the measurement of pros and cons (a.k.a., perceived benefits and perceived barriers) in Chapter 6 (on the health belief model) and Chapter 7 (on social cognitive theory). Thus, here I simply review an early study designed to assess the validity and reliability of decisional balance scales in the context of safe sex.

### *Measurement Validity*

Grimley et al. (1993) assessed the validity and reliability of scales designed to measure the pros and cons of safe sex for (1) pregnancy prevention and (2) disease prevention. To assess content validity Grimley et al. (1993) had three trained judges, who were familiar with the TTM and had expertise in contraceptive use, review a set of potential items. Only items with 100% agreement were retained for subsequent analysis. Next, Grimley et al. (1993) used exploratory factor analysis to organize the items into constructs. Their results suggested that the presence of two factors reflecting the pros and cons of contraceptive use for both pregnancy and disease prevention. In a subsequent study, Grimley et al. (1996) used confirmatory factor analysis to corroborate this finding using shorter and slightly revised versions of these scales and reported that results were consistent with expectations. Finally,

| | | TABLE 10.6    Continued | | | |
|---|---|---|---|---|---|
| Social Liberation | Self-Liberation | Counter-Conditioning | Helping Relationships | Reinforcement Management | Stimulus Control |
| .52 | – | .70 | .65 | .60 | .79 |
| .83 | .74 | .73 | .77 | .80 | .83 |
| .54 | – | .77 | .79 | .76 | .66 |
| .62 | .77 | .77 | .91 | .84 | .91 |
| .81 | .82 | .86 | .74 | .82 | .80 |
| .83 | .84 | .85 | .76 | .86 | .82 |

Grimley et al. (1993) interpret the significant main effects for stage of change on both pros (which tended to increase across stages) and cons (which tended to decrease across stages) as evidence of criterion-related validity.

| TABLE 10.7 | Sample Operational Definitions for Decisional Balance and Self-Efficacy |
|---|---|
| **Construct** | **Operational Definition** |
| Decisional Balance [1] | **Pros**<br>Here are some *advantages* of using condoms. How important is each one to you in your decisions to use condoms or not?<br>▶ It protects against sexually transmitted diseases.<br>▶ I would feel more responsible.<br>▶ It protects both me and my partner.<br>▶ It protects against unintended pregnancy. |
| | **Cons**<br>Here are some *disadvantages* of using condoms. How important is each one to you in your decisions to use condoms or not?<br>▶ Sex would feel less natural.<br>▶ My partner would be upset.<br>▶ I would have to rely on my partner's cooperation.<br>▶ My partner would think I do not trust them. |
| Self-Efficacy [2] | **Confidence**<br>How *confident* are you that you would use condoms in these situations?<br>▶ When you are really turned on.<br>▶ When I am under the influence of alcohol or drugs.<br>▶ When your partner does not want to use a condom.<br>▶ When I am depressed.<br>▶ When the risk seems low. |
| | **Temptation**<br>How *tempted* would you be to have unprotected sex (i.e., without condoms) in these situations?<br>▶ When you are really turned on.<br>▶ When I am under the influence of alcohol or drugs.<br>▶ When your partner does not want to use a condom.<br>▶ When I am upset.<br>▶ When the risk seems low. |

[1] Adapted from Grimley et al. (1996) and Prat et al. (2016). All decisional balance items measured using five-point scales ranging from "not important" to "extreme important."
[2] Adapted from Grimley et al. (1996) and Redding & Rossi (1999). All self-efficacy items measured using five-point scales ranging from "not at all confident/tempted" to "very confident/tempted."

## *Measurement Reliability*

Table 10.8 includes sample Cronbach's alphas for both the pros and cons components of decisional balance. Alphas range from .75 to .91 for pros, and from .72 to .80 for cons; all at or well above the .70 threshold. This holds true for a wide variety of topics and intended audiences.

## SELF-EFFICACY

Sample survey items for confidence and temptation are included in the bottom half of Table 10.7. I also discussed the measurement of self-efficacy in Chapters 6 through 9. However, given that the TTM conceptualizes self-efficacy a bit differently (i.e., as situational confidence and temptation), here I will summarize a study designed to assess the validity and reliability of these constructs in the realm of safer sex.

| TABLE 10.8 | Sample Alpha (α) Coefficients for Decisional Balance and Self-Efficacy | | | | |
|---|---|---|---|---|---|
| | | **Decisional Balance** | | **Self-Efficacy** | |
| **Study (Year)** | **Topic** | **Pros** | **Cons** | **Confidence** | **Temptation** |
| Velicer et al. (1990) [1] | Smoking | – | – | .93<br>.95<br>.92 | .84<br>.92<br>.83 |
| Grimley et al. (1993) [2] | Condom Use | .83<br>.88 | .87<br>.90 | – | – |
| Grimley et al. (1996) [3] | Condom Use | .75<br>.78 | .78<br>.78 | .88<br>.89 | |
| Redding & Rossi (1999) [4] | Safe Sex | – | – | .94<br>.93 | .95<br>.96 |
| Noar et al. (2001) | Condom Use | .84 | .80 | .86 | .85 |
| Blaney et al. (2012) | Exercise | .85 | .74 | .80 | – |
| Weller et al. (2014) [5] | Diet | .84 | .72 | .85<br>.83<br>.84 | – |

[1] Alphas for the positive/social, negative/affective, and habit/addictive dimensions of confidence and temptation.
[2] Alphas for pregnancy prevention and disease prevention.
[3] Alphas for women at high risk nonprimary partners (study 1) and college students nonprimary partners (study 2).
[4] Alphas for full scale (study 1) and full scale (study 2).
[5] Alphas for school self-efficacy, home self-efficacy, and combined self-efficacy scales.

## *Measurement Validity*

Redding and Rossi (1999) assessed the validity and reliability of scales developed to measure confidence in safer sex and temptation to engage in unprotected sex among college students in five different situations (i.e., sexual arousal, substance use, partner pressure, negative affect, and perceived low risk). To ensure content validity, they adapted their items from established measures in other domains (e.g., smoking), and had three doctoral level judges with relevant expertise classify the items into one of the five aforementioned situations. Confirmatory factor analysis results were consistent with expectations that both the confidence in safer sex (sub)scales and temptation for unprotected sex (sub)scales could each be scored either as five separate subscales or a single higher-order scale. Finally, Redding and Rossi (1999) interpret the significant main effects for stages of change on both confidence (which tended to increase across stages) and temptation (which tended to decrease across stages) as evidence of criterion-related validity.

## *Measurement Reliability*

Table 10.8 also includes sample Cronbach's alphas for both the confidence and temptation components of self-efficacy. As you can see, alphas for the Redding and Rossi's (1999) full confidence scale were .94 in study one and .93 in study two, and alphas for the full temptation scales were .95 in study one and .96 in study two. Not included in the table are the alphas for each of the confidence and temptation subscales, which ranged from .78 to .94 for the five confidence subscales and .77 to .96 for the five temptation subscales. Alphas for confidence and temptation from various other studies are also included in Table 10.8. As you can see, alphas range from .81 to .95 for confidence, and from .83 to .96 for temptation; all well above the .70 threshold. And, once again, this holds true for a wide variety of topics and intended audiences.

## THE TRANSTHEORETICAL MODEL: ADVANCES THROUGH META-ANALYSIS

In this section I will synthesize the results from six meta-analyses. Table 10.9 on the following page presents the number of subjects (*N*), number of studies (*k*), topic(s) studied, and a narrative summary of the key findings from each meta-analysis. With this in mind, here I examine what these meta-analyses teach us about (1) the effectiveness of stage of change interventions, (2) the relationship between the stages of change and the processes of change, (3) the relationship between stages of change and decisional balance, and (4) the relationship between stages of change and self-efficacy.

| | **TABLE 10.9** | **Key Findings From Transtheoretical Model Meta-Analyses** | |
|---|---|---|---|
| **Study** | **N (k)**[1] | **Topic** | **Key Findings** |
| Rosen (1999) | NA (47) | Various | ▶ "Use of the processes of change varies by stage, but the sequencing of the processes of change is not the same across health problems" (p. 593). |
| Marshal & Biddle (2001) | 68,580 (71) | Physical Activity | ▶ Level of physical activity increased across all stages of change. <br> ▶ Self-efficacy increased across all stage of change. <br> ▶ Perceived pros increased by 1.3 standard deviation (SD) and perceived cons decreased by 1.2 SD from the precontemplation to the action stages of change. <br> ▶ Both experiential and behavioral processes of change increased during both the earlier and later stages of change. |
| Hall & Rossi (2008) | 47,757 (120) | Various | ▶ Perceived pros increased by 1.00 standard deviation (SD) and perceived cons decreased by .56 SD from the precontemplation to the action stages of change. <br> ▶ Results were moderated by behavior. For pros, exercise had a considerably large effect size than the other behavior categories. For cons, medical screening and smoking showed slightly larger effect sizes than condom use and diet. |
| Di Noia & Prochaska (2010) | 20,402 (28) | Diet (various) | ▶ Perceived pros increased by .82 standard deviation (SD) and perceived cons decreased by .55 SD from the precontemplation to the action stages of change. |
| Krebs et al. (2018) | 25,918 (76) | Psychotherapy Outcomes (Various) | ▶ Pretreatment stage of change is associated with psychotherapy outcomes (i.e., the further along the stages of change a person is at the start of treatment, the better the treatment outcome). |
| Romain et al. (2018) | 10,350 (33) | Physical Activity | ▶ TTM-based interventions significantly improved physical activity behavior. <br> ▶ This effect was not moderated by stage-match interventions, selected by stage interventions, decisional balance, temptation, or processes of change. <br> ▶ This effect was moderated by self-efficacy and number of theoretical constructs included. |

[1] N = total number of participants included in the meta-analysis. k = total number of studies or independent samples included in the meta-analysis.

## THE EFFECTIVENESS OF TRANSTHEORETICAL MODEL INTERVENTIONS

The two most recent meta-analyses focused on the effectiveness of TTM-based interventions. As a reminder, when reporting effect sizes using Cohen's $d$, values of .20, .50, .80 are considered small, medium, and large effects, respectively (Cohen, 1988). With this in mind, Romain et al. (2018) report that TTM-based interventions had a small to medium effect on physical activity behavior ($d$ = .33). Next, they assessed how the use of five TTM constructs (i.e., stage of change, processes of change, decisional balance, self-efficacy, and temptation) moderated this effect. Results indicated that physical activity interventions were equally effective whether or not they were stage matched, selected participants by stage, used the process of change, used decisional balance, or used temptation. Moderator analyses also revealed that TTM-based interventions that used self-efficacy ($d$ = .48) were more effective than those that did not ($d$ = .19), and that interventions that used at least three of the five TTM constructs to tailor their interventions ($d$ = .49) were more effective than those that used two or fewer TTM constructs to do so ($d$ = .16).

Krebs et al. (2018) assessed the relationship between pretreatment readiness to change and psychotherapy outcomes. They report that baseline stage of change has a medium effect ($d$ = .41) on the amount of progress clients make during treatment. In other words, "patients beginning in the preparation and action stages (or with greater readiness scores) fare better than those beginning in precontemplation or contemplation (or those with lower readiness to change scores)" (p. 1969). This effect was not moderated by patient characteristics (i.e., age, gender, or race/ethnicity), treatment features (e.g., treatment setting, number of treatment sessions, treatment orientation, or outcome measures), or diagnostic category (eating disorder, substance use, or mood disorders).

## THE RELATIONSHIP BETWEEN STAGES OF CHANGE AND PROCESS OF CHANGE

The TTM posits that different processes of change are emphasized during different stages of change. Specifically, it suggests that people rely on experiential processes in the early stages of change and behavioral processes in the later stages of change. Rosen's (2000) meta-analysis tested this prediction. To do so, he looked at the relationships between the stages of change and the process of change across five health problems (i.e., smoking cessation, exercise adoption, diet change, substance abuse, and psychotherapy). Results indicated that the use of both experiential processes ($d$ = .70) and behavioral processes ($d$ = .80) varied by stage. However, the pattern was not consistent across health problems. To illustrate, consider these two examples. For smoking cessation, results were consistent with expectations—experiential processes peaked during the contemplation and preparation stages and behavioral processes peaked during the action stage. However, for exercise adoption, results were inconsistent with expectations—both experiential and behavioral process peaked during the action and maintenance stages (i.e., they increased together rather than sequentially). Rosen (2000) concludes that for some behaviors, such as smoking, experiential process should be emphasized before deciding to quit, whereas behavioral process should be emphasized after deciding to quit. However, for other behaviors, such as exercise, it may be best to emphasize both experiential and behavioral process for people in all stages of change.

These results were corroborated by findings from a meta-analysis conducted by Marshall and Biddle (2001). Amongst other things, they looked at the relationship between the stages of change and process of change in the area of physical activity and exercise. Results indicate that all 10 processes increased between (at least) the precontemplation and contemplation stages of change and between the preparation and action stages of change.

## THE RELATIONSHIP BETWEEN STAGES OF CHANGE AND DECISIONAL BALANCE

The TTM predicts that the pros of changing a given behavior should increase—and the cons of changing that behavior should decrease—as individuals move from precontemplation to action. More specifically, the TTM predicts that pros should increase by about one standard deviation from precontemplation to action (a.k.a., the strong principle of progress) and cons should decrease by about one-half a standard deviation from precontemplation to action (a.k.a., the weak principle of progress). Three meta-analyses examined these relationships, and results were generally consistent with expectations.

To illustrate, consider that pros increased by 1.3, 1.0, and .82 standard deviations from the precontemplation to the action stages in the Marshall and Biddle (2001), Hall and Rossi (2008), and Di Noia and Prochaska (2010) meta-analyses, respectively. Also consider that cons decreased by 1.2, .56, and .55 standard deviations from the precontemplation to the action stages in these same meta-analyses. Finally, consider Hall and Rossi's (2008) finding that "the principal moderator of ES [effect size] for both pros and cons was behavior" (p. 269). For example, for exercise the increase in pros was larger than for the other six topics under investigation, while for organ donation and smoking, the decrease in cons was greater than the decrease for condom use and diet. In sum, increasing pros and decreasing cons helps move people through the stages of change, though the amount of change necessary will vary for some behaviors.

## THE RELATIONSHIP BETWEEN STAGES OF CHANGE AND SELF-EFFICACY

The TTM predicts that confidence will increase, and temptation will decrease, as individuals progress from the earlier to the later stages of change. One TTM-based meta-analysis examined the relationship between self-efficacy (confidence) and stage of change (Marshall & Biddle, 2001). This meta-analysis, which focused on physical activity and exercise, reports medium to large increases in self-efficacy between each stage of change ($ds$ = .36 to .72).

## CONCLUSION

In Chapter 1, I noted that influencing behavior "is seldom, if ever, a one-message proposition; instead, people are constantly *in the process of* being persuaded" (Miller, 1980, p. 19). The TTM captures the essence of this idea by identifying five stages of change and providing a list of essential principles that help individuals move through these stages. The goal of this chapter was to provide an overview of the TTM. Toward this end, I began by reviewing the four key elements of the TTM (i.e., stages of change, process of change, decisional balance, and self-efficacy), and discussing the relationships between them. Next, I provided sample operational definitions for all TTM constructs, and summarized results from six meta-analyses that tested the critical assumptions of the TTM. Finally, and throughout, I included practical advice for planning and evaluating public health communication interventions guided by the TTM (most notably that interventions should be tailored to each individual's stage of change).

## REFERENCES

American College Health Association. (2019). *American College Health Association national college health assessment II: Spring 2019 reference group data report.*

Amoyal, N. R., Robbins, M. L., Paiva, A. L., Burditt, C., Kessler, D., & Shaz, B. H. (2013). Measuring the processes of change for increasing blood donation in black adults. *Transfusion*, *53*(6), 1280–1290. https://doi.org/10.1111/j.1537-2995.2012.03864.x

Blaney, C. L., Robbins, M. L., Paiva, A. L., Redding, C. A., Rossi, J. S., Blissmer, B., Burditt, C. & Oatley, K. (2012). Validation of the measures of the transtheoretical model for exercise in an adult African-American sample. *American Journal of Health Promotion*, *26*(5), 317–326. https://doi.org/10.4278/ajhp.091214-QUAN-393

Boswell, J. F., Sauer-Zavala, S. E., Gallagher, M. W., Delgado, N. K., & Barlow, D. H. (2012). Readiness to change as a moderator of outcome in transdiagnostic treatment. *Psychotherapy Research*, *22*(5), 570–578. https://doi.org/10.1080/10503307.2012.688884

Budd, R. J., & Rollnick, S. (1996). The structure of the Readiness to Change Questionnaire: A test of Prochaska & DiClemente's transtheoretical model. *British Journal of Health Psychology*, *1*, 365–376. https://doi.org/10.1111/j.2044-8287.1996.tb00517.x

Centers for Disease Control and Prevention. (2019). *STDs in adolescents and young adults.* https://www.cdc.gov/std/stats18/adolescents.htm

Centers for Disease Control and Prevention. (2020). *How you can prevent sexually transmitted diseases.* https://www.cdc.gov/std/prevention/default.htm

Cohen, J. (1988). *Statistical power analysis for the behavioral sciences* (2nd ed.). Laurence Erlbaum Associates.

de Oliveira, M. D. C. F., Anderson, J., Auld, G., & Kendall, P. (2005). Validation of a tool to measure processes of change for fruit and vegetable consumption among male college students. *Journal of Nutrition Education and Behavior, 37*(1), 2–11. https://doi.org/10.1016/s1499-4046(06)60253-4

DiClemente, R. J., Redding, C. A., Crosby, R. A., & Salazar, L. F. (2013). Stage models for health promotion. In R. J. DiClemente, L. F. Salazar, & R. A. Crosby (Eds.), *Health behavior theory for public health: Principles, foundations, and applications* (pp. 105–129). Jones & Bartlett Learning.

Di Noia, J., & Prochaska, J. O. (2010). Dietary stages of change and decisional balance: A meta-analytic review. *American Journal of Health Behavior, 34*(5), 618–632. https://doi.org/10.5993/ajhb.34.5.11

Dishman, R. K., Jackson, A. S., & Bray, M. S. (2010). Validity of processes of change in physical activity among college students in the TIGER study. *Annals of Behavioral Medicine, 40*(2), 164–175. https://doi.org/10.1007/s12160-010-9208-2

Dishman, R. K., Vandenberg, R. J., Motl, R. W., & Nigg, C. R. (2010). Using constructs of the transtheoretical model to predict classes of change in regular physical activity: A multi-ethnic longitudinal cohort study. *Annals of Behavioral Medicine, 40*, 150–163. https://doi.org/10.1007/s12160-010-9196-2

Epler, A. J., Kivlahan, D. R., Bush, K. R., Dobie, D. J., & Bradley, K. A. (2005). A brief readiness to change drinking algorithm: Concurrent validity in female VA primary care patients. *Addictive Behaviors, 30*(2), 389–395. https://doi.org/10.1016/j.addbeh.2004.05.015

Fernandez, A. C., Paiva, A. L., Lipschitz, J. M., Larson, H. E., Amoyal, N. R., Blaney, C. L., Sillice, M. A., Redding, C. A., & Prochaska, J. O. (2013). Disease prevention without relapse: Processes of change for HPV vaccination. *Open Journal of Preventive Medicine, 3*(3), 301–309. https://doi.org/10.4236/ojpm.2013.33041

Ferrer, R. A., Amico, K. R., Bryan, A., Fisher, W. A., Cornman, D. H., Kiene, S. M., & Fisher, J. D. (2009). Accuracy of the stages of change algorithm: Sexual risk reported in the maintenance stage of change. *Prevention Science, 10*(1), 13–21. https://doi.org/10.1007/s11121-008-0108-7

Grimley, D. M., Prochaska, G. E., & Prochaska, J. O. (1997). Condom use adoption and continuation: A transtheoretical approach. *Health Education Research, 12*(1), 61–75. https://doi.org/10.1093/her/12.1.61

Grimley, D. M., Prochaska, G. E., Prochaska, J. O., Velicer, W. F., Galavotti, C., Cabral, R. J., & Lansky, A. (1996). Cross-validation of measures assessing decisional balance and self-efficacy for condom use. *American Journal of Health Behavior, 2*, 406–416.

Grimley, D. M., Riley, G. E., Bellis, J. M., & Prochaska, J. O. (1993). Assessing the stages of change and decision-making for contraceptive use for the prevention of pregnancy, sexually transmitted diseases, and acquired immunodeficiency syndrome. *Health Education Quarterly, 20*(4), 455–470. https://doi.org/10.1177/109019819302000407

Hall, K. L., & Rossi, J. S. (2008). Meta-analytic examination of the strong and weak principles across 48 health behaviors. *Preventive Medicine, 46*(3), 266–274. https://doi.org/10.1016/j.ypmed.2007.11.006

Hammond, M. S., Mihael, T., & Luke, C. (2017). Validating a measure of stages of change in career development. *International Journal for Educational and Vocational Guidance, 17*(1), 39–59. https://doi.org/10.1007/s10775-016-9339-5

Kheawwan, P., Chaiyawat, W., Aungsuroch, Y., & Wu, Y. W. B. (2016). Patient readiness to exercise after cardiac surgery: Development of the readiness to change exercise questionnaire. *Journal of Cardiovascular Nursing, 31*(2), 186–193. https://doi.org/10.1097/JCN.0000000000000221

Kosma, M., & Ellis, R. (2010). Establishing construct validity of a stages-of-change algorithm for physical activity. *American Journal of Health Promotion, 25*(2), e11–e20. https://doi.org/10.4278/ajhp.090914-QUAN-296

Krebs, P., Norcross, J. C., Nicholson, J. M., & Prochaska, J. O. (2018). Stages of change and psychotherapy outcomes: A review and meta-analysis. *Journal of Clinical Psychology, 74*(11), 1964–1979. https://doi.org/10.1002/jclp.22683

LaBrie, J. W., Quinlan, T., Schiffman, J. E., & Earleywine, M. E. (2005). Performance of alcohol and safer sex change rulers compared with readiness to change questionnaires. *Psychology of Addictive Behaviors, 19*(1), 112. https://doi.org/10.1037/0893-164X.19.1.112

Lerdal, A., Moe, B., Digre, E., Harding, T., Kristensen, F., Grov, E. K., Bakken, L. N., Eklund, M. L., Ruud, I., & Rossi, J. S. (2008). Stages of change–continuous measure (URICA-E2): Psychometrics of a Norwegian version. *Journal of Advanced Nursing, 65*(1), 193–202. https://doi.org/10.1111/j.1365-2648.2008.04842.x

Marshall, S. J., & Biddle, S. J. (2001). The transtheoretical model of behavior change: A meta-analysis of applications to physical activity and exercise. *Annals of Behavioral Medicine, 23*(4), 229–246. https://doi.org/10.1207/S15324796ABM2304_2

McConnaughy, E. A., Prochaska, J. O., & Velicer, W. F. (1983). Stages of change in psychotherapy: Measurement and sample profiles. *Psychotherapy: Theory, Research & Practice, 20*(3), 368–375. https://doi.org/10.1037/h0090198

Miller, G. R. (1980). On being persuaded: Some basic distinctions. In M. E. Roloff & G. R. Miller (Eds.), *Persuasion: New directions in theory and research* (pp. 11–28). SAGE.

Noar, S. M., Morokoff, P. J., & Redding, C. A. (2001). An examination of transtheoretical predictors of condom use in late-adolescent heterosexual men. *Journal of Applied Biobehavioral Research, 6*(1), 1–26. https://doi.org/10.1111/j.1751-9861.2001.tb00104.x

Planned Parenthood. (2020). *STDs.* https://www.plannedparenthood.org/learn/stds-hiv-safer-sex

Prat, F., Planes, M., Gras, M. E., & Sullman, M. J. (2016). Perceived pros and cons of condom use as predictors of its consistent use with a heterosexual romantic partner among young adults. *Current Psychology, 35,* 13–21. https://doi.org/10.1007/s12144-015-9357-3

Prochaska, J. O., & DiClemente, C. C. (1983). Stages and processes of self-change of smoking: Toward an integrative model of change. *Journal of Consulting and Clinical Psychology, 51*(3), 390–395. https://doi.org/10.1037/0022-006X.51.3.390

Prochaska, J. O., Norcross, J. C., & DiClemente, C. C. (2013). Applying the stages of change. *Psychotherapy in Australia, 19,* 10–15. https://doi.org/10.1093/MED:PSYCH/9780199845491.003.0034

Prochaska, J. O, Redding, C. A., & Evers, K. E. (2015). The transtheoretical model and stages of change. In K. Glanz, B. K. Rimer, K. Viswanath (Eds.), *Health behavior: Theory, research, and practice* (5th ed. pp. 74–94). Jossey-Bass.

Prochaska, J. O., Velicer, W. F., DiClemente, C. C., & Fava, J. (1988). Measuring processes of change: Applications to the cessation of smoking. *Journal of Consulting and Clinical Psychology, 56*(4), 520–528. https://doi.org/10.1037/0022-006X.56.4.520

Redding, C. A., & Rossi, J. S. (1999). Testing a model of situational self-efficacy for safer sex among college students: Stage of change and gender-based differences. *Psychology & Health, 14*(3), 467–486. https://doi.org/10.1080/08870449908407341

Reed, G. R., Velicer, W. F., Prochaska, J. O., Rossi, J. S., & Marcus, B. H. (1997). What makes a good staging algorithm: Examples from regular exercise. *American Journal of Health Promotion*, *12*(1), 57–66. https://doi.org/10.4278/0890-1171-12.1.57

Rollnick, S., Heather, N., Gold, R., & Hall, W. (1992). Development of a short 'readiness to change' questionnaire for use in brief, opportunistic interventions among excessive drinkers. *British Journal of Addiction*, *87*(5), 743–754. https://doi.org/10.1111/j.1360-0443.1992.tb02720.x

Romain, A. J., Bortolon, C., Gourlan, M., Carayol, M., Decker, E., Lareyre, O., Ninot, G., Bioché, J., & Bernard, P. (2018). Matched or nonmatched interventions based on the transtheoretical model to promote physical activity. A meta-analysis of randomized controlled trials. *Journal of Sport and Health Science*, *7*(1), 50–57. https://doi.org/10.1016/j.jshs.2016.10.007

Rosen, C. S. (2000). Is the sequencing of change processes by stage consistent across health problems? A meta-analysis. *Health Psychology*, *19*(6), 593–604.

Timpson, S. C., Pollak, K. I., Bowen, A. M., Williams, M. L., Ross, M. W., McCoy, C. B., & McCoy, H. V. (2001). Gender differences in the processes of change for condom use: Patterns across stages of change in crack cocaine users. *Health Education Research*, *16*(5), 541–553. https://doi.org/10.1093/her/16.5.541

Velicer, W. F., Diclemente, C. C., Rossi, J. S., & Prochaska, J. O. (1990). Relapse situations and self-efficacy: An integrative model. *Addictive Behaviors*, *15*(3), 271–283. https://doi.org/10.1016/0306-4603(90)90070-e

Weinstein, N. D., Sandman, P. M., & Blalock, S. J. (2008). The precaution adoption process model. In K. Glanz, B. K. Rimer, B. K., K. Viswanath (Eds.), *Health behavior and health education: Theory, research, and practice* (4th ed., pp. 123–147). Jossey-Bass.

Weller, K. E., Greene, G. W., Redding, C. A., Paiva, A. L., Lofgren, I., Nash, J. T., & Kobayashi, H. (2014). Development and validation of green eating behaviors, stage of change, decisional balance, and self-efficacy scales in college students. *Journal of Nutrition Education and Behavior*, *46*(5), 324–333. https://doi.org/10.1016/j.jneb.2014.01.002

# SECTION 4

# Evaluation
# Research Methods

## CHAPTER 11

# Individual and Focus Group Interviews

## Chapter Outline

I.  Introduction
    A.   Semi-Structured Interviews
    B.   Individual and Focus Group Interviews
        1.   Choosing Between Individual and Focus Group Interviews
        2.   Example Uses of Individual and Focus Group Interviews in Public Health Communication
            a.   To Assess Needs
            b.   To Help Design an Intervention
            c.   To Supplement or Help Explain Quantitative Findings
II.  Collecting Interview Data
    A.   Drafting Questions and the Interview Guide
        1.   Common Types of Interview Questions
            a.   Discussion-Starter Questions
            b.   Primary and Secondary Questions
            c.   Wrap-Up Questions
        2.   Interview Protocol Refinement Framework
            a.   Phase 1: Ensuring Interview Questions Align With Research Questions
            b.   Phase 2: Constructing an Inquiry-Based Conversation
            c.   Phase 3: Receiving Expert Feedback on the Interview Protocol
            d.   Phase 4: Pilot Testing the Interview Protocol With Members of the Intended Audience
    B.   Selecting and Recruiting Participants
    C.   Setting the Stage and Conducting the Interviews
        1.   Setting the Stage
        2.   Conducting the Interviews
III.  Capturing, Coding, and Analyzing Interview Data
    A.   Capturing, Organizing, and Securing the Data
    B.   Codes, Coding, and Codebooks

## INTRODUCTION

As noted in Chapter 2, when you *evaluate* something, you examine or assess its value or usefulness (Roberto, 2014). The evaluation of a health communication intervention may occur before (i.e., formative evaluation), during (i.e., process evaluation), or after (i.e., outcome evaluation) the intervention is designed and implemented. The focus of this chapter is *formative evaluation*, which is used to improve the design and implementation of your intervention and to give it the greatest chance of success. More specifically, this chapter looks at two qualitative data-collection methods commonly used during the early stages or phases of intervention development: individual and focus group interviews. While all of the methods discussed in this last section of the book can provide useful data during the planning process, semi-structured interviews play a particularly important and prominent role because of the rich information they can provide about a topic and intended audience.

With this in mind, this chapter will begin by providing some general guidelines for choosing between individual and focus group interviews, and discussing example uses of these methods in a public health communication context. Subsequent sections will focus on collecting, analyzing, and reporting the results of interview data. Before moving on to those topics, however, I will provide some background information on semi-structured interviews in general and define individual interviews and focus group interviews in particular.

### SEMI-STRUCTURED INTERVIEWS

Generally speaking, an *interview* involves one person (i.e., the interviewer) asking one or more other people [i.e., the respondent(s)] to provide verbal answers to a series of questions. Interviews can be divided into three general categories based on the amount of control the interview has over the interaction (see Figure 11.1).

FIGURE 11.1    Interview Continuum of Control

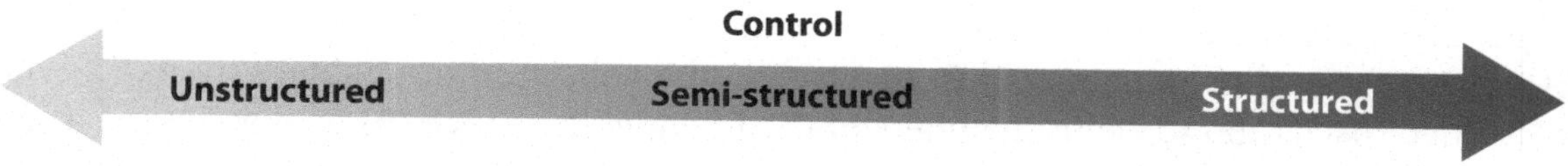

**Control**

Unstructured                    Semi-structured                    Structured

Adapted from Harrell and Bradley (2009).

At one end the continuum is the unstructured interview. As the name implies, an *unstructured interview* is a type of interview where specific questions are not prepared in advance. Instead, the interview guide may include a few general questions designed to engage the respondent in an open and spontaneous discussion. Then, subsequent questions may be asked based on responses to these general questions. In short, unstructured interviews include few guidelines or restrictions, and therefore offer little control over the interview in general or respondents' answers in particular. Gill et al. (2008) note that unstructured interviews are time-consuming, difficult to conduct, and difficult to participate in. Thus, they argue that unstructured interviews are most useful in situations where you want in-depth information about a topic where virtually nothing is known.

At the other end of the continuum is the structured interview. *Structured interviews* involve asking participants to respond to a predetermined and standardized set of items and response categories. As you will see, this is the same definition used to describe survey research in Chapter 12. That is because structured interviews "most closely approximate a survey being read aloud, without deviation from the script" (Harrell & Bradley, 2009, p. 28). Survey research (and by extension structured interviews) will be discussed in detail in the next chapter of this book.

Semi-structured interviews share some things in common with both unstructured and structured interviews, and therefore fall somewhere between those techniques on the continuum of control. That is, a *semi-structured interview* involves a predetermined set of key questions on a topic, but also allows the interviewer to probe for additional information and the respondents to answer in their own words. In this format, the key questions serve as a checklist to make sure the same general topics are covered with all respondents. But the interviewer may reword or reorder the questions to allow the discussion to flow more naturally, and both the interviewer and respondent are free to expand upon or clarify responses in more detail. This chapter focuses on semi-structured interviews, which can be conducted with one respondent at a time or with a small group of respondents (hereafter referred to as individual interviews and focus group interviews respectively).

## INDIVIDUAL AND FOCUS GROUP INTERVIEWS

Individual and focus group interviews share much in common (Adams & Cox, 2008; Gill et al., 2008; Harrell & Bradley, 2009; Lederman, 2014; Levitt, 2020; Morgan, 2019; Tong et al., 2007). To illustrate, they both involve (1) the collection of qualitative data (2) via a planned discussion (3) with members of the intended audience (4) who are asked a set of open-ended questions (5) in a permissive and non-threatening environment (6) that allows emerging topics to be discussed in more detail. In short, these six characteristics represent essential components of any good working definition for any semi-structured interviewing techniques.

The key differences between individual and focus group interviews concern the role and responsibilities of the person collecting the data and the number of participants involved. To illustrate, an *individual interview* is a one-on-one conversation where an interviewer asks questions to one respondent at a time. And, a *focus group interview* is a small group discussion lead by a moderator who asks questions, directs conversation, and encourages participation while multiple respondents interact. Given the aforementioned similarities and differences between individual and focus group interviews, you might wonder when to select one technique over the other. The following section reviews some of the key factors to consider when deciding which semi-structured interviewing technique is best for your particular situation.

### Choosing Between Individual and Focus Group Interviews

The available evidence comparing individual or focus group interviews is mixed at best. To illustrate, Guest et al. (2017) present results from 16 studies that compared individual interviews and focus groups along several important dimensions. The only consistent finding was that individual interviews and focus groups tend to lead to the same general conclusions. Further, results were evenly split regarding whether individual interviews or focus groups were more time-consuming. Otherwise, results tended to favor individual interviews over focus groups in terms of (1) number of ideas generated, (2) elaboration on ideas, (3) sensitivity of topics raised, and (4) cost effectiveness. However, in every case there were exceptions to these general patterns. That is, one or two studies always reported that focus groups performed the same as or better than individual interviews on each of these four outcomes.

Based on these findings it seems safe to conclude that you can select an interview method that best fits your practical circumstances. Your answers to the following questions will go a long way toward helping you decide whether individual or focus group interviews are most appropriate for a given situation (Adams, 2015; Krueger & Casey, 2015; Morgan, 2019; Stewart & Shamdasani, 2015).

First, what is the research objective? Individual interviews are typically a better option when you want to gain an in-depth understanding of each participant's responses or thought processes. During an individual interview, the interviewee has the undivided attention of the interviewer. This means each participant will typically have more time to speak, which means their answers can be explored in more detail and without group influence. Focus groups are best when you want to understand and explore the level of agreement or disagreement on a topic. Toward this end, a focus group moderator will typically encourage participants to express and discuss different positions for each key issue. And, this interaction can generate useful data regarding the various points of view on a topic.

Second, will you be discussing highly sensitive or personal topics? Individual interviews are particularly appropriate for discussing highly sensitive topics. For example, if you believe participants might be uncomfortable sharing their honest opinions about an issue in a group setting, or if you want to take extra steps to protect confidentiality, individual interviews will be the way to go. Alternatively, when asking about impersonal topics that participants will be comfortable discussing in a group setting, focus groups can work as well or better than individual interviews.

Third, how many different types of people do you want to interview? As noted in Chapter 3, *audience segmentation* involves dividing a population into relatively similar subgroups in strategically meaningful ways (i.e., based on geographic, demographic, psychographic, or behavioral characteristics). Individual interviews will typically be the most viable option when you need to gather information from many different segments, or when available participants are heterogenous and do not have much in common. Under these circumstances, it may not be possible to create just one or a few sets of questions that will be applicable or relevant to all participants. Alternatively, focus groups work best when you have identified fewer segments, or when potential participants are homogenous and have something relevant in common.

Finally, are there any other logistical restrictions or concerns that favor one method over another? As noted at the outset of this section, individual and focus groups may be more or less time-consuming or cost-effective depending on a variety of logistical considerations (Guest et al., 2017). On the one hand, individual interviews tend to be easier to organize when participants are geographically dispersed or when you are worried about getting enough participants to show up at the same place or at the same time. So, if it easier for an interviewer to travel to several respondents than the other way around, individual interviews may be the best choice. Focus groups, on the other hand, may be easier to coordinate when potential respondents are from the same general area or location (i.e., same town, workplace, school, community organization, etc.). So, if you are confident you can get 4–10 participants together at the same place and at the same time, focus groups will be a viable option.

For example, the first public health communication intervention I ever led was to develop a variety of gun-safety messages and materials for Michigan Department of Community Health (Meyer et al., 2003; Roberto et al., 2000; Roberto et al., 2002; Roberto et al., 1998). Early in the process we decided it was important to conduct formative evaluation with gun owners, gun store owners, and law enforcement officers. As it turned out, it was relatively easy to get enough gun owners together at the same time and same place to conduct focus groups with these individuals (I will say more on our recruitment strategy later in this chapter). However, we were unable to replicate this process for gun store owners or law enforcement officers who were scattered across the state, and thus ended up doing individual interviews with these participants.

In sum, individual interviews work best when you want an in-depth understanding of each participant's thought processes, will be covering highly sensitive topics, and when you must collect data from different types of participants at different times and places. Focus groups work best when trying to understand various points of view on a topic through interaction, will be discussing less personal topics, and when you are confident you can get enough homogenous participants together at the same place and time. But remember, individual and focus group interviews tend to yield similar conclusions (Guest et al., 2017), so you can confidently select the technique that best meets the needs of your intervention and intended audience.

### *Example Uses of Individual and Focus Group Interviews in Public Health Communication*

Individual and focus group interviews data can provide valuable information for making a wide variety of decisions. In the realm of public health communication, individual and focus group interviews are primarily used to (1) assess needs, (2) help design an intervention, and (3) supplement or help explain quantitative findings (Kreuger & Casey, 2015; Morgan, 2019; Rubin & Rubin, 2012; Seidman, 2013; Stewart & Shamdasani, 2015). These three tasks are discussed in detail elsewhere in this book (see Chapters 2 through 4) and are briefly reviewed here as a reminder.

**To assess needs.** The early stages or phases of the health communication program cycle (Chapter 3) and PRECEDE-PROCEED Model (Chapter 4) emphasize the importance of understanding a health issue from the intended audience's perspective. They also stress the importance of gaining community input on how to best address a health issue. Individual and focus group interviews represent one important way to gather rich, qualitative data from the intended audience that can inform the overarching goal of an intervention.

**To help design an intervention.** Individual and focus group interviews play an important role in many different aspects of intervention development. For example, they are often used during preproduction formative evaluation to identify and better understand the behavioral and environmental factors that influence health-related decisions (and the predisposing, enabling, and reinforcing factors that impact them). They are also used to generate ideas for an intervention, obtain feedback on rough concepts, or provide guidance about what theory or theories might be most appropriate for a given topic and intended audience. Further, individual and focus group interviews are commonly used during postproduction formative evaluation to gather feedback on draft messages and materials before they are finalized. In sum, individual and focus group interviews provide valuable information for developing intervention strategies and objectives.

**To supplement or help explain quantitative findings.** Health behavior is complex and therefore difficult to fully understand using information gathered from a single research method. Collecting data using both qualitative and quantitative methods allows intervention developers to gain a more comprehensive understanding of a problem and how to address it than either method alone. A mixed-method approach also helps compensate for the limitations of a single method, and when results from different methods converge you can have more confidence in your findings (John & McNeal, 2017). Thus, individual and focus group interviews are often conducted in conjunction with surveys (see Chapter 12) and experiments (see Chapter 13).

For example, if you wish to create an intervention guided by the reasoned action approach (see Chapter 9), you could start by conducting a series of individual or focus group interviews to identify a comprehensive list of behavioral, normative, and control beliefs for your topic and intended audience. Then, you could conduct a larger-scale survey to identify and select the most important beliefs you will need to change with your intervention. Also, for example, you might conduct an experiment to determine if the intervention worked as intended, followed by individual or focus group interviews to make sense of any puzzling results or unintended consequences.

So far, this chapter has introduced semi-structured interviews in general, and individual and focus groups in particular. It also offered some recommendations for choosing between the individual and focus group interviews and reviewed some common uses of these techniques in a public health communication context. The remainder of this chapter reviews the four main steps for gathering information using these research methods: (1) collecting interview data, (2) analyzing interview data, (3) estimating theoretical saturation, and (4) reporting the results. A visual representation of this process is presented in Figure 11.2.

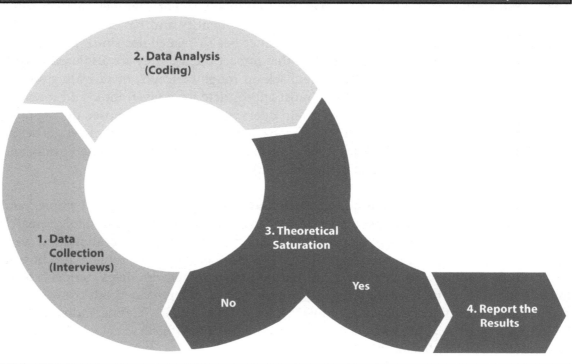

FIGURE 11.2    An Iterative Framework for Qualitative Data Collection and Analysis

## COLLECTING INTERVIEW DATA

The first step in the planning process is to carefully explicate the research question you want to answer. Having a clear idea about the decisions that must be made and the information you will need to make them serves at least two important purposes. First, it will tell you what type of data you need and who you need to collect it from. This will help you determine if semi-structured interviews in general, or individual interviews or focus groups in particular, are the best method for gathering the desired information. Second, it will inform the types of questions you ask during the interviews. For example, your interview guide will be quite different when assessing needs, versus generating ideas for a new intervention, versus obtaining feedback on existing messages before they are finalized. This section focuses on three practical aspects of the interview planning process: (1) drafting questions and the interview guide, and (2) selecting and recruiting participants, and (3) arranging and conducting the interviews.

## DRAFTING QUESTIONS AND THE INTERVIEW GUIDE

Individual and focus group interviews use a series of open-ended questions and probes to generate and guide discussion. Collectively, these questions make up the interview guide, or interview protocol. Here, I review some common types of interview questions, along with a useful strategy for developing questions and the question route.

### Common Types of Interview Questions

Three general categories of questions make up the core of any interview guide: (1) discussion starter questions, (2) primary and secondary questions, and (3) wrap-up questions (Brinkmann & Kvale, 2018; Castillo-Montoya, 2016; Krueger & Casey, 2015; Morgan, 2019; Rubin & Rubin, 2012). Here and elsewhere in this chapter I will refer to a series of focus groups conducted to determine what factors influence whether or not college students and other young adults use active transportation (Simons et al., 2014). Just so you know, active transportation is any mode of transportation that uses physical activity to get around (e.g., walking and cycling, using a skateboard or scooter, rollerblading, etc.). With this in mind, Table 11.1 includes an example for each of the three types of questions that make up most interview guides.

**Discussion-starter questions.** Generally speaking, *discussion-starter questions* are designed to get everyone talking early in the discussion and to introduce the general topic of the interview. More specifically, Kreuger and Casey (2015) draw a distinction between two types of discussion starter questions. An *opening question* is designed to get participants talking and to help people feel comfortable. To illustrate, notice how the opening questions in Table 11.1 simply asks for some general information about participants and may only be tangentially related to the main purpose of the study. Also notice that all participants are asked to answer this question, even when conducting focus group interviews. The opening question is followed by one or more *introductory questions*, which are designed to introduce the general topic under investigation and provide everyone with a common point of reference for the remainder of the interview. In Table 11.1 this takes the form of asking participants, "what comes to mind when you hear the term 'active transportation'?" This discussion should conclude by making sure everyone has the same general understanding of what is meant by the main topics under investigation.

**Primary and secondary questions.** The main reason for the interview will be covered in a series of three to six *primary questions* (sometimes called *key questions*), which are designed to gather information for each main topic under investigation. Krueger and Casey (2015) note that these are usually "the first questions to be developed . . . and the ones that require the greatest attention in the analysis" (p. 45). Each primary question will

| TABLE 11.1 | Common Types of Interview Questions |
|---|---|
| **Type of Question** | **Example** |
| **Discussion Starter Questions** | |
| Opening Question | 1. *(Note: Ask all participants to answer this question.)* What is your first name, how long have you been a student at ASU, and do you live on or off campus? |
| Introductory Question | 2. What comes to mind when you hear the term "active transportation"? |
| **Primary and Secondary Questions** | |
| Primary Question | 3a. What do you see as the key *advantages or benefits* of using active transportation? <br> 3b. What do you see as the key *disadvantages or barriers* of using active transportation? |
| Secondary Question | 4a. How would you go about *increasing* the perceived advantages or benefits of using active transportation? <br> 4b. How would you go about *decreasing* the perceived disadvantages or barriers of using active transportation? |
| **Wrap-up Questions** | |
| All Things Considered Question | 5. *(Note: Ask all participants to answer this question.)* Of all the issues we talked about today, which do *you* feel is the most important? |
| Summary Question | 6. *(Note: Provide short summary of the focus group discussion here.)* Did we miss anything important? |
| Final Question | 7. *(Note: Provide a short description of the main purpose of the focus group here.)* Is there anything else that we did not discuss that you feel is important for this topic; something we should ask about in future interviews? |

Adapted from Krueger and Casey (2015), Morgan (2019), and Simons et al. (2014).

typically be followed by a set of *secondary questions* (sometimes called *follow-up questions*), which are designed to collect more in-depth information about a topic. For example, the primary questions in Table 11.1 focus on the advantages and disadvantages of using active transportation, while the corresponding secondary questions focus on ways to increase the perceived advantages and decrease the perceived disadvantages of this behavior.

Morgan (2019) draws a distinction between secondary questions (which are a pre-planned aspect of the primary question) and probes (which are a more spontaneous way to encourage discussion). Common probes include questions like, "can you say something more about that?" "can you provide an example?", "does anyone have a different thought?", or "what do others think about this issue?" Silence or pauses can also serve as effective probes. On the one hand Kreuger and Casey (2015) recommend using a few probes early in the interview to communicate the importance of elaboration. On the other hand, Morgan (2019) notes, "if a group is sustaining its own discussion, there may be little need for the moderator to probe" (p. 66).

**Wrap-up questions.** Finally, *wrap-up questions* create a sense of closure, allow participants to reflect on previous comments, and provide participants with an opportunity to identify something that was especially meaningful or important to them (Krueger & Casey, 2015; Morgan, 2019). Thus, be sure to allow enough time for one or more of the following three types of wrap-up questions. First, *all things considered questions* provide participants with the opportunity to identify what they view as the key issue(s) raised during the interview (e.g., "Of all the issues we talked about today, which one do you feel is the most important?"). For focus groups, all participants are asked to answer this question. Thus, it may be worthwhile to ask participants to first write down their answers on a note card to help ensure that later responses are not impacted by earlier ones. Second, *summary questions* begin with a short summary of the session followed by a question designed to assess if this synopsis was complete and accurate (e.g., "Did we miss anything important?"). Notice that both of these techniques have the advantage of aiding subsequent data analysis. Third, *final questions* begin by providing a short description of the main purpose of the interview and asking a question intended to make sure nothing important was missed (e.g., "Is there anything else that we did not discuss that you feel is important for this topic; something we should ask about in future interviews?"). In addition to providing useful information for the researcher, these sorts of wrap-up questions provide participants with an opportunity to raise any issues they were thinking or worrying about during the interview but have not yet been raised (Brinkmann & Kvale, 2018).

In short, discussion starter questions get people talking and introduce the general topic, primary and secondary questions are used to gather the information needed to meet the main objectives of the study, and wrap-up questions conclude the interview in a way that allows you to make sure nothing important was missed. Now that you understand the three main types of interview questions, I will discuss some of the basics for crafting good questions and developing a question route.

### Interview Protocol Refinement Framework

Crafting a good interview guide can be more challenging than it appears. Amongst other things, you must decide what and how many questions to ask, which probes and activities to include, how to sequence everything, and how much time to spend on each topic; all while staying true to the research questions that led to the decision to conduct the interviews in the first place. To help manage the process, this section reviews Castillo-Montoya's (2016) interview protocol refinement framework for systematically developing and refining an interview guide (a.k.a., interview protocol). This framework is comprised of four phases:

1. Ensuring interview questions align with research questions,

2. Constructing an inquiry-based conversation,

3. Receiving expert feedback on the interview protocol, and

4. Pilot testing the interview protocol with members of the intended audience.

A discussion of each of these phases follows.

**Phase 1: Ensuring interview questions align with research questions.** In the beginning, it is a good idea to meet with a small group of people who are familiar with the purpose of your study to help you brainstorm possible questions for your interviews (Kreuger & Casey, 2015). After that, the one or two individuals responsible for developing the interview guide should spend some time combining related questions, eliminating redundant ones, and selecting and prioritizing the most important questions from those that remain. Even after these initial steps, however, you will likely find yourself in a situation where you have more questions to ask than you have time to ask them (i.e., typically 20–30 minutes per individual interview and 75–90 minutes per focus group; Coenen et al., 2012). At this point you will want to use a systematic process to determine which interview questions have the potential to elicit information for which research questions. To do this, Castillo-Montoya (2016) recommends creating an interview protocol matrix to explicitly connect each interview question to one or more of your research questions (see Table 11.2). This process will help you confirm the purpose and justify the necessity of each question in your interview protocol and allow you to determine if any gaps exist before data collection begins.

**Phase 2: Constructing an inquiry-based conversation.** You will probably not be surprised to learn that the *how the* questions are asked can significantly impact the answers that are given. Here, I offer three general guidelines for constructing an inquiry-based conversation.

| TABLE 11.2 | Example Interview Protocol Matrix | | | |
| --- | --- | --- | --- | --- |
| | Background Information | Research Question 1 | Research Question 2 | Research Question 3 |
| Interview Question 1 | ✓ | | | |
| Interview Question 2 | ✓ | | | |
| Interview Question 3 | | ✓ | | |
| Interview Question 4 | | ✓ | | |
| Interview Question 5 | | ✓ | ✓ | |
| Interview Question 6 | | | ✓ | |
| Interview Question 7 | | | | ✓ |
| Interview Question 8 | | ✓ | ✓ | ✓ |

Adapted from Castillo-Montoya (2016).

These guidelines focus on (1) phrasing the questions, (2) sequencing the questions, and (3) estimating the time for each question.

In terms of phrasing, interviews use open-ended questions that allow respondents to answer in any way that they chose (including ways that the researcher might not have anticipated). Thus, you should avoid biased or leading questions that encourage respondents to answer in a particular way. Further, the questions should be expressed using the everyday language of the interviewees (Brinkman & Kvale, 2018) and follow the social rules that apply to ordinary conversation (Rubin & Rubin, 2012). For example, you should "ask only one question at a time, try not interrupting participants when they are speaking, indicate understanding through nodding and other gestures, ask clarifying questions, transition from one topic to another, express gratitude," etc. (Castillo-Montoya, 2016, p. 822). In short, the goal is to evoke conversation and engage participants via questions that are relevant, interesting, and accessible.

Unless there is a good reason to do otherwise, the interview guide will typically follow a funnel-shaped sequence (Brinkman & Kvale, 2018; Krueger & Casey, 2015; Morgan, 2019; Rubin & Rubin, 2012). The *funnel-shaped sequence* starts with a broad question and gradually gets more specific as the interview progresses. For example, you might begin with a general opening question to get participants talking, followed by an introductory question to provide a common point of reference, followed by primary questions to get information on a key topic under investigation, followed by secondary questions to collect more in-depth information about the topic.

On a related note, it is typically best to ask uncued questions before cued questions (Krueger & Casey, 2015). *Uncued questions* are more general than cued questions and ask about a topic while providing little or no specific information about how a participant might respond.  A sample uncued question from Table 11.1 would be, "what comes to mind when you hear the term 'active transportation'?"  Respondents can answer any way they chose, and whether or not a particular topic naturally arises will tell you something interesting and important about the topic. *Cued questions* ask about more specific topics. For example, active transportation includes a variety of different behaviors such as walking and cycling, using a skateboard or scooter, and rollerblading. So, if a particular mode of active transportation is important to your research question but does not arise naturally in response to your uncued question, you can ask the appropriate cued question(s) as needed. In sum, starting with cued questions is potentially problematic as it can negatively impact participants' range of answers, whereas starting with uncued questions opens up many possibilities that you may not have previously considered.

Finally, you should estimate the amount of time you want to spend on each question. To make sure you use your time wisely, Morgan (2019) suggests thinking of time as a budget and allocating a likely length to each question. For example, for a 30-minute individual interview this might translate to 3 minutes for the discussion-starter questions, 8 minutes to cover each of your three primary questions (24 minutes total), and 3 minutes for your wrap-up questions. Or, for a 90-minute focus group you might allot 15 minutes for your discussion-starter questions, 20 minutes for each of your three primary questions (60 minutes total), and 15 minutes for your wrap-up questions. However, these time budgets should serve as a general guide rather than a strict timeline (Morgan, 2019). Thus, another best practice for sequencing your questions is to ask your most important questions earlier to make sure you do not run out of time to answer them.

**Phase 3: Receiving expert feedback on the interview protocol.** Gathering expert feedback involves having several individuals with relevant knowledge or experience critique your interview protocol. For example, interview experts can provide guidance about the content and order of your questions, and content experts can help ensure that your language choices are appropriate for your topic and intended audience. In short, expert reviews are a relatively simple way to gather recommendations for improving your interview protocol before pilot testing it with members of your intended audience or fully implementing it in the field.

**Phase 4: Pilot testing the interview protocol with members of the intended audience.** As a reminder, a *pilot test* is a small-scale study designed try something out before using it on a larger scale. Here, that "something" is your interview protocol, and the pilot test entails administering it to a few members of your intended audience to assess how well it works before fully implementing it in the field. The goal here is to simulate an actual interview as closely as possible to ensure the questions are understandable, engaging, and properly sequenced. A pilot test also provides an excellent way to estimate completion times, identify potentially problematic questions, and to make sure the interview protocol is generating the type of information necessary to answer your research questions.

## SELECTING AND RECRUITING PARTICIPANTS

Whom to recruit will be dictated by the research objective, which will typically involve learning something about the intended audience. Participants should have something in common related to the purpose of the study and have the experience and knowledge necessary to provide rich information on the topic (Krueger & Casey, 2015). You should develop a detailed screening criterion that each respondent must meet, and carefully document the number of participants and the important characteristics of the sample for any written or oral reports. A related consideration is the types of comparisons you will want to make during data analysis. For example, if you wish to compare the beliefs, attitudes, and motivations of people from different segments (i.e., age, gender, race, ethnicity, stage of change, etc.), you must be sure to conduct enough individual or focus group interviews with members of each segment.

As for how many individuals you should recruit, it is ideal to continue data collection until little or no new information is being generated (see discussion of theoretical saturation later in this chapter). This will typically occur somewhere between 8–16 individual interviews or 3–5 focus groups (Coenen et al, 2012; Namey et al., 2016); sometimes for each type of participant when gathering information from participants or intended audiences that differ from one another in meaningful ways (Krueger & Casey, 2015; Stewart & Shamdasani, 2015). For focus groups you must also consider how many individuals to include in each group. Generally speaking, focus groups can include anywhere from 4–10 participants. Your main goal is to find the right balance between generating a variety of ideas and providing all participants with an opportunity to contribute. More specifically, Krueger and Casey (2015) recommend smaller, 5–6 person focus groups when the topic is complex, the participants have considerable experience with the topic, or when you plan to ask a larger number of primary questions. Conversely, they recommend larger, 7–10 person focus groups for simpler topics, with less experienced participants, or a smaller number of primary questions.

You must also develop and document the procedures you used to select and recruit participants. In terms of sample selection, individual and focus group interviews typically rely on *purposive samples*, where participants are chosen with a specific reason in mind. For example, interviewing members of the intended audience who are knowledgeable, available, and willing to participate often provides the most time- and cost-effective way to meet your research objective. Alternatively, *snowball sampling* involves interviewing the members of the intended audience that you are able to locate, then asking these individuals to recommend other potential participants that also meet your inclusion criteria, and so on. In other words, a snowball sample gets bigger and bigger as you accumulate more participants. Snowball sampling is especially useful when collecting data from small or hard-to-find populations.

Once you know who you want to interview, you have to figure out the best way to recruit them. In some cases, you or your organization may already have a relationship with the intended audience, in which case you can recruit participants directly. For example, perhaps potential participants have used your programs or services in the past. Alternatively, if you do not have direct access to members of the intended audience, you can partner with an individuals or organizations that do and ask them to help you recruit participants. For example, when developing gun-safety materials for Michigan Department of Community Health, we partnered with an instructor who taught hunter safety classes for the Michigan Department of Natural Resources to help us recruit and host a series of focus groups with individuals who owned guns primarily for hunting purposes (Roberto et al., 1998). Similarly, when asked by National Kidney Foundation of Ohio to develop messages targeting 40- to 60-year-old Hispanics (Roberto et al., 2009), we partnered with the Ohio Hispanic Coalition to help us recruit and host a series of focus groups with members of this intended audience. It may even be possible to set up (or "piggyback") your interviews in conjunction with another event, meeting, or occasion (Krueger & Casey, 2015). If neither of these options is available to you, you can attempt to recruit participants by posting flyers on noticeboards, advertising on social networking or other websites, approaching people in public spaces, etc.

Finally, once you have selected participants and they have agreed to participate, there are a number of steps you can take to make sure they show up. First, you should aim to increase benefits and decrease costs of participation as much as possible. Thus, you should select times and locations that are convenient for participants, provide a worthwhile incentive to those who participate, and cover transportation and childcare expenses when applicable. Second, you must establish trust. Partnering with an organization that is familiar to and highly valued by the intended audience can go a long way toward establishing trust, as can conducting the interviews in a location where participants feel safe, sharing how the results will be used, and promising confidentiality to the fullest extent possible. Third, the recruitment process should incorporate multiple, personalized, and strategically timed contacts. Examples include but are not limited to the initial contact and all reminder emails, letters, or phone calls.

## SETTING THE STAGE AND CONDUCTING THE INTERVIEWS

Once you have created your interview guide and set up the interviews, you will want to make sure you get the best information possible from the participants. Thus, this section provides guidance on setting the stage and conducting the interviews. An overarching principle to keep in mind is that issues of confidentiality and consent should be addressed at the beginning of the interview and guided by your organization's Institutional Review Board (Harrell & Bradley, 2009). While a detailed description of the ethical principles and guidelines for the protection of human subjects is beyond the scope of this chapter, a link to *The Belmont Report* is included in the reference section for those not already familiar with these practices (National Commission for the Protection of Human Subjects of Biomedical and Behavioral Research, 1979).

### Setting the Stage

Setting the stage is a four-part process that involves (1) welcoming participants, (2) providing an overview of the topic, (3) reviewing some important ground rules, and (4) asking the discussion starter questions (Kreger & Casey, 2015). This process is designed to build rapport, familiarize participants with the study's procedures, and help participants feel comfortable joining the discussion. Toward this end, you can use your opening statement to welcome participants, thank them for coming, introduce yourself (and the assistant moderator when applicable), and to review any remaining confidentiality and consent issues that have not already been addressed. Second, you should state the general purpose of the interview for the respondent(s). The goal here is to provide participants with enough information to focus the discussion, but not so much information that it dramatically impacts their responses. Third, it is important to present any important ground rules. For example, you should inform participants that that there are no right or wrong answers, that all views are welcome, and that you value different opinions. Further, for focus group interviews in particular, explicitly mentioning that you want to hear from everyon equally can go a long way toward preemptively preventing a few members from dominating the discussion and encouraging quiet individuals to participate (Kreuger & Casey, 2015). Finally, you will begin the interview by asking the discussion-starter questions from your interview protocol. Recall that the reasons for these questions are to get participants talking about the general topic of the interview.

### Conducting the Interviews

The interviewer's task is to get the best possible data. To do this the interviewer must understand the purpose of the study and be able to generate discussion without leading it. A good interviewer is able to create a permissive and nonthreatening environment and will likely have something in common with the respondents, such as their age, sex, race, ethnicity, or language (Powell & Single, 1996). For focus groups, it is helpful to have an assistant moderator take notes and document important aspects of the group's interaction so the moderator can concentrate on the discussion (Kreuger & Casey, 2015).

The bulk of the interview will address the primary and secondary questions from the interview guide (discussed previously). But, as a reminder, interviewer may reword or reorder the questions to allow the discussion to flow more naturally. Interviewers are also free to use additional pauses and probes to expand upon or clarify any issues that seem important to the purpose of the study. However, when collecting interview data it is generally advisable to "listen more, talk less" (Seidman, 2013, p. 78) and to "follow up, but don't interrupt" (p. 87).

## CAPTURING, CODING, AND ANALYZING INTERVIEW DATA

As is the case for information gathered using any research method, the analysis of individual and focus group interview data should be guided by the study's purpose. This can be particularly challenging with interview data which yield vast amounts of information, thus making it easy to become overwhelmed and distracted by the details (Kreuger & Casey, 2015; Tracy, 2020). Remember, not all questions and responses are equally important, and continually revisiting the purpose of the study will make data collection and analysis more manageable.

Unlike quantitative research where data collection and analysis traditionally represent distinct and sequential steps in the research process, qualitative research often involves collecting and analyzing data at the same time (Brinkmann & Kvale, 2018; Kreuger & Casey, 2015; Tracy, 2020). In other words, the collection and analysis of qualitative data is an iterative process that continues until theoretical saturation is achieved. For the purposes of this chapter the goal of qualitative content analysis is to categorize responses and identify themes across interviews. In this section I review the key factors involved capturing, coding, and analyzing interview data.

### CAPTURING, ORGANIZING, AND SECURING THE DATA

Audio recording and note taking are the best and most common ways of capturing interview data (Kreuger & Casey, 2015; Morgan, 2019). Audio recordings are an obvious necessity when you plan to conduct transcript-based analysis. However, even if you plan to conduct note-based or memory-based analyses, audio recordings provide a useful way to verify one's recollections and to identify direct quotes to illustrate key findings. Kreuger and Casey (2015) recommend using multiple strategies to capture data. In focus groups in particular participants are often asked to engage in a variety of different tasks. For example, participants may be asked to complete a short survey, write on index cards, or engage in sorting, brainstorming, or other types of activities. Thus, any physical documents generated during an interview—surveys, index cards, flip charts, etc.—should be collected and organized for subsequent analysis.

As Johnson et al. (2010) note, even small qualitative research projects generate "mountains of words" (p. 648). Thus, it is helpful to organize this information in a manner that will allow you to effectively and efficiently manage, store, retrieve, and analyze your data. The first step is to identify the topic, participant(s), interviewer, date, time, and location of the interview on each document (i.e., notes, recordings, transcripts, etc.) to prevent them from getting mixed up. Second, you should create a clear and descriptive folder and document naming system. When creating folder and document names, you should use keywords or abbreviations that describe the essential elements of what is in the folder or document. For example, if your first focus group on active transportation was conducted with college freshmen on June 18, 2021, the document name might look like this: "FG01_AT_Freshmen_061821." For computer directory and file names, this has the added advantage of helping you find the folder or document again when searching. Third, you should consider creating a "Read Me" document for each folder to more thoroughly describe the information or abbreviations contained within. Finally, you should have a central repository where all of the data (including the original raw data) are stored and readily available by everyone with permission to access them (Johnson et al., 2010).

In terms of security, it is vital that you carefully follow all procedures approved by your organization's Institutional Review Board and promised to participants. The general goal is to protect the rights, welfare, and privacy of participants by preventing their personal information and individually identifiable responses from being accessed by unauthorized individuals. This typically involves storing physical documents under lock and key (e.g., in a locked file cabinet or in a locked room). For digital materials this typically involves password protecting or encrypting files, computers, external hard drives, or remote servers. In all cases it is advisable that two or more individuals have full access to the data to prevent it from becoming inaccessible. On a related note, consider backing up your data regularly and in multiple locations. For example, you can store digital documents locally on a personal computer or on an external hard drive, or remotely using cloud storage.

## CODES, CODING, AND CODEBOOKS

Put simple, a *code* is label; it is a word or phrase designed to capture the essence of an important idea from your data. Codes and coding schemes (i.e., sets of codes) can be based on previous theory and research or the data itself (more on this below). Regardless of how your coding scheme is created, you will eventually have to analyze your data using a process called coding. *Coding* is the process of comparing, sorting, and categorizing your interview data (Charmaz, 2014; Tweed & Charmaz, 2012). For example, you might categorize a response using an already existing code when appropriate, or you might have to create a new code when necessary. Finally, a *codebook* provides detailed information about your codes and coding procedures so that all decisions are well documented and consistently applied. At a minimum, your codebook should provide an appropriate name, clear definition, and relevant examples for each code.

Given that coding is a fundamental aspect of qualitative data analysis, it requires that you use a systematic, verifiable, and continuous process to categorize your qualitative data (Kreuger & Casey, 2015). That is, you should use established procedures to ensure that results accurately reflect what was learned from the interviews. Further, your procedures should be well documented so that other researchers can replicate them. Finally, qualitative data analysis is a continuous process that requires careful consideration before, during, and after the interviews are conducted. For example, all questions should be written with data analysis in mind, probes and wrap-up questions should be used during the interviews to generate additional information when needed, and you should debrief and begin your analysis shortly after each interview.

## ANALYZING INTERVIEW DATA

Many decisions must be made when interpreting qualitative data. Some of these decisions will be made before data collection or analysis begin. For example, how will you analyze your data? What type of analysis will you conduct? And, how will you develop your coding scheme? Many other decisions will be made when coding your data. For example, you must determine if a response answers the question that was asked, says something important about the topic, or is similar to something that was said before. Next, I will review some common answers to each of the three questions posed above. After that, I will review how to manually conduct transcript-based analysis using an inductive coding scheme—a common and useful approach for coding and analyzing qualitative data.

### Manual and Computer-Aided Data Analysis

First, you must decide how to analyze your data (i.e., will you code it manually or use computer-aided qualitative data analysis software). The *manual approach* involves someone reviewing the qualitative data and categorizing it by hand. This approach will be discussed in more detail below. *Computer-aided qualitative data analysis software* (CAQDAS) are computer programs specifically created to facilitate qualitative data analysis. The key word in this definition is "facilitate"; just as a word-processor does not write papers on its own, CAQDAS does not analyze data on its own (Tracy, 2020). Popular examples include ATLAS.ti (www.atlasti.com) and NVivo (www.qsrinternational.com). In short, CAQDAS can help you organize, code, and retrieve your data, but they can be costly and take a while to learn (Krueger & Casey, 2015; Tracy, 2020). As noted above, this chapter will focus on how to manually code qualitative data using an inductive coding scheme. Those interested in learning more about CAQDAS are referred to Silver and Lewins' (2014) *Using Software in Qualitative Research: A Step-by-Step Guide.*

### Transcript-Based, Notes-Based, and Memory-Based Analysis

Second, you must decide what type of analysis to conduct (i.e., will you conduct transcript-based, note-based, or memory-based analysis?). As noted previously, multiple forms of data can be collected during the interview process. Common examples include audio recordings of the participants, notes taken by the interviewer or other observers, and information recalled by the interviewer or other observers. Thus, early on you will need to decide if transcript-based, note-based, or memory-based analysis best fits the circumstances of the study. For example, if the risk of being wrong is high you should conduct *transcript-based analysis*, which involves creating and analyzing complete transcripts from the audio recordings of each interview (Kreuger & Casey, 2015). This is the most rigorous method of analyzing data, but it is also the costliest and most time-consuming. You can also use abridged transcripts where the researcher makes some preliminary decisions while listening to the recordings and transcribes only those comments that might be useful when performing subsequent analysis. Alternatively, if decisions are low stakes, easily reversible, or must be made quickly, note-based or memory-based analyses might suffice (Kreuger & Casey, 2015). *Note-based analysis* involves analyzing the field notes and debriefing sessions from the interviews, while *memory-based analysis* centers around what the interviewer recalls from the interviews. Note-based and memory-based analyses should be used with caution as they are inexact and difficult to perform well (Kreuger & Casey, 2015). Also keep in mind that regardless of which data analytic strategy you plan to use, it is wise to always record your interviews in case you need to supplement your notes or memory, select direct quotes for written reports, or decide to conduct more rigorous analyses in the future.

### Inductive and Deductive Coding Schemes

Third, you must decide how to develop your coding scheme (i.e., will you use an inductive, deductive, or hybrid approach?) (Brinkman & Kvale; 2018; Tracy, 2020). The *inductive approach* is data driven; it categorizes responses using codes that arise naturally from the data. The inductive approach is particularly valuable during is in the early stages of intervention development (e.g., when conducting pre-production formative evaluation). To illustrate, if you are unsure about what theories will help you make sense of your data, or if you want a completer and more unbiased look at your data, the inductive approach will be the way to go (Tracy, 2020). The *deductive approach* is concept driven; it categorizes responses using predetermined codes derived from previous theory and research.

For example, a deductive approach based on the extended parallel process model (EPPM; see Chapter 8) would identify and code responses as they relate to perceived threat (i.e., severity and susceptibility) and efficacy (i.e., response-efficacy and self-efficacy). Finally, the *hybrid approach* starts with a preset coding scheme based on previous theory and research and expands it as needed while examining the data. For example, and returning to the EPPM example mentioned under the deductive approach, as you place responses into the perceived threat category, you might realize they can be further subdivided in other meaningful ways (i.e., threat to self vs. threat to other, physical threats vs. social threats, etc.). The hybrid approach allows you to revise and (re)code your data using this expanded coding scheme.

### *Conducting Manual Transcript-Based Analysis Using an Inductive Coding Scheme*

In this section I will review a simple but effective way to manually code qualitative data using an inductive scheme. This approach, which closely follows recommendations from numerous experts on qualitative data analysis (e.g., Charmaz, 2014; Kreuger & Casey, 2015; Morgan, 2019; Seidman, 2013; Tracy, 2020), involves (1) preparing the transcripts for analysis, (2) immersing yourself in the data, (3) developing and applying the coding scheme, and (4) identifying patterns or themes in the data. It is helpful to have someone familiar with the purpose of the study conduct the analyses, and to regularly revisit the research question(s) so they do not become overwhelmed and distracted by the details.

That said, the first step is to prepare the transcripts for analysis. Kreuger and Casey (2015) recommend you print out two hard copies of each transcript (one to cut up and an original for reference), on a different color paper for each type of participant (so you can tell them apart), with each line numbered (so you can locate a statement within the original transcript), and eventually cut and place similar responses into piles (see below). They go on to note that the manual approach is low-tech, but it works; "and if you've never done qualitative analysis before, this is a great way to start" (Krueger & Casey, 2015, pp. 151–152).

The second step in qualitative data analyses involves immersing yourself in the data. The goal here is to familiarize yourself with the data by reading and re-reading all of your transcripts. You can also write down some notes or mark anything that seems particularly important or interesting as you do, but you should not start coding (yet). Immersing yourself in the data will help you clarify, contextualize, connect, interpret, and generate potential ideas for your analysis. And, as Seidman (2013) notes, "there is no substitute for total immersion in the data" (p. 128).

Third, and once you have familiarized yourself with the data, you can condense and describe it by developing and applying your coding scheme. As a reminder, an inductive coding scheme categorizes responses using codes that arise naturally from the data. A common way to do this is to use the constant comparative method introduced by Glaser and Strauss (1967). To do so, Kreuger and Casey (2015) suggest using scissors to literally cut up your transcripts and place similar responses into piles using procedures summarized in Table 11.3. Each pile represents a different code and therefore should include a clear label and definition so subsequent statements can more easily be compared to codes that already exist (or to help you determine if you need to create new codes). In short, this process of *primary-cycle coding* (sometimes called *open coding* or *initial coding*) involves "examining the data and assigning words or phrases that capture their essence" (Tracy, 2020, p. 234). Keep in mind that these labels and definitions are tentative and may change as new statements are compared and categorized. For example, some codes may die out while new ones may appear, some may be merged into a single code while others may be separated into multiple codes, etc.

The final step is to perform *secondary-cycle coding* (sometimes called *thematic coding*), which involves identifying and interpreting patterns or themes in your data (Tracy, 2020). This step involves reviewing your primary-cycle codes and grouping them together into higher-order categories. To illustrate, Simons et al. (2014) conducted focus groups to better understand the factors that impact whether or not young adults use active transportation. A few of the reasons they identified during primary-cycle coding included (1) autonomy, (2) finances, (3) comfort, (4) health, (5) access to facilities, (6) weather, (7) perceived safety,

### TABLE 11.3    How to Manually Conduct Transcript-Based Analysis Using an Inductive Coding Scheme and the Constant Comparative Method

Step 1:  Does the comment answer the question that was asked?

IF YES → Go to Step 3
IF NO → Go to Step 2.

Step 2:  Does the comment answer a different question?

IF YES → Move it to that question.
If NO → Set aside for possible later use.

Step 3:  Does the comment say something important about the topic?

IF YES → Go to Step 4.
IF NO → Set aside for possible later use.

Step 4:  Is the comment similar to something that has been said before?

IF YES → Group like answers together.
IF NO → Start a new group.

Adapted from Kreuger and Casey (2015).

and (8) ecology. They then used secondary-cycle coding to collapse these codes into two higher-level themes they labeled personal factors (made up of codes 1–4) and physical environmental factors (made up of codes 5–8).

## ESTIMATING THEORETICAL SATURATION

By now, you have probably already asked yourself, "how many individual interviews or focus groups should I conduct?" Ideally, data collection and analysis will continue until theoretical saturation is achieved. Theoretical saturation (sometimes called data saturation or thematic saturation) has been conceptualized and operationalized in a variety of different ways in qualitative research (Saunders et al., 2018). For our purposes, *theoretical saturation* is the point in data collection and analysis where little or no new information on the research topic is being generated. Theoretical saturation represents one important way to assess the quality of qualitative research; it suggests you have performed a comprehensive examination of the topic and intended audience under investigation (Faulkner & Trotter, 2017; Levitt, 2020; Tong et al., 2007).

Practically, theoretical saturation will typically occur somewhere between 8 and 16 individual interviews and three to five focus groups. To illustrate, Coenen et al. (2012) collected data from patients with rheumatoid arthritis in an effort to determine how many individual interviews or focus groups were necessary to achieve theoretical saturation. They report that saturation was achieved after 13 individual interviews and five focus groups. In another study, Namey et al. (2016) conducted 40 individual interviews and 40 focus groups to learn about health-seeking behaviors of African American men. They conclude that eight individual interviews and three focus groups were required to achieve 80% saturation, and 16 individual interviews and five focus groups were needed to reach 90% saturation. Aldiabat and Le Navenec (2018) identified a number of factors that can impact how quickly saturation is reached. For example, saturation will typically be achieved more quickly (1) when answering less complex research questions, (2) when collecting data from homogenous samples, or (3) for data collected by experienced qualitative researchers.

In sum, and as you may recall from Figure 11.2, you should continue to collect and analyze additional data until you have achieved an adequate level of theoretical saturation for the purposes of your study. Eventually, you will reach a point of diminishing returns with respect to theoretical saturation. You will know this has happened when you keep hearing the same things over and over again from participants, or when no new codes or themes are being generated. At this point it is generally safe to stop collecting and analyzing your data and move on to reporting the results.

## REPORTING THE RESULTS

Once data collection and analysis are complete you will want to summarize your findings in a written or oral report. One key purpose of the report is to clearly convey the most important lessons learned about the topic and intended audience to your research team and all relevant stakeholders. Another purpose of the report is to create a historical record of the study to facilitate the retrieval of key findings throughout the planning, implementation, and evaluation processes. Written reports typically use a narrative or bulleted format (Krueger & Casey, 2015). A *narrative report* provides an in-depth description of the study's method and results, and typically includes numerous direct quotes from participants to illustrate and support the report's conclusions and recommendations. A *bulleted report* uses a list or outline format to quickly and clearly convey the most important information from the study. Regardless of how you ultimately chose to report your results, here are some general guidelines to consider (Brinkmann & Kvale, 2018; Kreuger & Casey, 2015; Levitt, 2020; Tong et al, 2007).

First, clearly state the general purpose of the study and the specific research questions the interviews were designed to answer. For example, why did you conduct the study? And, why did you select individual interviews or focus groups to answer these questions? Answers to these and similar questions will help you create an outline for the report and allow you to communicate your findings more clearly.

Second, provide information about the research team. For example, who conducted interviews? How much experience or training did they have? Were the interviewers demographically similar to or different from the individuals they interviewed? Did the interviewer have a prior relationship to the participants that might impact their responses?

Third, describe the method and procedures you used to collect and analyze the data. Begin by describing the participants and the setting. For example, how many participants were interviewed? How were participants selected and recruited? Where and when did the interviews take place? Next, provide information about data collection procedures. For example, what primary and secondary questions were asked? How long did the interviews last? Were the interviews recorded or transcribed? Lastly, review how the data were analyzed. That is, did you code it manually or use computer-aided qualitative data analysis software? Did you conduct a transcript-based, note-based, or memory-based analysis? Did you create the coding scheme using an inductive, deductive, or hybrid approach? What level of theoretical saturation was achieved?

Fourth, review the results of the study and provide recommendations to improve the intervention. For example, did any consistent themes emerge across topics or intended audiences? Were there any unanticipated but important findings? How can this feedback be used to improve the intervention? What questions remain unanswered? Is any additional qualitative or quantitative research needed to answer these unanswered questions? You will typically organize your results and recommendations around the primary questions that were asked or the main themes that emerged during data collection and analysis. It is generally a good idea to include at least a few relevant and insightful quotations to document and illustrate your key findings. Most importantly, you should summarize, synthesize, and prioritize your findings and conclusions in a way that will be most interesting and beneficial to the report's end user.

Finally, written reports will typically include an abstract (for academic reports) or executive summary (for non-academic ones) that briefly presents the key research questions, method, results, and conclusions from the study. As always, this summary should focus on the issues that are most relevant to the people who will see and make decisions based on the report. And, keep in mind that although the abstract or executive summary are placed first in a written report, they are often written last to ensure they represent the full report as accurately as possible.

## CONCLUSION

In conclusion, semi-structured interviews are commonly used during the early stages or phases of intervention development. This chapter reviewed how to (1) draft an interview guide using the interview protocol refinement framework, (2) conduct manual transcript-based analysis using an inductive coding scheme, (3) estimate theoretical saturation, and (4) report the results for individual interview or focus group data. Further, it stressed that collection and analysis of qualitative data is a multi-step and iterative process that involves reading and re-reading, coding and re-coding, analyzing and re-analyzing, and collecting and re-collecting data until theoretical saturation is achieved (Moser & Korstjens, 2018). When it comes to gaining a rich understanding of respondents' point of view, there is no substitute for semi-structured interviews.

## REFERENCES

Adams, W. (2015). Conducting semi-structured interviews. In K. E. Newcomer, H. P. Hatry, & J. S. Wholey (Eds.), *Handbook of practical program evaluation* (4th ed., pp. 492–506). Jossey-Bass.

Adams, A., & Cox, A. L. (2008). Questionnaires, in-depth interviews and focus groups. In P. Cairns & A. L. Cox (Eds.), *Research methods for human computer interaction* (pp. 17–34). Cambridge University Press.

Aldiabat, K. M., & Le Navenec, C-L. (2018). Data saturation: The mysterious step in grounded theory methodology. *The Qualitative Report, 23*(1), 245–261. https://nsuworks.nova.edu/tqr/vol23/iss1/18

Brinkmann, S., & Kvale, S. (2018). *Doing interviews* (2nd ed.). SAGE.

Castillo-Montoya, M. (2016). Preparing for interview research: The interview protocol refinement framework. *Qualitative Report, 21*(5), 811–831. https://nsuworks.nova.edu/tqr/vol21/iss5/2

Charmaz, K. (2014). *Constructing grounded theory* (2nd ed.). SAGE.

Coenen, M., Stamm, T. A., Stucki, G., & Cieza, A. (2012). Individual interviews and focus groups in patients with rheumatoid arthritis: A comparison of two qualitative methods. *Quality of Life Research, 21*(2), 359–370. https://doi.org/10.1007/s11136-011-9943-2

Faulkner, S. L., & Trotter, S. P. (2017). Theoretical saturation. In J. Matthes, C. S. Davis, & R. F. Potter (Eds.), *The international encyclopedia of communication research methods* (pp. 1–2). Wiley.

Gill, P., Stewart, K., Treasure, E., & Chadwick, B. (2008). Methods of data collection in qualitative research: Interviews and focus groups. *British Dental Journal, 204*(6), 291–295. https://doi.org/10.1038/bdj.2008.192

Glaser, B. G., & Strauss, A. L. (1967). *The discovery of grounded theory: Strategies for qualitative research.* Aldine.

Guest, G., Namey, E., Taylor, J., Eley, N., & McKenna, K. (2017). Comparing focus groups and individual interviews: Findings from a randomized study. *International Journal of Social Research Methodology, 20*(6), 693–708. https://doi.org/10.1080/13645579.2017.1281601

Harrell, M. C., & Bradley, M. A. (2009). *Data collection methods: Semi-structured interviews and focus groups.* RAND Corporation.

John, K. S., & McNeal, K. S. (2017). The strength of evidence pyramid: One approach for characterizing the strength of evidence of geoscience education research (GER) community claims. *Journal of Geoscience Education, 65*(4), 363–372. https://doi.org/10.5408/17-264.1

Johnson, B. D., Dunlap, E., & Benoit, E. (2010). Structured qualitative research: Organizing "mountains of words" for data analysis, both qualitative and quantitative. *Substance Use and Misuse, 45*(5), 648–670. https://doi.org/10.3109/10826081003594757

Krueger, R. A., & Casey, M. A. (2015). *Focus groups: A practical guide for applied research* (5th ed.). SAGE.

Lederman, L. C. (2014). Focus groups. In T. Thompson (Ed.), *Encyclopedia of health communication* (pp. 503–505). Sage.

Levitt, H. M. (2020). *Reporting qualitative research in psychology: How to meet APA style journal article reporting standards* (Revised Ed.). American Psychological Association.

Meyer, G., Roberto, A. J., & Atkin, C. K. (2003). A radio-based approach to promoting gun safety: Process and outcome evaluation implications and insights. *Health Communication, 15*(3), 299–318. https://doi.org/10.1207/S15327027HC1503_3

Morgan, D. L. (2019). *Basic and advanced focus groups.* SAGE.

Moser, A., & Korstjens, I. (2018). Practical guidance to qualitative research. Part 3: Sampling, data collection and analysis. *European Journal of General Practice, 24*(1), 9–18. https://doi.org/10.1080/13814788.2017.1375091

Namey, N., Guest, G., & McKenna, K. (2016). Evaluating bang for the buck: A cost-effectiveness comparison between individual interviews and focus groups based on thematic saturation levels. *American Journal of Evaluation, 37*(3), 425–440. https://doi.org/10.1177/1098214016630406

National Commission for the Protection of Human Subjects of Biomedical and Behavioral Research. (1979). *The Belmont report: Ethical principles and guidelines for the protection of human subjects of research.* U.S. Department of Health and Human Services. https://www.hhs.gov/ohrp/sites/default/files/the-belmont-report-508c_FINAL.pdf

Powell, R. A., & Single, H. M. (1996). Focus groups. *International Journal for Quality in Health Care, 8*(5), 499–504. https://doi.org/10.1093/intqhc/8.5.499

Roberto, A. J. (2014). Evaluation methods, quantitative. In T. L. Thompson (Ed.), *Encyclopedia of health communication* (pp. 456–461). SAGE.

Roberto, A. J., Johnson, A. J., Meyer, G., Robbins, S. L., & Smith, P. K. (1998). The Firearm Injury Reduction Education (FIRE) Program: Formative evaluation insights and implications. *Social Marketing Quarterly, 4*(2), 25–35. https://doi.org/10.1080/15245004.1998.9960994

Roberto, A. J., Meyer, G., Johnson, A. J., & Atkin, C. K. (2000). Using the parallel process model to prevent firearm injury and death: Field experiment results of a video-based intervention. *Journal of Communication, 50*(4), 157–175. https://doi.org/10.1111/j.1460-2466.2000.tb02867.x

Roberto, A. J., Meyer, G., Johnson, A. J., Atkin, C. K., & Smith, P. K. (2002). Promoting gun trigger-lock use: Insights and implications from a radio-based health communication intervention. *Journal of Applied Communication Research, 30*(3), 210–230. https://doi.org/10.1080/00909880216584

Roberto, A. J., Raup-Krieger, J. L., & Beam, M. A. (2009). Enhancing web-based kidney disease prevention messages for Hispanics using targeting and tailoring. *Journal of Health Communication, 14*(6), 525–540. https://doi.org/10.1080/10810730903089606

Rubin, H. J., & Rubin, I. S. (2012). *Qualitative interviewing: The art of hearing data* (3rd ed.). SAGE.

Saunders, B., Sim, J., Kingstone, T., Baker, S., Waterfield, J., Bartlam, B., Burroughs, H., & Jinks, C. (2018). Saturation in qualitative research: Exploring its conceptualization and operationalization. *Quality and Quantity, 52,* 1893–1907. https://doi.org/10.1007/s11135-017-0574-8

Seidman, I. (2013). *Interviewing as qualitative research: A guide for researchers in education and the social sciences* (4th ed.). Teachers College Press.

Silver, C., & Lewins, A. (2014). *Using software in qualitative research: A step-by-step guide.* SAGE.

Simons, D., Clarys, P., De Bourdeaudhuij, I., de Geus, B., Vandelanotte, C., & Deorche, B. (2014). Why do young adults choose different transport modes? A focus group study. *Transport Policy, 36,* 151–159. https://doi.org/10.1016/j.tranpol.2014.08.009

Stewart, D. W., & Shamdasani, P. N. (2015). *Focus groups: Theory and practice* (3rd ed.). SAGE.

Tong, A., Sainsbury, P., & Craig, J. (2007). Consolidated criteria for reporting qualitative research (COREQ): A 32-item checklist for interviews and focus groups. *International Journal for Quality in Health Care, 19*(6), 349–357. https://doi.org/10.1093/intqhc/mzm042

Tracy, S. J. (2020). *Qualitative research methods. Collecting evidence, crafting analysis, communicating impact* (2nd ed.). Wiley.

Tweed, A., & Charmaz, K. (2012). Grounded theory methods for mental health practitioners. In A. R. Harper & D. Thompson (Eds.), *Qualitative research methods in mental health and psychotherapy: A guide for students and practitioners* (pp. 131–146). Wiley.

## Chapter Outline

## INTRODUCTION

The previous chapter reviewed how to collect and analyze qualitative data using semi-structured interviews. In that chapter, I compared semi-structured interviews (which rely mostly on open-ended questions that allow both the interview and the respondent to clarify and probe) with structured interviews (which rely mostly on closed-ended questions that make respondents select an answer from a list of alternatives provided by the researcher). In this chapter, I will focus on *survey research* (and by extension *structured interviews*), which involves asking participants to respond to a predetermined and standardized set of items and response categories. Surveys are commonly used during the planning process to better understand a health issue from the intended audience's perspective, and to measure the intended audience's beliefs, attitudes, intentions, and behaviors when assessing the effectiveness of an intervention. However, crafting good survey items is fraught with potential pitfalls. That is because even minor changes in how questions or response options are worded, formatted, or ordered can result in major changes in the answers provided.

To illustrate this point, consider the following example. Smyth et al. (2007) conducted an experiment to see how different response options impacted college students' answers to questions like, "How many hours per day do you typically spend on a computer?" All students received the exact same questions. One group, however, received six response options ranging from "½ hour or less" to "more than 2½ hours," while another group received six response options ranging from "2½ hours or less" to "more than 4½ hours." As you can see in Figure 12.1 these two sets of response options are logically equivalent. So, in theory, the same percentage of students should select one of the "2½ hours or less" and one of the "more than 2½ hours" options in both conditions. But that is not what happened. In fact, 37% more students selected one of the "more than 2½ hours" options when higher-frequency response options were used.

**FIGURE 12.1 How Questions Shape Answers:
The Effect of Low Frequency vs. High Frequency Scale**

| Low Frequency Scale | High Frequency Scale |
|---|---|

**How many hours per day do you typically spend on a computer?**

| | Low Frequency Scale | High Frequency Scale | |
|---|---|---|---|
| | ½ hour or less | | |
| | From ½ to 1 hour | | |
| | From 1 to 1½ hours | | |
| | From 1½ to 2 hours | | |
| 71% | From 2 to 2½ hours | 2 ½ hour or less | 34% |
| 29% | More than 2 ½ hours | From 2½ to 3 hours | 66% |
| | | From 3 to 3½ hours | |
| | | From 3½ to 4 hours | |
| | | From 4 to 4½ hours | |
| | | More than 4½ hours | |

Notice how the percentage of students reporting spending 2½ hours or more on a computer was significantly greater when the high frequency scale was used (66%) than when the low frequency scale was used (29%). That is a 37% difference!
Source: Smyth et al. (2007).

So, what is it about these two sets of response options that caused participants to respond differently? It seems participants use the response options as a source of information when answering questions. In this instance, as Schwarz (1999) explains:

> Essentially, respondents assume that the researcher constructs a meaningful scale, based on his or her knowledge of, or expectations about, the distribution of the behavior in the "real world." Accordingly, respondents assume the values in the middle range of the scale reflect the "average," or "usual" behavior frequency, whereas the extremes on the scale correspond to the extremes of the distribution (pp. 97–98).

In short, participants used the extra information from the response options as a point of reference when estimating their own behavior.

Fortunately, there are a number of practical steps you can take to improve survey items and formatting. Towards that end, this chapter begins by introducing four common types of survey research methods. Next, it provides an overview of the tailored design method, which involves customizing survey procedures for your topic and intended audience. Then, it reviews the most common types of survey items, provides 10 specific recommendations for crafting good survey items, and notes how an item's level of measurement impacts data analysis and the interpretation of results. This chapter concludes with an overview of three well-regarded methods for testing and evaluating survey items and formatting.

## COMMON TYPES OF SURVEY RESEARCH

Survey research can be grouped into four main categories based on (1) whether or not the survey is completed in person (i.e., in the presence of the researcher) and (2) whether or not the survey is self-administered. When crossed, these two factors capture the most common survey modes: in-person self-administered surveys, mail or internet surveys, telephone interview surveys, and in-person interview surveys (see Figure 12.2).

Each survey mode comes with a unique set of advantages and disadvantages. To illustrate, here are just three of the many issues to consider. *Cost* refers to the amount of money that has to be spent to complete the survey. The primary expenses for conducting survey research include designing the survey, administering the survey (i.e., printing, programming, postage, interviewers, incentives for participants, etc.), and data-entry. *Speed* refers to the amount of time necessary to collect the data. In other words, once everything is set up and ready to go, how long does it take to complete data collection? This is particularly important given that data analysis typically does not start until all expected responses are in. Generally speaking, *response rate* refers to "the proportion of sampled individuals that respond to the survey" (Dillman et al., 2014, p. 5). Also, generally speaking, response rate is calculated by dividing the number of people who completed the survey by the total sample of people that were asked to complete the survey (American Association for Public Opinion Research, 2015). So, for example, if you sent out mail (or internet) surveys to 1000 members of your intended audience and 320 of these individuals completed and returned the survey, your response rate would be 32% (i.e., 320/1000 = .32). Similarly, if you approached (or called) 100 members of your intended audience to ask them to complete an interview survey and 49 individuals agreed, your response rate would be 49% (i.e., 49/100 = .49).

**FIGURE 12.2    Modes of Survey Delivery**

|  |  | In-Person | |
|---|---|---|---|
|  |  | Yes | No |
| Self-Administered | Yes | In-Person Self-Administered | Mail; Internet Self-Administered |
|  | No | In-Person Interview | Telephone Interview |

Regardless of which mode or modes are chosen, there are a number of important issues to consider when conducting survey research (Dillman et al., 2014). The balance of this chapter will review a variety of issues to consider when crafting or evaluating how surveys and survey items are worded, formatted, and ordered based on the tailored design method.

## THE TAILORED DESIGN METHOD

Consider all the processes involved in accurately responding to a survey item. These processes include (1) *comprehension*—respondents must interpret and understand the question, (2) *retrieval*—respondents must remember and recall the relevant information, (3) *judgment*—respondents must estimate their final decision or answer, and (4) *response*—respondents must select the most appropriate response option from the alternatives provided (Tourangeau et al., 2000). Each part of the process represents a potential pitfall in survey research. For example, respondents may misinterpret or misunderstand a question (poor comprehension), forget important information (poor retrieval), reach incorrect conclusions based on what they do remember (poor judgment), or be unable or unwilling to select a correct response option (poor response).

The *tailored design method* is a set of procedures intended to reduce survey errors by customizing survey procedures and creating positive social exchange (Dillman et al., 2014). The tailored design method takes a scientific approach to survey design that includes three guiding principles and hundreds of practical recommendations. This section reviews the three guiding principles of the tailored design method: reducing survey error, customizing survey procedures, and creating positive social exchange.

### REDUCING SURVEY ERROR

Generally speaking, *survey error* refers to anything that negatively impacts the quality of the answers provided. As noted at the outset of this chapter, many factors can impact the accuracy of a survey's responses. Indeed, Weisberg (2005) identifies three general categories and nine specific types of survey error (see also Groves et al., 2009). The first general category focuses on respondent selection, which includes sampling error, coverage error, and nonresponse error at the unit level. These types of errors all relate to who responds to the survey, which can limit how representative the results are to the population of interest. The second general category focuses on response accuracy, which includes nonresponse error at the item level, measurement error due to the respondents, and measurement error due to the interviewers. These types of errors all relate to the accuracy or completeness of the provided information. The third general category focuses on survey administration, which includes post-survey error and mode effects. These types of errors all relate to how the data is processed (e.g., coding errors, data entry errors, etc.) and collected (e.g., in-person, self-administered, etc.).

A detailed discussion of all nine types of survey error is beyond the scope of this chapter. Instead, this section will review two general types of survey error: nonresponse error and measurement error. These types of errors were selected because the vast majority of the guidelines and recommendations offered by the tailored design method focus on these types of survey error (Dillman et al., 2014). Further, these two types of error also happen to be particularly relevant to the types of surveys that are typically conducted when planning and evaluating public health communication interventions. However, different types of survey error are important under different circumstances. So, readers who believe that one or more of the other types of survey error may be relevant to their specific circumstances are referred to Weisberg's (2005) book: *The Total Survey Error Approach*.

With this general overview in mind, *non-response error* occurs when those who do and do not respond to a survey or item are different in a way that is important to a study. It is not uncommon for people to refuse or forget to respond to a survey or item. However, this becomes a problem when certain types of individuals are more inclined to respond than others. For example, students who are struggling in college may be less likely to respond to a survey about their college experience than students who are not. Employees who exercise regularly may be more willing to answer questions about health and wellness than employees who exercise less frequently (or not at all). Community members who believe a particular health topic is important and personally relevant to them and their families may be more likely to respond to a survey regarding that issue than community members who do not. In all of these instances those who responded to the survey would be different from those who did not respond in some meaningful way, which raises concerns that the results may have been different under other circumstances. Minimizing non-response error involves developing a set of survey procedures that increase participants' motivation and ability to respond. As will be discussed in more detail below, this includes using multiple survey modes, using multiple contacts, personalizing all contacts, carefully and strategically timing all contacts, and sending a token of appreciation with the survey request (Dillman et al., 2014).

Generally speaking, *measurement error* occurs when participants are unable or unwilling to provide accurate information. Measurement error can take many forms, including misunderstanding a question, forgetting important information, providing socially desirable answers, etc. For example, a respondent may interpret a question or response option differently than the surveyor intended; in which case they may accidentally provide incorrect information. Similarly, if a respondent cannot correctly recall the necessary information, they will be forced to guess or skip the questions. Further, if a respondent wishes to be viewed favorably, they may over-report a "good" behavior or under-report a "bad" one.

Minimizing measurement error can be done by crafting good survey items and response options, carefully formatting and ordering items and response options, testing and evaluating every aspect of your survey and survey procedures, and selecting an appropriate survey mode (Dillman et al., 2014).

## CUSTOMIZING SURVEY PROCEDURES

As the name implies, the tailored design method avoids a one-size-fits-all approach to survey research. Instead, the second guiding principle of the tailored design method involves customizing survey procedures for different situations. Put somewhat differently, what works well for one topic, intended audience, type of intervention, budget, or timeline might not work well for others. Many different survey features or procedures can be customized (Dillman et al., 2014). For example, how will the survey be completed? Do you need a random sample, or will a convenience sample do? How many times, and how many different ways, will you contact participants? What, if any, type of incentive will you provide? How long is the survey and what does it look like? What types of questions will be asked and how will they be organized? In short, a non-exhaustive list of survey features or procedures that can be tailored include:

- ▶ Survey mode or modes
- ▶ Type of sample and sample size
- ▶ Number, timing, mode, wording, and visual design of contact(s)
- ▶ Type, amount, and timing of incentive
- ▶ Survey length, layout, organization, and visual design
- ▶ Question type, organization, wording, and visual design

To illustrate, in some circumstances the best possible option may be telephone interviews (mode) with 500 randomly selected members of the intended audience (random sample) that you attempt to reach up to four times (number of contacts) with no inducements (incentives) to answer a dozen (survey length) closed-ended questions (question type). While in other circumstances the best possible option may be to conduct in-person self-administered surveys (mode) with individuals who happen to participate in the intervention (convenience sample) and are offered one opportunity (number of contacts) to receive $5 (incentive) to complete a 50-item survey (survey length) containing both open- and closed-ended questions (question type).

In sum, customizing surveys and procedures based on your specific circumstances is one important way to reduce non-response and measurement error. It also provides important guidance regarding how to decrease the perceived costs of participation, increase the perceived benefits of participation, and establish trust with the intended audience. Which brings us to the third and final guiding principle of the tailored design approach: creating positive social exchange.

## CREATING POSITIVE SOCIAL EXCHANGE

The third and final guiding principle of the tailored design method involves creating positive social exchange. As a reminder (see Chapter 3), *exchange theory* posits that people are more likely to comply with a request when they trust that the benefits will eventually outweigh the costs (Blau, 1964; Homans, 1958; Thibaut & Kelley, 1959). In the realm of survey research, *benefits* include any advantages of completing a survey or anything that makes the completing a survey easier to perform; while *costs* include any disadvantages of completing the survey or anything that makes completing the survey more difficult to perform. So, creating positive social exchange involves increasing the benefits of participation, decreasing the costs of participation, and establishing trust.

Given that the direct or immediate benefits of responding to a survey are limited, Dillman et al. (2014) provide two general strategies for increasing the perceived benefits of participation. First, since people often find helping others to be rewarding, you can ask participants for their assistance and advice. Tell them how the results will be used to guide practical decisions that benefit the organizations or communities to which they belong. Highlight how only a small number of people have been asked to participate, and that the requested information is not available anywhere else. Second, when possible, include a token cash incentive with the survey request to encourage reciprocity. This recommendation is based on the facts that, regardless of survey mode selected, (1) incentives significantly increase response rates, (2) monetary incentives increase response rates more than gifts, and (3) prepaid incentives increase response rates more than promised incentives or lotteries (Singer & Ye, 2013).

While most of the benefits of completing a survey are likely to be indirect and long term, the costs are direct and immediate. For example, filling out a survey takes time and effort, can be inconvenient, and may make the respondent uncomfortable by asking for personal or sensitive information that they are reluctant to share. Dillman et al. (2014) make the following recommendations for decreasing the perceived costs of participation. First, keeping survey procedures short and simple and using design principles that make the survey easier to complete can help minimize the time and effort it takes to complete the survey. Second, selecting a survey mode that is preferred by and comfortable for the intended audience can go a long way towards easing convenience concerns. Third, you should minimize requests for personal or sensitive information. But, when such information is absolutely necessary, you might (1) use a self-report survey as it provides more privacy, (2) ask sensitive questions later in the survey after trust has been built, (3) briefly explain why the information is important and how it will be protected, and (4) carefully word questions and response options to be as unobtrusive as possible

Finally, it is important to establish trust; participants must believe that their privacy will be protected and that the promised benefits will be realized (Dillman et al., 2014). For example, *anonymous data* is collected in such a way that it is impossible for anyone—including the researcher—to link individual responses to a particular participant. *Confidential data*, on the other hand, is collected in such a way that it is possible for the researcher—but no one else—to potentially link individual responses to a particular participant. So, to establish trust you should not collect information that can be linked to a specific person (i.e., name, address, phone number, social security number, student identification number, IP addresses, etc.) unless absolutely necessary. And, when it is necessary to collect individually identifiable information, it is important to tell participants the steps that will be taken to prevent anyone else from connecting them to their responses.

Another way to establish trust includes being clear about the purpose of the survey (e.g., "your responses to this survey will help us better understand . . ."). It is also important to provide a way for participants to assess the authenticity of the survey and ask questions about it (e.g., "if you have any questions about this survey, please feel free to contact . . ."). Further, "if the survey sponsor is generally viewed in a good light, seen as legitimate, and trusted by the target population, that sponsorship should be emphasized" (Dillman et al., 2014, p. 39).

In sum, this section examined the three guiding principles of the tailored design method, which include reducing survey error, customizing survey procedures, and creating positive social exchange. The following sections will build upon these general principles by providing several specific recommendations for crafting good survey items.

## COMMON TYPES OF SURVEY ITEMS

### OPEN-ENDED ITEMS

*Open-ended items* let respondents answer in any way they choose. As the following examples illustrate, open-ended items can be used to solicit numbers, lists, or detailed descriptions:

Sample Open-Ended Items

**Please indicate the number of fitness classes you have taken at the Sun Devil Fitness Complex in the past seven days.**

☐ # of Classes

**Please list what you see as the three main advantages of taking fitness classes at the Sun Devil Fitness Complex.**

Advantage #1 [_____]
Advantage #2 [_____]
Advantage #3 [_____]

**Your answer to this question is very important for our understanding of what brings people to the Sun Devil Fitness Complex. How would you describe your experiences at the Sun Devil Fitness Complex to a friend?**

The key advantages of open-ended items are that respondents can provide in-depth answers in their own words, which can yield rich and useful data that a researcher might not have anticipated. The key disadvantages are that they take longer for participants to answer, and responses must first be interpreted and coded (which can be difficult and time-consuming) before they can be analyzed and reported.

The three examples provided above were purposefully selected to illustrate some important points regarding the use of text boxes to encourage respondents to provide more complete and accurate information (Dillman et al., 2014). First, when appropriate, label the answer box(es) to indicate the type of response that is required. To illustrate, in the first example the answer box is followed by "# of Classes," which highlights that a numeric response is desired. The second example includes "Advantage #" before the answer boxes to remind respondents that this question focuses on the advantages of taking fitness class at the Sun Devil Fitness Complex.

Second, the number of answer boxes should match the number of answers sought. To illustrate, the first example requires a single numeric response so only one answer box is provided (same for the third example where a single general description is sought). However, in the second example participants are being asked to list three advantage of taking fitness class at the Sun Devil Fitness Complex, so three answer boxes are provided.

Finally, answer boxes should be sized to match the type of answer to be provided. To illustrate, for the first example most people will provide a single or double-digit number, so a small answer box that can accommodate only a couple of characters is provided. In the second example key words or short sentences are desired, so larger answer boxes are provided. And, in the third example a very large answer box is provided to indicate that a longer narrative response is desired.

## CLOSED-ENDED ITEMS

*Closed-ended items* require respondents to select an answer from a list of alternatives provided by the researcher. For example, the first open-ended behavior item asked above can easily be converted to the following closed-ended item:

Sample Closed-Ended Item

**Please indicate the number of fitness classes you have taken at the Sun Devil Fitness Complex in the past seven days.**

O 0      O 1      O 2      O 3      O 4      O 5      O 6 or more

Closed-ended items typically make it easier for participants to respond quickly, and participants are more likely to answer questions about sensitive topics when asked using a closed-ended format. For the researcher, closed-ended items are easier to code, compare, and statistically analyze. The key disadvantage of closed-ended items is that there is no way for a respondent to express a thought or opinion that is not included as a closed-ended choice, which could lead to measurement errors or the loss of valuable information. A discussion of two specific types of closed-ended items that are commonly used by public health communication practitioners follows.

### Likert and Likert-Type Items

A *Likert item* (Likert, 1932) consists of a statement that a respondent is asked to evaluate using a set of continuous responses (usually strongly disagree to strongly agree). To illustrate, consider the following intention item:

Sample Likert Item

**I will attend a fitness class at the Sun Devil Fitness Complex in the next seven days.**

- ○ Strongly disagree
- ○ Disagree
- ○ Neither disagree nor agree
- ○ Agree
- ○ Strongly agree

*Likert-type items* are those that use the general format of a Likert item (i.e., a statement followed by a continuous set of responses), but that assess something other than agreement or that are not completely symmetrical (Uebersax, 2006). Here is an example using a revised version of the above intention measure:

Sample Likert-Type Item

**How unlikely or likely is it that you will attend a fitness class at the Sun Devil Fitness Complex in the next seven days.**

- ○ Very unlikely
- ○ Unlikely
- ○ Neither unlikely nor likely
- ○ Likely
- ○ Very likely

Likert and Likert-type items are popular and can be used to measure a wide variety of concepts including agreement (i.e., strongly disagree—strongly agree), likelihood (i.e., very unlikely—very likely), importance (i.e., very unimportant—very important), frequency (i.e., never—more than once a day), satisfaction (very unsatisfied—very satisfied), opposition/support (i.e., strongly oppose—strongly support), and more.

### Semantic Differential Items

Generally speaking, *semantics* refers to the study of meaning. Thus, *semantic differential items* (Osgood et al.,1957) were designed to assess positive or negative meanings participants assign to an idea, concept, object, person, or event. For example, how do members of the intended audience feel or react when they think about a recommended behavior, such as attending an aerobics class at the Sun Devil Fitness Complex in the next seven days? Semantic differential items begin with a statement, and then ask participants to rank that statement along some bi-polar dimension(s). For example, here is a sample semantic differential item:

Sample Semantic Differential Items

**For me, attending a fitness class at the Sun Devil Fitness Complex in the next seven days would be:**

Unimportant     O     O     O     O     O     Important

Given that semantic differential items focus on meanings, associations, feelings, or emotional reactions, they are commonly used to measure instrumental attitude (i.e., one's assessment of the value of performing the behavior; is it unimportant—important, bad-good, etc.) and experiential attitude (i.e., one's feelings or emotional reactions to the idea of performing the behavior; is it boring—interesting, unpleasant—pleasant, etc.) towards a behavior (Fishbein & Ajzen, 2010).

## ITEMS VERSUS SCALES

*Items* are single statements or questions that a respondent is asked to respond to or answer. And, as Uebersax (2006) notes, a single statement or question, regardless of its format, should not be called a scale. A *scale*, on the other hand, is a set of multiple items designed to measure a single variable (i.e., there is some logical or empirical relationship between them; Babbie, 2010). To illustrate, we expect these four individual attitude items to be related in such that we can combine them into a single instrumental attitude scale (Fishbein & Ajzen, 2010):

302 Chapter 12 Survey Research

Four Individual Attitude Items for an Overall Attitude Scale

**For me, attending a fitness class at the Sun Devil Fitness Complex in the next seven days would be:**

| | | | | | | |
|---|---|---|---|---|---|---|
| Unimportant | $O_1$ | $O_2$ | $O_3$ | $O_4$ | $O_5$ | Important |
| Bad | $O_1$ | $O_2$ | $O_3$ | $O_4$ | $O_5$ | Good |
| Harmful | $O_1$ | $O_2$ | $O_3$ | $O_4$ | $O_5$ | Beneficial |
| Worthless | $O_1$ | $O_2$ | $O_3$ | $O_4$ | $O_5$ | Valuable |

If results indicate that these four items do, in fact, measure the same thing, we can combine these four individual items to form a single scale. This can be done by assigning each point along the continuum a number (i.e., from 1 to 5), and summing up the responses to all items in the scale. For example, an individual's score on this four-item attitude scale would range from 4 (if they selected the most negative option for all four items, i.e., 1 + 1 + 1 + 1 = 4) to 20 (if they selected the most positive option for all four items, i.e., 5 + 5 + 5 + 5 = 20). However, it is often easier to work with *mean-item scores*, which simply takes the sum of all responses and divides it by the number of items. So, if someone selected the most negative option for all four items, they would end up with a mean item score of 1 (4/4 = 1), whereas someone who selected the most positive option for all four items would end up with a mean item score of 5 (20/4 = 5). Using mean item scores keeps the scale score within the range of the original items (e.g., 1 to 5), which makes the scores easier to understand and interpret.

In sum, this section provided an overview of the most common types of survey items. It defined and provided examples of both open-ended and closed-ended items in general, and Likert, Likert-type, and semantic differential items in particular. It also made an important distinction between individual items and multi-item scales. However, good scales start with good survey items, so the next section provides 10 specific recommendations for crafting good survey items (with an emphasis on closed-ended survey items).

## CRAFTING GOOD SURVEY ITEMS

Regardless of the survey mode or types of items selected, there are many guidelines to keep in mind both when creating your own items or when evaluating other's items. For example, Dillman et al. (2014) provide 178 specific recommendations for several survey modes (e.g., telephone, web, mail, and mixed mode surveys) and questions (e.g., open-ended,

---

**TABLE 12.1    Recommendations for Crafting Good Survey Items**

1. Ask one question at a time.
2. Avoid biased or leading items or response categories.
3. Develop response options that are exhaustive.
4. Develop response options that are mutually exclusive.
5. Use 5- to 7-point measures with a "neutral" middle category.
6. Use construct-specific response options.
7. Avoid vague quantifiers.
8. Verbally label all response options.
9. Maintain equal spacing between response options.
10. Use force-choice items instead of check-all-that-apply items.

Adapted from Dillman et al. (2014) and Artino et al. (2018).

---

closed-ended, nominal, ordinal, etc.). In this section I review 10 important, yet relatively easy, recommendations for improving survey items (these recommendations are also summarized in Table 12.1). As simple as these recommendations may seem, they still represent common issues among even the most experienced survey researchers. For example, Artino et al. (2018) content analyzed 37 surveys from studies published in top-tier journals and report that 95% of the surveys they analyzed violated one or more of these best practices.

## RECOMMENDATION 1: ASK ONE QUESTION AT A TIME

It is important to avoid *double-barreled items*, or those that ask more than one question at a time. To illustrate, consider the following double-barreled item:

The Problem: Double-Barreled Items

**For me, participating in aerobics or strength training classes at the Sun Devil Fitness Complex in the next seven days is:**

- ○ Very difficult
- ○ Somewhat difficult
- ○ Neither difficult nor easy
- ○ Somewhat easy
- ○ Very easy

The problem is that this one item asks about both aerobic and strength training classes. This will make it difficult or impossible for people who feel differently about these two activities to respond accurately. For example, someone might feel it is very difficult to participate in an aerobics class and very easy to participate in a strength training class (or vice versa). This person would be unable to accurately answer this item as worded. The solution is to ask one question at a time:

The Solution: Ask One Question at a Time

**For me, participating in *aerobics classes* at the Sun Devil Fitness Complex in the next seven days is:**

- O Very difficult
- O Somewhat difficult
- O Neither difficult nor easy
- O Somewhat easy
- O Very easy

**For me, participating in *strength training* classes at the Sun Devil Fitness Complex in the seven days is:**

- O Very difficult
- O Somewhat difficult
- O Neither difficult nor easy
- O Somewhat easy
- O Very easy

Whenever a conjunction (e.g., and, but, or, etc.) appears in a survey item, it is important to make sure you have not inadvertently created a double-barreled item.

## RECOMMENDATION 2: AVOID BIASED OR LEADING ITEMS OR RESPONSE CATEGORIES

*Biased or leading items* are those that encourage respondents to select a particular option. A survey question may be biased because of the way it is worded or because of the response options that are provided. For example, consider the following item:

The Problems: Biased or Leading Items or Response Categories

**How positively would you rate the aerobics class you most recently attended at the Sun Devil Fitness Complex?**

      ○ Poor
      ○ Slightly positive
      ○ Moderately positive
      ○ Very positive

The first problem is with the questions itself. That is, it leads participants by providing them with a sense of how the researcher wants them to answer the question (i.e., positively). This might cause some respondents to provide the answer they think the researcher wants to hear rather than how they actually feel. A second problem is the unbalanced response options (i.e., it provides more positive than negative options). The solution is to remove or replace any biased or leading language in an item itself, and to make sure the response categories include an equal number of positive and negative options:

The Solutions: Avoid Biased or Leading Items or Response Categories

**How negatively or positively would you rate the aerobics class you most recently attended at the Sun Devil Fitness Complex?**

      ○ Very negative
      ○ Negative
      ○ Neither negative nor positive
      ○ Positive
      ○ Very positive

## RECOMMENDATION 3: DEVELOP RESPONSE OPTIONS THAT ARE EXHAUSTIVE

It is important to make sure the response categories are *exhaustive*, which means they include all possible response options that might be expected. For example, suppose a researcher asked the following question:

The Problem: Missing Response Options

**During the past seven days, how many aerobics classes did you attend at the Sun Devil Fitness Complex?**

○ 1–2 classes
○ 3–4 classes
○ 5–6 classes
○ 7 or more classes

The problem is that these response categories are not exhaustive since there is no "0" option. Therefore, a respondent who did not attend any aerobics classes in the past two weeks would be unable to answer the question or be forced to pick an incorrect answer (two undesirable outcomes). The solution is to make sure all possible options are represented, or to ask an open-ended question where participants can write in their own answer:

The Solution: Develop Response Options That Are Exhaustive

**During the past seven days, how many aerobics classes did you attend at the Sun Devil Fitness Complex?**

○ 0 classes
○ 1–2 classes
○ 3–4 classes
○ 5–6 classes
○ 7 or more classes

**During the past seven days, how many aerobics classes did you attend at the Sun Devil Fitness Complex?**

☐ # of Classes

Also, if you ever have any doubt about whether or not you have fully captured all possible responses or do not feel an open-ended item is appropriate, it is best to include an "other" option so everyone can answer as accurately as possible (and perhaps a "please specify" option if it may be important to the study).

## RECOMMENDATION 4: DEVELOP RESPONSE OPTIONS THAT ARE MUTUALLY EXCLUSIVE

Response options should also be *mutually exclusive*, which means respondent should not be able to select more than one correct answer. This is most likely to be a problem when using ranges as response categories. Suppose, for example, a researcher asked:

The Problem: Overlapping Response Options

**During the past seven days, how many aerobics classes did you attend at the Sun Devil Fitness Complex?**

- ○ 0–2 classes
- ○ 2–4 classes
- ○ 4–6 classes
- ○ 6 or more classes

The problem is that someone who attended 2, 4, or 6 aerobics classes would be forced to choose between one of the two correct answers. This may lead to inaccurate responses that could easily have been avoided by either letting people fill in the blank with the correct number, or by using the mutually exclusive response options similar to the following instead:

The Solution: Develop Response Options That Are Mutually Exclusive

**During the past seven days, how many aerobics classes did you attend at the Sun Devil Fitness Complex?**

- ○ 0–1 classes
- ○ 2–3 classes
- ○ 4–5 classes
- ○ 6 or more classes

**During the past seven days, how many aerobics classes did you attend at the Sun Devil Fitness Complex?**

☐ # of Classes

## RECOMMENDATION 5: USE 5- TO 7-POINT MEASURES WITH A "NEUTRAL" MIDDLE CATEGORY

Two related questions often arise when developing Likert, Likert-type, or semantic differential items. The first question has to do with length of the continuum; for example, is it best to provide three, four, five, six, or seven or more response options? The second question has to do with the inclusion of a middle category; for example, is it better or worse to include a neutral option (i.e., "neutral," "unsure," "neither _____ nor _____," etc.).

The Problem: Too Few or Too Many Response Options

**It is likely that I will attend an aerobics class at the Sun Devil Fitness Complex in the next seven days.**

- O No
- O Unsure
- O Yes

**How unlikely or likely is it that you will attend an aerobics class at the Sun Devil Fitness Complex in the next seven days?**

- O Extremely unlikely
- O Very unlikely
- O Moderately unlikely
- O Slightly unlikely
- O Slightly unlikely
- O Moderately likely
- O Very likely
- O Extremely likely

The problem is that research indicates that including too few response categories negatively impacts measurement reliability and validity, as does the omission of a neutral category. Similarly, too many response options can make it difficult for respondents to differentiate between options. The solution is to provide enough response options that respondents are able to describe themselves fully and accurately, but not so many options that the categories begin to lose their meaning or become ambiguous (Dillman et al., 2014).

The Solution: Provide Five to Seven Response Options with a "Neutral" Middle Category

**How unlikely or likely is it that you will attend an aerobics class at the Sun Devil Fitness Complex in the next seven days?**

○ Very unlikely
○ Unlikely
○ Neither unlikely nor likely
○ Likely
○ Very likely

To illustrate the effects of number of response options and the inclusion of a neutral middle category on measurement reliability and validity, consider the following two meta-analyses. Saris and Gallhofer (2007) assessed 1023 measures from 87 samples, and Hamby and Peterson (2016) assessed 2813 measures from 481 samples. Generally speaking, both meta-analyses conclude that increasing the number of response options increases measurement reliability and validity. This is especially true when all response categories were labeled (Hamby & Peterson, 2016) and include a natural middle category (Saris & Gallhofer, 2007). In sum, research suggests that unless there is a very good reason to do otherwise, it is best to use five or seven fully labeled response options that include a middle category (Dillman et al., 2014; Hamby & Peterson, 2016; Lietz, 2010; Saris & Gallhofer, 2007).

## RECOMMENDATION 6: USE CONSTRUCT-SPECIFIC RESPONSE OPTIONS

As noted earlier in this chapter, Likert items consist of a statement that respondents are asked to evaluate using a set of continuous responses (typically ranging from strongly disagree to strongly agree). For example:

The Problem: Response Options That Do Not Emphasize the Construct Being Measured

**It is likely that I will attend an aerobics class at the Sun Devil Fitness Complex in the next seven days.**

○ Strongly disagree
○ Disagree
○ Neither disagree nor agree
○ Agree
○ Strongly Agree

One problem with this format is that it requires respondents to process an extra concept by first having to decide how likely it is that they will exercise and then converting that judgment into a different concept (i.e., how much they agree or disagree; Dillman et al., 2014). Another problem with this format is that it is more prone to *acquiescence*, or the tendency to agree with any assertion made in an item, regardless of its content (Artino et al., 2018). The solution is to use *construct-specific response options*, or those that match or emphasize the construct being measured. Notice that in the following example both the item and the response options focus on the same construct of interest (i.e., likelihood):

The Solution: Use Construct-Specific Response Options

**How unlikely or likely is it that you will attend an aerobics class at the Sun Devil Fitness Complex in the next seven days?**

○ Very unlikely
○ Unlikely
○ Neither unlikely nor likely
○ Likely
○ Very likely

In sum, agreement items remain very common in public health communication research, likely because they can be presented efficiently using a matrix format which can save space over stand-alone items. But, when possible, using construct-specific items is recommended as they reduce acquiescence, cognitive burden, and measurement error (Artino et al., 2018; Dillman et al., 2014).

## RECOMMENDATION 7: AVOID VAGUE QUANTIFIERS

Consider the following frequency item:

The Problem: Vague Response Options are Open to Interpretation

**How often do you attend aerobics classes at the Sun Devil Fitness Complex?**

○ Never
○ Rarely
○ Sometimes
○ Often
○ Always

The problem is that the terms "never," "rarely," "sometimes," "often," and "always" are vague and open to interpretation. To illustrate, I recently asked students in my graduate health communication class to indicate the percentage of time each of these words meant that something occurred. Here are their ranges of responses: never (0–5% of the time), rarely (1–30% of the time), sometimes (11–79% of the time), often (36–99% of the time), and always (61–100% of the time). These results are consistent with more formal research indicating that individuals assign a wide variety of meanings to these terms (Bocklisch et al., 2012; Hakel, 1968; Pace & Friedlander, 1982; Simpson, 1944). The solution is to use a more concrete time metric, preferably over a naturally occurring time frame such as seven days (one week) or 30 days (one month), or one year (Dillman et al., 2014), similar to the following:

The Solutions: Use a More Concrete Time Metric

**How often do you attend aerobics classes at the Sun Devil Fitness Complex?**

- O Never
- O A few times per year
- O About once a month
- O Two or three times a month
- O About once a week
- O More than once a week

**How many times did you attend aerobics classes at the Sun Devil Fitness Complex in the past seven days?**

O 0    O 1    O 2    O 3    O 4    O 5    O 6 or more

**How many times did you attend aerobics classes at the Sun Devil Fitness Complex in the past seven days?**

[ ] # of Times

## RECOMMENDATION 8: VERBALLY LABEL ALL RESPONSE OPTIONS

*Polar-point response options* only provide verbal labels for the endpoints of a continuum. To illustrate, consider the following item:

The Problem: Unlabeled Response Options

**How unlikely or likely is it that you will attend an aerobics class at the Sun Devil Fitness Complex in the next seven days?**

| Very Unlikely | | | | Very Likely |
|---|---|---|---|---|
| ○ | ○ | ○ | ○ | ○ |

The problem is that the unlabeled categories are open to interpretation, and different respondents may interpret them differently. Further, the labeled options have a different visual weight than the unlabeled options; and options that stand out more are more likely to be selected (Dillman et al., 2014). The solution is to use *fully labeled response options*, which provide a verbal label for every point on the continuum:

The Solution: Verbally Label All Response Options

**How unlikely or likely is it that you will attend an aerobics class at the Sun Devil Fitness Complex in the next seven days?**

| Very Unlikely | Unlikely | Neither Unlikely nor Likely | Likely | Very Likely |
|---|---|---|---|---|
| ○ | ○ | ○ | ○ | ○ |

**How unlikely or likely is it that you will attend an aerobics class at the Sun Devil Fitness Complex in the next seven days?**

○ Very unlikely
○ Unlikely
○ Neither unlikely nor likely
○ Likely
○ Very likely

Fully labeled response options provide more control over how all points on the continuum are interpreted and increases the likelihood that respondents will interpret the options similarly. Further, recent meta-analysis results indicate that fully labeled response options significantly increase measurement reliability (Hamby & Peterson, 2016).

## RECOMMENDATION 9: MAINTAIN EQUAL SPACING BETWEEN RESPONSE OPTIONS

Unequal spacing between response options is problematic for a variety of reasons. For example, consider the following items:

The Problem: Unequal Spacing Between Response Options

**How many times did you attend aerobics classes at the Sun Devil Fitness Complex in the past seven days?**

| 0 | 1 | 2 | 3 | 4 | 5 | 6 or more |
|---|---|---|---|---|---|-----------|
| O | O | O | O | O | O | O |

One problem is that this spacing provides different visual weight to different options. Also, as was the case with polar-point response options discussed above, people are more likely to select categories with greater visual weigh. Another problem is that this unequal spacing shifts the visual midpoint of the continuum (i.e., it *looks* like the midpoint of the continuum is 4). The solution is to maintain equal spacing between response options:

The Solution: Maintain Equal Spacing Between Response Options

**How many times did you attend aerobics classes at the Sun Devil Fitness Complex in the past seven days?**

| 0 | 1 | 2 | 3 | 4 | 5 | 6 or more |
|---|---|---|---|---|---|-----------|
| O | O | O | O | O | O | O |

**How many times did you attend aerobics classes at the Sun Devil Fitness Complex in the past seven days?**

○ 0
○ 1
○ 2
○ 3
○ 4
○ 5
○ 6 or more

As Dillman et al. (2014) note, respondents rely heavily on the visual midpoint of a continuum when interpreting the meaning of the continuum's other options. So, it is important to make sure that the visual midpoint matches the conceptual midpoint.

## RECOMMENDATION 10: USE FORCE-CHOICE ITEMS INSTEAD OF CHECK-ALL-THAT-APPLY ITEMS

Some surveys use *check-all-that-apply items*, where respondents are provided with a list of options and asked to select any or all that pertain to them. For example:

The Problem: Check-All-That-Apply Questions

**In the past seven days, which of the following types of exercise classes have you attended at the Sun Devil Fitness Complex?** *Please check all that apply.*

❏ Aerobic
❏ Strength
❏ Flexibility
❏ Balance

The problem with check-all items is that participants are less likely to process all of the options For example, participants tend to select fewer options, and are more likely to endorse the options in the top half of the list regardless of what those items are (Dillman et al., 2014). Further, check-all questions make it difficult to know why a participant did not respond to a particular option, which can result in measurement error. For example, was it left blank because the answer was "no," because the participant chose not to respond, or because the participant did not process the option? The solution is to use *forced-choice questions*, which require respondents to consider and make an explicit judgment about every option. For example:

The Solution: Use Forced-Choice Questions

**In the past seven days, have you attended any of the following types of exercise classes at the Sun Devil Fitness Complex?**

| Yes | No | |
|-----|-----|---|
| O | O | Aerobic |
| O | O | Strength |
| O | O | Flexibility |
| O | O | Balance |

Forced-choice questions encourage participants to focus on one item at a time, which increases the likelihood that they will process each item, and that they will endorse more items throughout the entire list rather than just those in the top half of the list.

## LEVELS OF MEASUREMENT

One important issue to keep in mind when developing items or scales is their level of measurement (Stevens, 1958). Remember that closed-ended survey items provide *quantitative data*, which involve the collection and statistical analysis of numerical data. *Level of measurement* tells us how these numbers relate to one another. There are four levels of measurement: nominal, ordinal, interval, and ratio. Table 12.2 provides an easy way to remember the properties of each level of measurement. Notice that each level of measurement has the properties of all previous levels, plus one additional quality.

| TABLE 12.2 | Information Provided by Each of the Four Levels of Measurement | | | |
|---|---|---|---|---|
| | **Nominal** | **Ordinal** | **Interval** | **Ratio** |
| Classification | ✓ | ✓ | ✓ | ✓ |
| Rank order | | ✓ | ✓ | ✓ |
| Equal intervals | | | ✓ | ✓ |
| True zero | | | | ✓ |

## NOMINAL LEVEL

The *nominal* level of measurement classifies objects into different categories. The values assigned each category are labels (names) only; they have no quantitative meaning. Consider the following survey item:

Sample Nominal Item:

**What sex were you assigned at birth, on your original birth certificate?**

○ Male
○ Female

This measure of biological sex is a classic example of a nominal variable since we will have to assign an arbitrary number to each category to analyze this data (i.e., "1" for "Male" and "2" for "Female"). However, since the assignment of numbers to categories is arbitrary, and since there is no real order between them, we could just as easily assign a "2" for "Male" and a "1" for "Female." Other common examples of nominal items include marital status, religion, race, and occupation.

## ORDINAL LEVEL

The *ordinal* level of measurement classifies objects into categories and provides a rank order to those categories. In other words, the different values represent relatively more or less of something. However, the numbers do not indicate absolute quantities, nor do they indicate that the interval between numbers are equal. Consider the following survey item:

Sample Ordinal Item:

**What is your current class in college?**

○ Freshman
○ Sophomore
○ Junior
○ Senior
○ Other

Here, an individual is both classified into a category (i.e., freshman, sophomore, junior, senior, etc.), and rank ordered along some dimension (i.e., number of credit hours completed). However, the distance between categories is not necessarily equal (i.e., the exact number of credits hours is unknown). Thus, there is no way to determine exactly how much the individuals in these groups differ. For example, there is little difference between a freshman with 27 credits and a sophomore with 33 credits, but a great difference between an incoming freshman with zero credits and a second-semester sophomore with 57 credits. Nonetheless, anyone with less than 30 credits would be considered a "freshman," and anyone with between 30 and 59 credits would be considered a "sophomore." So, while this item clearly allows us to rank order individuals, it does not allow us to determine whether or not the distance between categories is equal. Other examples of ordinal items include many individual Likert, Likert-type, and semantic differential items.

## INTERVAL LEVEL

The *interval* level of measurement classifies objects into categories, rank orders the categories along some dimension, and the distances between the intervals are either known or assumed to be equal. Consider the following survey item:

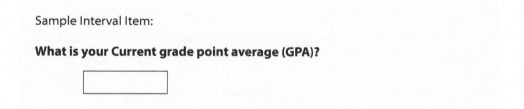

Sample Interval Item:

**What is your Current grade point average (GPA)?**

This item allows researchers to divide participants into categories based on their actual GPA (e.g., each option ranging from 0.0 to 4.0 represents its own category). It also ranks these categories (e.g., 2.4 GPA is lower than a 3.0 GPA, and a 3.0 GPA is lower than a 3.7 GPA, etc.). Finally, and this is important, the distances between each category are equal (e.g., the distance between 2.4 and 2.5 and the distance between 3.0 and 3.1 is the same in both cases—they both represent a change of .1). It is also important to note that interval measures do *not* contain a true zero point (i.e., zero does not represent the absence of a variable under investigation). Instead, zero on an interval measure typically signifies the smallest measurable quantity of a variable. For example, someone with a 0.0 GPA still has a GPA, it is just a very bad one.

## RATIO LEVEL

Finally, the *ratio* level of measurement classifies objects into categories, rank orders the categories along some dimension, has equal intervals between categories, and has a true zero point. It is only at this level of measurement that you can say someone, or something has none of the property being measured. Consider the following survey item:

Sample Ratio Item

**In the seven days, how many days did you attend an aerobics class at the Sun Devil Fitness Complex?**

☐ Days (0 to 7)

Here, a response of "0" means that the respondent did not attend an aerobics class at the Sun Devil Fitness Complex for the past seven days (or the absence of aerobics classes at the Sun Devil Fitness Complex in the past week). Many frequency items are measured at the ratio level of measurement (i.e., number of male friends, number of times married, number of sexual partners in the past year, how many servings of fruits and vegetables you had yesterday, number of text messages sent the last time you drove, etc.).

## IMPORTANT NOTES REGARDING LEVELS OF MEASUREMENT

Two final, but important notes regarding levels of measurement. First, it is generally preferable to measure a variable at the highest possible level since a variable measured at a higher level of measurement can easily be collapsed into a lower level of measurement (but not vice versa). For example, let us revisit the following item:

Higher Level of Measurement

**In the seven days, how many days did you attend an aerobics class at the Sun Devil Fitness Complex?**

☐ Days (0 to 7)

Since this is a ratio level item, it can easily be collapsed in a number of different ways. For example, though dichotomous data should be used with caution (Norman, 2010), it would be possible to compare individuals who have not (i.e., "0") to those who have (i.e., "1–7") attended an aerobics class at the Sun Devil Fitness Complex in the past seven days. It would also be possible to compare those who never (i.e., "0"), sometimes (i.e., "1–3"), or often (i.e., "4–7") attended an aerobics class at the Sun Devil Fitness Complex in the past seven days.

However, the opposite is *not* true. To illustrate, consider the following items which measure the same variable but using lower levels of measurement:

Lower Levels of Measurement

**In the seven days, did you attend an aerobics class at the Sun Devil Fitness Complex?**

　　O No
　　O Yes

**In the seven days, how often did you attend aerobics classes at the Sun Devil Fitness Complex?**

　　O Never (0 days)
　　O Sometimes (1–3 days)
　　O Often (4–7 days)

In both cases, it would be impossible to convert these items into an exact number of days should it ever become necessary to do so. So, again, as a general rule it is better to err on the side of caution and measure all variables of interest at the highest possible level.

Second, and in theory, level of measurement impacts which statistical analyses can be conducted and the type of conclusions that can be made with one's data. For example, Pearson correlation ($r$), regression, factor analysis, structural equation modeling (SEM), $t$-tests, and analysis of variance (ANOVA) assume interval- or ratio-level data are being analyzed. In practice, however, decades of research indicate that these and similar statistics are very robust (i.e., resistant to errors) for ordinal variables with at least five categories (Johnson & Creech, 1983; Norman, 2010; Sullivan & Artino, 2013; Zumbo & Zimmerman, 1993). This is yet another reason to use 5- or 7-point measures Likert, Likert-type, or semantic differential items (see Recommendation 5). Further, and as noted earlier, when you sum or calculate mean item scores from multiple items into a single scale the number of categories will be much greater than any of the items used to create them.

In sum, crafting good survey items and selecting the appropriate level of measurement will go a long way toward reducing nonresponse and measurement error. However, it is important to obtain feedback from experts and the intended audience before finalizing your survey and administering it on a large scale. Three common methods for testing and evaluating survey items include expert feedback, cognitive interviews, and pilot tests. An introduction to each of these methods follows.

## METHODS FOR TESTING AND EVALUATING SURVEYS

In the realm of survey design, numerous studies have been conducted to better understand "how the questions shape the answers" (Schwartz, 1999, p. 93). This research clearly indicates that a number of seemingly inconsequential decisions can dramatically impact participants' responses to survey items. Examples include, but are not limited to, decisions about how a question is worded, how questions are ordered, the response options that are provided, and how the responses options are formatted (Dillman et al., 2014; Hamby & Peterson, 2016; Lietz, 2010; Saris & Gallhofer, 2007; Schwarz, 1999). Fortunately, there are a number of ways to identify and correct potential pitfalls. The final section of this chapter reviews three proven methods for testing and evaluating survey items (Dillman et al., 2014; Presser et al. 2004): expert reviews, cognitive interviews, and pilot tests.

### EXPERT REVIEWS

As the name implies, *expert reviews* involve having several individuals with relevant knowledge or experience evaluate and provide feedback on your survey. For example, survey experts can offer advice regarding question wording or survey design, theory experts can provide feedback regarding how well items measure the intended constructs (i.e., content validity), and content experts can provide information about appropriate language for a specific topic and intended audience.

Each of the theory chapters provides at least one excellent examples of the ways in which public health communication experts have used expert reviews to assess and improve the survey items and scales used to measure various theoretical constructs. For example, González et al. (2012) obtained expert reviews from seven professionals with extensive knowledge in the theory of planned behavior or survey construction. Also, for example, Priest (2015) obtained expert reviews from seven researchers and practitioners with expertise in measurement development, the human papillomavirus vaccine, the theory of planned behavior, and college students (i.e., the intended audience)

### COGNITIVE INTERVIEWS

*Cognitive interviewing* involves collecting information about how participants respond to survey items (i.e., are the survey items generating the intended information?). In short, the objective of cognitive interviewing "is to reveal the thought process involved in interpreting a question and arriving at an answer. These thoughts are then analyzed to diagnose problems with the question" (Presser et al., 2004, p. 112). For example, do participants skip any questions, make any comments, ask any questions, provide incorrect information, hesitate, look confused, change their answers, etc.? In short, cognitive interviews can help you understand the survey from the respondent's perspective, which is particularly important

| TABLE 12.3    Common Cognitive Probes | |
|---|---|
| **Type of Probe** | **Example** |
| Comprehension | What does the phrase "fitness class" mean to you? |
| Paraphrasing | Can you repeat the question I just asked in your own words? |
| Confidence | How sure are you that you took _____ fitness classes at the Sun Devil Fitness Center in the past seven days? |
| Recall | How do you remember that you took _____ fitness classes at the Sun Devil Fitness Center in the past seven days? |
| Specific | Why do you think that _____ is an advantage of taking fitness classes at the Sun Devil Fitness Center? |
| General | How did you arrive at that answer? Was the question easy or hard to answer? I notice that you hesitated when answering the question. Can you tell me what you were thinking? |

Adapted from Willis (1999).

when planning and evaluating public health communication interventions for new topics or intended audiences.

Cognitive interviews can follow a variety of formats (Beatty & Willis, 2007; Dillman et al., 2014; Presser et al., 2004; Willis, 1999). The *"think aloud" technique* asks participants to verbally express their thought process while responding to each item, so the survey designer can better understand the processes participants used to arrive at an answer. Alternatively, the *verbal probing technique* asks participants to read and respond to the item(s), and then asking follow-up probes about each question and the answer given. Examples of common cognitive probes are provided in Table 12.3.

It is also worth noting that the "think aloud" technique is a current technique as it asks respondents to provide a verbal account of their thought process in real time (i.e., as they are answering each question). The verbal probing technique can be done either concurrently (i.e., as the participant answers each question) or retrospectively (i.e., after the participant responds to all questions). However, as Willis (1999) notes, when using the retrospective technique there is "a significant danger that subjects may no longer remember what they were thinking as they answered a question, and will instead fabricate an explanation" (p. 7).

## PILOT TESTS

As a reminder, a *pilot test* is small-scale investigation designed to try out part of an intervention (including the survey used to evaluate it) before it is fully implemented on a larger scale. Also, as a reminder, pilot testing usually takes part during the formative evaluation stages or phases of the planning process. A pilot test is a useful way to identify potentially problematic survey items or procedures. For example, a pilot test can provide guidance for selecting reliable and valid items for the final survey. Also, for example, a pilot test can provide insight into completion times, response rates, variable distributions, and how well the study procedures work in practice (Dillman et al., 2014). Finally, if there are any questions or concerns regarding how item wording, order, response options, or formatting might impact participants' responses, it may be worthwhile to conduct a small experiment (see Chapter 13) to determine the effects of different options and to select the option that works best.

## CONCLUSION

The primary goals of this chapter were to demonstrate how survey items and procedures can impact non-response and measurement error, and to provide some practical recommendations to minimize the likelihood that such errors will occur. Survey research plays a prominent role during both the formative and outcome evaluation stages of public health communication interventions. Thus, it is essential that all items and procedures be developed with care. This includes selecting the appropriate procedures for your topic and intended audience, following best practices for crafting good survey items, measuring all variables at the appropriate level of measurement, and using expert reviews, cognitive interviews, and pilot tests to evaluate survey procedures and items. In the end, and all other things being equal, the more carefully you craft your survey, the more confidence you will have in the decisions you make and the conclusions you draw from your data.

## REFERENCES

American Association for Public Opinion Research. (2015). *Standard definitions: Final dispositions of case codes and outcome rates for surveys* (8th ed.). Author.

Artino, A. R., Phillips, A. W., Utrankar, A., Ta, A. Q., & Durning, S. J. (2018). "The questions shape the answers": Assessing the quality of published survey instruments in health professions education research. *Academic Medicine, 93*, 456–463. https://doi.org/10.1097/ACM.0000000000002002

Babbie, E. (2010). *The practice of social research* (12th ed.). Wadsworth.

Beatty, P. C., & Willis, G. B. (2007). Research synthesis: The practice of cognitive interviewing. *Public Opinion Quarterly, 71*, 287–311. https://doi.org/10.1093/poq/nfm006

Blau, P. M. (1964). *Exchange and power in social life*. John Wiley.

Bocklisch, F., Bocklisch, S. F., & Krems, J. F. (2012). Sometimes, often, and always: Exploring the vague meanings of frequency expressions. *Behavior Research Methods, 44*, 144–157. https://doi.org/10.3758/s13428-011-0130-8

Dillman, D. A., Smyth, J. D., & Christian, L. M. (2014). *Internet, phone, mail, and mixed-mode surveys: The tailored design method* (4th ed.). Wiley.

Fishbein, M., & Ajzen, I. (2010). *Predicting and changing behavior: The reasoned action approach*. Psychology Press.

González, S. T., López, M. C. N., Marcos, Y. Q., & Rodríguez-Marín, J. (2012). Development and validation of the theory of planned behavior questionnaire in physical activity. *The Spanish Journal of Psychology, 15*(2), 801–816. https://doi.org/10.5209/rev_SJOP.2012.v15.n2.38892

Groves, R. M., Fowler, F. J., Jr., Couper, M. P., Lepkowski, J. M., Singer, E., & Tourangeau, R. (2009). *Survey methodology* (2nd ed.). John Wiley & Sons.

Hakel, M. D. (1968). How often is often? *American Psychologist, 23*(7), 533–534. https://doi.org/10.1037/h0037716

Hamby, T., & Peterson, R. A. (2016). A meta-analytic investigation of the relationship between scale-item length, label format, and reliability. *Methodology, 12*(3), 89–96. https://doi.org/10.1027/1614-2241/a000112

Homans, G. C. (1958). Social behavior as exchange. *American Journal of Sociology, 63*, 597–606. https://doi.org/10.1086/222355

Johnson, D. R., & Creech, J. C. (1983). Ordinal measures in multiple indicator models: A simulation study of categorization error. *American Sociological Review, 48*(3), 398–407. https://doi.org/10.2307/2095231

Lietz, P. (2010). Research into questionnaire design: A summary of the literature. *International Journal of Market Research, 52*(2), 249–272. https://doi.org/10.2501/S147078530920120X

Likert, R. (1932). A technique for the measurement of attitudes. *Archives of Psychology, 140*, 1–55.

Norman, G. (2010). Likert scales, levels of measurement and the "laws" of statistics. *Advances in Health Sciences Education, 15*(5), 625–632. https://doi.org/10.1007/s10459-010-9222-y

Osgood, C. E., Suci, G., & Tannenbaum, P. (1957). *The measurement of meaning*. University of Illinois Press.

Pace, C. R., & Friedlander, J. (1982). The meaning of response categories: How often is "occasionally," "often," and "very often"? *Research in Higher Education, 17*, 267–281. https://doi.org/10.1007/BF00976703

Presser, S., Couper, M. P., Lessler, J. T., Martin, E., Martin, J., Rothgeb, J. M., & Singer, E. (2004). Methods for testing and evaluating survey questions. *Public Opinion Quarterly, 68*(1), 109–130. https://doi.org/10.1093/poq/nfh008

Priest, H. M. (2015). *Development and validation of a theory of planned behavior-based instrument to predict human papillomavirus vaccination intentions of college males at a southeastern university* [Unpublished doctoral dissertation]. University of Alabama, Tuscaloosa.

Saris, W. E., & Gallhofer, I. (2007). Estimation of the effects of measurement characteristics on the quality of survey questions. *Survey Research Methods, 1*(1), 29–43. https://doi.org/10.18148/srm/2007.v1i1.49

Schwarz, N. (1999). Self-reports: How the questions shape the answers. *American Psychologist, 54*(2), 93–105. https://doi.org/10.1037/0003-066X.54.2.93

Simpson, R. H. (1944). The specific meanings of certain terms indicating differing degrees of frequency. *Quarterly Journal of Speech, 30*, 328–330. https://doi.org/10.1080/00335634409381009

Singer, E., & Ye, C. (2013). The use and effects of incentives in surveys. *The ANNALS of the American Academy of Political and Social Science, 645*(1), 112–141. https://doi.org/10.1177/0002716212458082

Smyth, J. D., Dillman, D. A., & Christian, L. M. (2007). Context effects in internet surveys. In A. Joinson, K. McKenna, T. Postmes, & U. Reips (Eds.), *The Oxford handbook of Iiternet psychology* (pp. 430–445). Oxford University Press.

Stevens, S. S. (1958). Problems and methods of psycho-physics. *Psychological Bulletin, 55*(4), 177–196. https://doi.org/10.1037/h0044251

Sullivan, G. M., & Artino, A. R., Jr. (2013). Analyzing and interpreting data from Likert-type scales. *Journal of Graduate Medical Education, 5*(4), 541–542. https://doi.org/ 10.4300/JGME-5-4-18

Thibaut, J. W., & Kelley, H. H. (1959). *The social psychology of groups.* John Wiley.

Tourangeau, R., Rips, L. J., & Rasinski, K. (2000). *The psychology of survey response.* Cambridge University Press.

Uebersax, J. S. (2006). *Likert scales: Dispelling the confusion.* John Uebersax PhD. http://john-uebersax.com/stat/likert.htm

Weisberg, H. F. (2005). *The total survey error approach: A guide to the new science of survey research.* University of Chicago Press.

Willis, G. B. (1999). *Cognitive interviewing: A "how to" guide.* Research Triangle Institute.

Zumbo, B. D., & Zimmerman, D. W. (1993). Is the selection of statistical methods governed by level of measurement? *Canadian Psychology, 34(4),* 390–400. https://doi.org/10.1037/h0078865

## CHAPTER 13

# Practical Experimental Design

## Chapter Outline

## INTRODUCTION

This chapter focuses on *outcome evaluation*, which is used to assess whether or not an intervention met its goals and objectives. To illustrate, public health communication experts often develop message strategies based on one or more of the theories discussed in Chapters 6 through 10 to change an intended audiences' beliefs, attitudes, and behaviors regarding an important health issue. Then, they implement the intervention, or show their message(s) to members of the intended audience. Finally, they assess, or evaluate, what effect the intervention had on these individuals via experiments. In short, the main goal of outcome evaluation is to establish a cause-effect relationship between your intervention and changes in the intended audience. This can only be accomplished via a strong experimental or quasi-experimental design.

### INDEPENDENT AND DEPENDENT VARIABLES

*Experiments* are used to identify cause-effect relationships between independent and dependent variables. An *independent variable* is the variable you have control over and can change in an experiment. A *dependent variable* is a variable that is dependent on, or is caused by, another variable (i.e., the independent variable). In short, the independent variable would be the cause and the dependent variable would be the effect in a cause-effect relationship. For example, imagine you were asked to develop a health communication intervention to increase exercise behavior among college students. In this instance, the intervention would be the independent variable and exercise behavior would be the dependent variable because the intervention is being designed to cause changes in exercise behavior. You might also track the effects of your independent variable on other dependent variables such as beliefs, attitude, and intention, just to name a few of the many possible dependent variables public health communication interventions might attempt to change (see Chapters 6 through 10).

## THREE WAYS TO GAIN CONTROL IN EXPERIMENTS

The goal of outcome evaluation in general, and experiments in particular, is to be able to confidently state that any observed changes in the dependent variable were caused by the independent variable and not something else. But anything that happens during an experiment represents a possible alternative explanation for the cause-effect relationship you wish to test. Thus, in the realm of practical experimental design, *control* means (1) taking steps to minimize or prevent potential alternative explanations, or (2) including design features that allow you to estimate or rule out plausible alternative explanations. In other words, it is important to do everything you can to prevent variables other than the independent variable from causing changes in the dependent variable. For example, participants in all groups should be similar to each other and be treated the same as each other in all important ways other than your independent variable. In addition, you might want to sequester participants to prevent outside events from causing changes in the dependent variable. Alternatively, you can keep your procedures short to prevent changes in participants that occur naturally over time from causing changes in the dependent variable.

Unfortunately, researchers may not have as much control over the situation or environment in a field setting, so it is especially important that they identify relevant threats and rule them out using various design features. For example, using a control group, a pretest, and randomization are important design features that help assess or rule out many common plausible alternative explanations. There are three ways to gain control in an experiment to help determine if a relationship is indeed causal: (1) manipulating exposure to the independent variable, (2) ruling out initial differences between groups, and (3) minimizing or preventing the effects of extraneous variables (Cook & Campbell, 1979; Frey et al., 2000). A discussion of each follows.

### *Manipulating Exposure to the Independent Variable: Experimental and Control Groups*

The first way a researcher can exercise control in experiments is by manipulating exposure to the independent variable (i.e., they control who is exposed to the independent variable and who is not). For example, to determine if your intervention to increase exercise behavior among college students worked, you might randomly divide your sample of college students into two groups: one that is exposed to the intervention and one that is not. If the intervention worked, you would expect those who were exposed to the intervention to exercise more in the future than those who were not. In experiments, each of these groups, or conditions, has a name. The *experimental or treatment group* includes the individuals that are exposed to the independent variable (in this case the intervention), while the *control group* consists of the individuals that are not exposed to the independent variable. The main purpose of a control group is to provide reliable baseline data to which the experimental group data can be compared.

Sometimes you may also want to include a comparison group in your evaluation design, either instead of or in addition to a control group. A *comparison group* is a group that receives a different level of your independent variable (i.e., a different intervention) rather than no intervention. For example, you may not only want to know if your intervention works (i.e., versus a no intervention control group), but also know how well it works compared to another intervention (i.e., versus a comparison group exposed to a different intervention). To keep things simple, we will use control groups for most of the examples discussed in this chapter. But you could easily add a comparison group, or replace the control group with a comparison group, in all the relevant examples and designs discussed below (and a few examples will be presented in the Collecting Data from Additional Groups or at Additional Points in Time section toward the end of this chapter).

### Ruling Out Initial Differences Between Groups: Pretests and Randomization

A second way a researcher can exercise control in experiments is by ruling out initial differences between groups to make sure the groups were similar at the start of the experiment. To continue with our exercise intervention example, suppose that instead of randomly assigning participants to groups, a researcher compared students recruited from the student recreation center who were exposed to the program (the experimental group), to students recruited from the student center who were not shown the program (the control group). This would clearly not be a fair comparison as people recruited at the student recreation center are probably more likely to exercise than those recruited at the student center to begin with. In this case any observed differences in the dependent variables are likely the result of initial difference between the groups, and not to students' exposure to the exercise intervention. So, how do you assess or rule out initial differences between groups? Fortunately, there are at least two ways to do this: pretesting and randomization.

**Pretesting.** A *pretest* measures the dependent variable in all groups before exposing the experimental group to the independent variable. In our example, you might ask participants how much they currently exercise, their current weight and height, and how they feel about exercise before the intervention is implemented. This way the researcher can assess how similar or different the groups are at the start of the experiment.

**Randomization.** Another way to rule out initial differences between groups is with randomization. *Randomization,* or *random assignment,* means that each participant has an equal chance of being assigned to each condition in an experiment. Randomization could be as complex as using a computerized random number generator, or as simple as asking each participant to flip a coin when they arrive and randomly assigning those that came up heads to the experimental group and tails to the control group (or vice versa). In theory (especially with a large enough sample), randomization should minimize or eliminate the likelihood of initial differences between groups. However, if doubts remain, the researcher can and should still include a pretest in the study.

### Minimizing or Preventing the Effects of Extraneous Variables: Internal Validity

A third way researchers exercise control in experiments is by minimizing or preventing the effects of extraneous variables (Campbell & Stanley, 1963; Cook & Campbell, 1979; Shadish et al., 2002). *Extraneous variables* are those besides your independent variable that might also influence the dependent variable. Extraneous variables are problematic as they negatively impact *internal validity*, or your ability to draw accurate conclusions about the cause-and-effect relationship under investigation. In other words, were changes in your dependent variable really caused by your independent variable, or could they have been caused by something else? There are several categories of extraneous variables that are common and worrisome enough that you must be especially careful about them when designing an experiment. A discussion of each of these extraneous variables, or alternative explanations, follows.

Seven basic threats to internal validity have been identified: selection, attrition, regression, history, maturation, testing, and instrumentation. These seven basic threats can be classified in a couple of different ways to help make them easier to remember. For example, Trochim (2001) identifies the first one—selection—as a threat in multiple group designs, and that the other six—attrition, regression, history, maturation, testing, and instrumentation—as threats in single group designs. That is not to say these latter six alternative explanations cannot occur in multiple-group designs, but most of the multiple-group designs discussed below control for these threats by adding one or more design elements that allow you to estimate or rule out these alternative explanations (whereas single-group designs do not allow you to estimate or rule out such threats).

Craig and Hannum (2007) place these seven basic threats into three general categories (which will be used to guide the discussion of these seven threats below). The first three threats to internal validity—selection, attrition, and regression—all concern factors that make it look like the dependent variable changed, when in fact it did not; or vice versa. The next two threats—history and maturation—both concern actual changes in the dependent variable that are not caused by the independent variable (i.e., the change is caused by something other than the independent variable). The final two threats—testing and instrumentation—both concern problems associated with measuring the dependent variable. Table 13.1 provides a definition for these threats to internal validity, and a detailed discussion of each threat is provided next.

| TABLE 13.1    Threats to Internal Validity | |
|---|---|
| **Threat** | **Definition** |
| Selection | When initial differences between participants in the experimental and control groups cause differences or changes in the dependent variable. |
| Attrition (Mortality) | When the number or characteristics of participants that drop out of the study cause differences or changes in the dependent variable. |
| Regression to the Mean | When random variance from participants selected based on extreme scores causes differences or changes in the dependent variable. |
| History | When events outside the study cause differences or changes in the dependent variable. |
| Maturation | When physiological or psychological changes in participants that occur naturally over time cause differences or changes in the dependent variable. |
| Testing | When earlier measurements of the dependent variable (i.e., a pretest) cause differences or changes to a later measurement of the dependent variable (i.e., the posttest). |
| Instrumentation | When modifications in how the dependent variable is measured cause differences or changes in the dependent variable. |
| Additive or Interaction Effects | When the impact of multiple threats can be added together (additive effects); or when the effects of one threat depend on the level of another threat (interaction effects). |

## Systematic Differences Between Experimental and Control Groups

*Selection.* Any time you have more than one group in your experiment, such as an experimental and control group, you need to be concerned about the selection threat. A *selection threat* to internal validity occurs when initial differences between participants in the experimental and control groups causes differences or changes in your dependent variable. In other words, groups that are different in ways related to your dependent variable at the beginning of your study are also likely to be different at the end of the study for reasons unrelated to your independent variable. I have already introduced one example of a selection threat to internal validity above, when I talked about assigning students to condition based on location (i.e., students recruited from the student recreation center were assigned to the experimental group and students recruited from the student center were assigned to the control group). That is, it is plausible that students recruited at the student recreation center will exercise more than students recruited from the student center even in the absence of an intervention. As a result, attributing any observed differences to the intervention is problematic.

A selection threat also exists whenever researchers allow participants to self-select into groups. In these and similar instances the question becomes, were differences in exercise behavior (your dependent variable) caused by your intervention (your independent variable) or by how participants were assigned to, or selected for, groups (the extraneous variable)?

Using an experimental design with proper randomization to conditions is the best defense against the selection threat to internal validity. Thus, selection is always a concern for quasi-experimental designs (and especially nonexperimental designs) with multiple groups since participants in such studies are not randomly assigned to conditions. Pretests make it possible to estimate the likelihood of a selection threat for all measured variables, but it is always possible that participants in non-randomized groups differ in some unforeseen but important way. In short, when conducting an experiment, it is important to randomly assign participants to conditions whenever possible, and to use a pretest when random assignment to conditions is not possible.

*Attrition.* An *attrition threat* to internal validity occurs when the number or characteristics of participants that drop out of the study cause differences or changes in the dependent variable. When conducting an experiment, it is common for some participants to drop out before the study is completed. Attrition represents a potential threat to internal validity when those who drop out of the study are systematically different from those who do not.

In the single group designs, the concern is that those who drop out of the study differ from those who remain in a way that is systematically related to the dependent variable. For example, if only those who regularly exercised stayed in the study, and those who did not regularly exercise dropped out, it might appear as though your intervention caused participants to exercise more. However, had those who did not regularly exercise remained in the study, the results would have looked very different.

In a multiple-group design the concern is that groups that were the same at the beginning of a study will end up being different at the end of the study for reasons unrelated to your independent variable. For example, imagine the experimental condition in our exercise promotion intervention involved three mandatory exercise sessions designed to demonstrate some effective exercise routines. Imagine further that the least physically fit individuals in the experimental group dropped out of the study (leaving only the most physically fit individuals left in the experimental group to complete the posttest at the end of the study). If the individuals remaining in the experimental group outperformed the individuals in the control group on your dependent measures at the posttest, you might conclude that your intervention was successful. However, this would be a faulty conclusion as the difference was really caused by systematic and differential attrition in the experimental group (i.e., the average score of the remaining participants in the experimental group was higher than it otherwise might have been had those who dropped out also completed the study). Whenever you experience a substantial loss of participants in an experiment, especially a differential loss of participants from the experimental and control groups, you need to be wary of the attrition threat to internal validity.

The best defenses against an attrition threat to internal validity involve keeping procedures short (so there is little reason or opportunity for participants to drop out) and offering financial or other incentives (so participants are motivated to complete the study). Also, attrition is less of a concern when participants drop out of the study for non-systematic reasons, or when dropout rates across conditions are comparable. Thus, designs that include a pretest can help estimate the extent to which attrition might be a threat, as it allows you to compare pretest scores for individuals who did and did not remain in the study.

*Regression.* A *regression*, or *regression to the mean*, threat to internal validity occurs when random variance in participants selected based on extreme scores causes differences or changes in the dependent variable. Regression to the mean is likely to occur when you select participants based on extreme scores (i.e., people who score particularly high or low on some measure administered before the study). And the more extreme the scores, the more likely these scores are to move (or regress) toward the mean when they are measured a second time. Put somewhat differently, when participants are selected based on extremely high or low scores, they will naturally score closer to the mean when they are measured a second time even in the absence of a public health communication intervention. Trochim (2001) refers to this as the "you can only go up (or down) from here phenomenon" (p. 177). That is, when participants are selected based on extreme scores, they can only stay the same or improve; they cannot get worse.

For example, imagine weight loss is a dependent variable for our exercise promotion intervention. A researcher might be tempted to study students reporting that their weight recently reached a new high in hopes of halting or reversing this trend. Alternatively, students may sign up for (or self-select into) your exercise promotion study when their weight is at its peak, such as after gaining weight over the holidays. In both cases, participating students may lose some weight over time for reasons that have nothing to do with the exercise promotion intervention, and more to do with the natural tendency for weight to fluctuate on its own over time.

The best way to prevent or reduce regression to the mean is to not select or assign participants to conditions based on extreme scores. However, what if selecting participants based on extreme scores is an integral part of the intervention? For example, students who are the most overweight or who exercise the least may be your intended audience. In this case it is important to first recruit many individuals with extreme scores, and then to randomly assign these individuals to your experimental and control conditions. That way, if regression to the mean does occur, it should occur equally for each group. Another option is to conduct two pretest measurements, and then select participants based on either the mean of both measurements or the second measurement. As Barnett et al., (2005) note, "this method can be thought of as an attempt to get a better estimate of each subject's true mean before the intervention" (p. 218).

### Changes in the Dependent Variable That Are Not Caused by the Independent Variable

*History.* A *history threat* to internal validity is when events outside the study causes differences or changes in the dependent variable. For example, suppose the student health center happens to sponsor a highly regarded motivational speaker to talk about the importance of exercise while you are conducting your experiment. It is quite possible that any changes in the dependent variable were caused by this motivational speaker and not your intervention. Without a strong experimental design, it would be impossible to parcel out the effects of your independent variable and the history threat.

Keeping your study short or sequestering your participants during the study are two good ways to minimize or eliminate the likelihood that a history threat will occur. Both options will often be possible when studying the short-term effects of a public health communication intervention under more controlled circumstances. However, neither is usually a viable option in field experiments designed to assess long-term effects of larger interventions. For example, if the message is short enough (say a pamphlet that takes 15 minutes to read, a video that takes 25 minutes to watch, or a presentation that takes one hour to attend), it will often be possible to randomly divide individuals into two groups, give the experimental group the message in one room, not give the control group the message in another room, and then administer the posttest to both groups. Under such circumstances, outside events are less likely to occur (i.e., because your procedures were so short), and even if any events do occur, they are unlikely to impact your participants (i.e., because participants were sequestered and therefore not exposed to such events until after the experiment is over).

Unfortunately, neither of these precautions will be possible in field experiments designed to assess the long-term effects of an intervention. For example, the effects of some campaigns may be assessed over a few months to several years (Snyder & Hamilton, 2002), so they are not short by definition. Further, it is usually impractical or impossible to sequester participants for such a long period of time. While it may not be possible to prevent participants from being exposed to outside events under such circumstances, a strong experimental design will still allow you to rule out or estimate the effects of any events that do occur. For example, if an outside event does occur, it should similarly affect both the experimental and control group. For this to be true, however, it is important to recruit participants from the same areas, and to administer the pretests and posttest to both groups at the same time. Finally, it is always a good idea to keep track of and document outside events that could influence participants during the study (Shadish et al., 2002).

*Maturation.* A *maturation threat* to internal validity is when psychological or physiological changes in participants that occur naturally over time causes differences or changes in the dependent variable. For example, as people age (or mature), they naturally gain more knowledge, wisdom, and experience, which can cause changes in your dependent variable. Further, as people age, muscle-to-fat ratios change, as do metabolism rates. Thus, experiments evaluating interventions for children need to be especially concerned about the maturation threat to internal validity since children naturally change so rapidly over time. Similarly, if your study was conducted over a long period of time (such as over four years of college), it would be reasonable to expect all sorts of psychological and physiological changes in your participants that were not due to your intervention. For example, most students gain some weight during their four years of college (Lloyd-Richardson et al., 2009). Thus, a poor experimental design may make it seem like your intervention failed (i.e., as though people gained rather than lost weight). However, a strong experimental design might tell a very different story. That is, while everyone in the study may indeed have gained weight (the maturation threat), those individuals exposed to your intervention may have gained less weight than those who were not.

Fortunately, many of the precautions used to protect against a history threat to internal validity also work for the maturation threat. For example, keeping the experiment short can minimize or eliminate the likelihood of a maturation threat. Also, if you have a good reason to expect maturation may be an issue, you could take the extra precautions to make sure that participants in the experimental and control groups are the same age or maturation status at the start of the study so that they will be similarly affected by naturally occurring changes during the study. As always, a strong experimental design will allow you to estimate or rule out the possibility of a maturation threat to internal validity.

## Problems Associated With Measurement of the Dependent Variable

*Testing.* A *testing threat* to internal validity occurs when earlier measurements of the dependent variable (i.e., a pretest) causes differences or changes to a later measurement of the dependent variable (i.e., the posttest). As Campbell and Stanley (1963) note, "it has long been a truism in the social sciences that the process of measuring may change that which is being measured" (p. 9). A testing threat can manifest in a few different ways. First, a pretest might sensitize participants to the behavior being investigated (i.e., exercise), and might cause them to behave differently in the future. That is, simply asking participants questions about exercise might cause participants to think about exercise differently or to exercise more than they otherwise might.  For example, if weight loss is a dependent variable in our exercise promotion intervention, the initial weigh-in might be the stimulus for weight reduction even in the absence of the independent variable (Campbell & Stanley, 1963). Second, the pretest might cue participants to pay more attention to certain parts of the public health communication message than they would have otherwise (causing the message to have a greater effect than it otherwise might). Finally, one should be particularly concerned about a testing threat any time knowledge or skills are being assessed (two key dependent variables for many public health communication interventions). As the old saying goes, "practice makes perfect"; and, it is not unreasonable to suspect that the pretest practice might help perfect the posttest scores.

As noted earlier, a pretest represents one key we measure and control for initial differences between groups, so any time you use a pretest you need to make sure you use a strong experimental design that controls for this threat to internal validity. Another way to help reduce the possibility of a testing threat is to increase the amount of time between the pretest and the posttest. However, this may come at the cost of increasing the likelihood of the attrition, history, and maturation threats.

*Instrumentation.* An *instrumentation* threat to internal validity is when changes in how the dependent variable is measured causes differences or changes in the dependent variable. Such change can be intentional or unintentional. For example, when knowledge is a dependent variable, a researcher may intentionally decide not to use the exact same items on the pretest and the posttest (to avoid a testing threat, for example).  Instead, alternate forms of the test are typically designed to be equivalent but not identical. In such cases, the presence or extent of an instrumentation threat depends on how successful the researcher is at creating equivalent alternative measures of the dependent variable. Other times such changes are unintentional. For example, when measuring weight, a scale may be incorrectly or differentially calibrated at the pretest or the posttest (or for the experimental or control group). Also, for example, perhaps scores on the dependent variable involve subjective grading or coding. Using different coders at different points in time could result in an instrumentation threat if all coders are not very carefully and similarly trained. Even when using the same coders throughout a study, however, one can easily imagine them getting more tired, bored, or careless (or more skilled, proficient, or experienced) as time passes. Each of these possibilities represents a potential instrumentation threat to internal validity.

The best way to prevent the possibility of an instrumentation threat is to avoid changing a measure during a study. If changes are required, it is important to do extensive pilot testing to make sure the alternative forms are, in fact, equivalent. Also, when possible, it is worth retaining both the original and new items to calibrate one against the other (Shadish et al., 2002). When using coders, adopt procedures (such as keeping coding sessions short) that minimize the likelihood that they will get tired, bored, or careless. Campbell and Stanley (1963) suggest using a control technique, such as shuffling all pretest and posttest measures together and coding everything at the same time. Finally, when the dependent measures involve things like measuring weight with scales, time with stopwatches, etc., it is important to make sure such instruments are properly calibrated at the start of each session (and to double check that they remain so at the end of each session).

### Additive or Interaction Effects of Threats to Internal Validity

Up to this point, the discussion has focused on the individual effects of seven basic threats to internal validity. Sometimes, however, each of these basic threats may be added to or interact with one or more of the other basic threats to produce a more complex threat. For example, *additive effects*, or *main effects*, occur when the impact of two or more threats can be aggregated together (i.e., they combine additively). For example, participants in an experiment might both be exposed to some outside event (a history threat) and change naturally over time (a maturation threat). The combined effects are additive when the impact of each threat is independent and not affected by the level of another threat.

*Interaction effects*, on the other hand, occur when the impact of one threat depends on the level of another threat (i.e., they combine multiplicatively). While it is possible for any of the basic threats to internal validity to interact with each other, most of the time we are concerned about interactions between selection and one of the other basic threats (Cook & Campbell, 1979; Shadish et al., 2002; Trochim, 2002).

For example, a *selection-history interaction* occurs when nonequivalent groups formed at the start of experiment (selection threat) are also exposed to different outside events during the experiment (history threat). As we have already seen, we would have a selection threat if students recruited from the student recreation center were assigned to the experimental group, and students recruited from the student center were assigned to the control group. Also, we would have a history threat if the student health center hired a motivational speaker to talk about the importance of exercise during your experiment. However, suppose the motivational speaker spoke at the student recreation center. In this case, only the experimental group will experience the history threat (i.e., whether or not a participant is exposed to the history threat depends on what group they are in).

## Summary

In sum, strong experimental designs manipulate exposure to the independent variable, rule out initial differences between groups, and control for the effects of extraneous variables (i.e., threats to internal validity). The next section in this chapter will review three categories of research designs: nonexperimental designs, full experimental designs, and quasi-experimental designs.

## RESEARCH DESIGNS

A *research design* provides a detailed description of how a study will be conducted to answer a research question as clearly as possible (de Vaus, 2001). When conducting an outcome evaluation, the question we want to answer is: Did the independent variable (i.e., your intervention) cause changes in the dependent variable(s) (i.e., beliefs, attitude, intention, and behavior)? As the preceding discussion on internal validity illustrates, answering this question is no easy task as many factors besides an independent variable can also cause changes in a dependent variable. Thus, the goal of experimental research design is to gather information in such a way that any changes in the dependent variable can be confidently attributed to your intervention. This is achieved using the various design features introduced earlier in this chapter to prevent, minimize, or estimate plausible alternative explanations.

The remainder of this chapter focuses on three categories of designs: (1) nonexperimental, (2) experimental, and (3) quasi-experimental. Nonexperimental designs are offer few protections against incorrect causal inferences. However, they offer a useful point of reference for discussing the other designs reviewed in this chapter and can provide other useful information under certain circumstances (Hornik, 2002). For example, they can let you know if results are consistent with expectations, if recalled exposure to the independent variable is associated with the dependent variables, etc. Answers to these and similar questions can be indicative of success, but they do not provide the information necessary to make strong causal inferences. Experimental designs, which randomly assign participants to conditions, are considered the gold standard for evaluation research as they remove many sources of bias from the research process (Shadish & Ragsdale, 1996; Shadish et al., 2002; Shadish et al., 2008). Unfortunately, random assignment to conditions is not always possible, in which case evaluators can turn to quasi-experimental designs (which typically lack random assignment to conditions or some other feature of an experimental design).

Quasi-experimental designs have some potential limitations (i.e., selection, and interactions between selection and the other threats to internal validity). However, research indicates that "studies using nonrandom assignment may produce acceptable approximations to results from randomized experiments under some circumstances" (Shadish & Ragsdale, 1996, p. 1290). These circumstances will be discussed in more detail when we review quasi-experimental designs toward the end of this chapter.

All the research designs discussed in the chapter are also included in Table 13.2. Here is a description of each notation included in these designs:

- ▶ X indicates exposure the independent variable. This distinguishes between an experimental group that is exposed to an independent variable (X present) and the control group, which is not (X absent).

- ▶ O represents the observation of the dependent variable; or the pretest and/or posttest measures of the dependent variable (often a survey). The subscripts after the observations are used to note sequential order (e.g., observations marked $O_1$ happen at the same time and before anything marked $O_2$).

- ▶ NR indicates that participants were nonrandomly assigned to the experimental or control conditions. This is typically also accompanied by a dashed line (i.e., -----) to further indicate that the groups were nonrandomly formed.

- ▶ R indicates participants were randomly assigned to the experimental and control conditions.

Please keep this notation in mind as you read the following discussion on nonexperimental, experimental, and quasi-experimental designs.

## NONEXPERIMENTAL DESIGNS

*Nonexperimental designs* (sometimes called *pre-experimental designs*) lack most or all of the design features necessary to gain control in an experiment. For example, nonexperimental designs may lack a control group (i.e., they do not manipulate exposure to the independent variable), or they may include a control group but provide no way to rule out initial differences between groups (i.e., there is no randomization or pretesting). Thus, nonexperimental designs offer few protections against the major threats to internal validity, and therefore do not allow you to confidently draw conclusions about a cause-effect relationship between the independent and dependent variables. Thus, they should be avoided when strong causal inference is necessary. With this in mind, consider the following three nonexperimental designs.

| TABLE 13.2 | Nonexperimental, Quasi-Experimental, and Experimental Designs [1,2] |
|---|---|

**Nonexperimental Designs**

      Design A:  One-Group Posttest-Only Design

$$X \qquad O_1$$

      Design B:  One-Group Pretest-Posttest Design

$$O_1 \qquad X \qquad O_2$$

      Design C:  Posttest-Only Control-Group Design Without Random Assignment

$$NR \qquad X \qquad O_1$$
$$\text{----------}$$
$$NR \qquad\qquad O_1$$

**Experimental Designs**

      Design D:  Posttest-Only Control-Group Design With Random Assignment

$$R \qquad X \qquad O_1$$
$$R \qquad\qquad O_1$$

      Design E:  Pretest-Posttest Control-Group Design With Random Assignment

$$R \qquad O_1 \qquad X \qquad O_2$$
$$R \qquad O_1 \qquad X \qquad O_2$$

      Design F:  Factorial Design With Random Assignment

$$R \qquad X_{A1B1} \qquad O_1$$
$$R \qquad X_{A1B2} \qquad O_1$$
$$R \qquad X_{A2B1} \qquad O_1$$
$$R \qquad X_{A2B2} \qquad O_1$$

**Quasi-Experimental Designs**

      Design G: Pretest-Posttest Control-Group Design Without Random Assignment

$$NR \qquad O_1 \qquad X \qquad O_2$$
$$\text{------------------}$$
$$NR \qquad O_1 \qquad\qquad O_2$$

      Design H: Interrupted Time Series Design With a Nonequivalent Control Group

$$NR \qquad O_1 \quad O_2 \quad O_3 \ X \ O_4 \quad O_5 \quad O_6$$
$$\text{------------------------------}$$
$$NR \qquad O_1 \quad O_2 \quad O_3 \qquad O_4 \quad O_5 \quad O_6$$

      Design I:  Separate-Sample Pretest-Posttest Design With Random Assignment

$$R \qquad O_1 \qquad (X)$$
$$R \qquad\qquad X \qquad O_2$$

[1] NR = nonrandom assignment; R = random assignment; O = observation (i.e., the posttests and/or pretests); X = independent variable (e.g., public health communication intervention)

[2] All designs originally presented in Campbell and Stanley (1963), Cook and Campbell (1979), or Shadish et al. (2002).

### One-Group Posttest-Only Design

The posttest-only design has one group of participants view an intervention (X), and then complete a posttest measuring the dependent variables under investigation ($O_1$). This non-experimental design is diagramed as follows:

#### Design A

One-Group Posttest-Only Design

$$X \quad O_1$$

Note that this design contains no comparison points (i.e., there is no pretest and no control group), so there is no way to know if any change occurred or what would have happened without the intervention. Further, nearly all the threats to internal validity potentially apply to this design (Shadish et al., 2002). Thus, it is not possible to conclude with any certainty that the independent variable caused changes to the dependent variable.

### One-Group Pretest-Posttest Design

The one-group pretest-posttest design has a single group of participants complete a pretest ($O_1$), view an intervention (X), and then complete a posttest ($O_2$). This nonexperimental design is diagramed as follows:

#### Design B

One-Group Pretest-Posttest Design

$$O_1 \quad X \quad O_2$$

The addition of a pretest represents a slight improvement over one-group posttest-only design (i.e., you can now compare scores on the pretest to scores on the posttest to see if there were any changes over time). Further, in my experience, some organizations are tempted to use this design as they are confident their intervention will work and do not want to prevent some participants from getting it by assigning them to a control group. However, this design does not rule out many different alternative explanations for any observed changes between the pretest and the posttest. Consequently, this design does not control for most major threats to internal validity.

### Posttest-Only Control-Group Design Without Random Assignment (a.k.a., Posttest-Only Control-Group Design With Nonequivalent Groups)

The posttest-only control-group design without random assignment typically incorporates two preexisting groups (i.e., two classrooms, two schools, two organizations, two cities, etc.) or people recruited via two different locations (i.e., the student center and the student recreation center). In other words, the two groups are nonrandomly (NR) formed or assigned. Then, the experimental group is shown the intervention (X present), while the control group is not shown the intervention (X absent). Finally, both groups complete the posttest measure of the dependent variables under investigation ($O_1$). This pre-experimental design is diagramed as follows:

**Design C**

Posttest-Only Control-Group Design Without Random Assignment

$$NR \quad X \quad O_1$$
$$\text{--------}$$
$$NR \qquad\quad O_1$$

However, the lack of a pretest means there is no way to know if the two groups were similar in important ways at the start of the experiment, and the lack of random assignment means it is not safe to assume that they were. For example, it is quite possible that the two groups were different in ways related to your dependent variable before the study began (i.e., body mass index, frequency of exercise, etc.). Therefore, any observed posttest differences may have already existed before the intervention and not have been caused by the independent variable (making selection a plausible threat to internal validity with this design).

As noted previously, selection may interact with any of the other six basic treats to internal validity. Further, since there is no way to know how similar or different the groups were before the intervention, there is no way to know for sure if the groups may have changed differently over time based on their initial composition. For example, a group of younger individuals may change at a different rate than a group of older individuals (representing a potential selection × maturation threat to internal validity). Similarly, groups recruited from different locations may be exposed to different outside events (representing a potential selection × history threat to internal validity).

In sum, these three nonexperimental designs provide little confidence that an intervention caused any observed changes in the dependent variables. Not only do these designs fail to control for the effects of important extraneous variables, Designs A and B do not manipulate exposure to the independent variable (i.e., everyone is exposed to the intervention and there is no control group), and Design C does not rule out initial differences between groups (i.e., there is no random assignment and no pretest). The full experimental designs discussed next represent significant improvements in these criteria.

## EXPERIMENTAL DESIGNS

*Experimental designs* have all of the features necessary to gain control in an experiment (i.e., a control group and randomization) and therefor control for all major threats to internal validity. Such designs are commonly referred to as "randomized control trials," and each of the three words in this phrase represents an important element of experimental design (Oakley, 2010, p. 918). *Randomized* means that participants are divided into groups by chance. For example, this means that everyone has an equal opportunity of being assigned to the experimental group or control group, and that neither the researcher nor the participants get to choose which individuals are placed in which group. Randomization is important because it increases the likelihood that variables related to the independent variable (i.e., *confounding variables*) are equally distributed across conditions, which allows you to rule them out as a plausible alternative explanation for your results. *Controlled* means one or more comparison groups are included to check one's inferences or conclusions (i.e., that the independent variable, and not something else, caused changes in the dependent variable). Finally, *trial* means the independent variable is being tested or judged to see if it is effective at causing changes in one or more dependent variables.

Randomized control trials are one of the most powerful tools for evaluating the effectiveness of public health communication interventions. Indeed, randomized control trials are considered the gold standard for assessing causal relationships as they give researchers a great deal of control over all aspects of the research design. For example, the only difference between Design C above and Design D below is that participants are randomly assigned to conditions. However, this is a very important difference. To illustrate, Design C is a weak nonexperimental design, whereas Design D is a strong experimental design. In sum, random assignment means that each participant has an equal chance of being assigned to each condition in an experiment and is an important method for ruling out initial differences between conditions and alternative explanations for your results.

### Posttest-Only Control-Group Design With Random Assignment

The most basic experimental design begins by randomly assigning (R) a pool of participants to conditions. Then, the experimental group is exposed to the intervention (X present), and the control group is not (X absent). Finally, both groups complete a posttest measuring the dependent variables under investigation at the end of the study ($O_1$). This experimental design is diagramed as follows:

**Design D**

Posttest-Only Control-Group Design with Random Assignment

$$R \quad X \quad O_1$$
$$R \quad \quad O_1$$

The primary threat to this design is attrition, so the lack of a pretest can be risky if there is any likelihood of attrition in your study (Shadish et al., 2002). No pretest means there is no way to determine if those who drop out of the study are systematically different from those who do not. No pretest also means there is no way to make sure that groups that were the same at the beginning of a study remained that way by the end of the study. As noted previously, keeping procedures short can reduce or eliminate attrition as it provides little reason or opportunity for participants to drop out. Therefore, this design will be most useful when pilot testing individual intervention components (i.e., when X and O are administered in single session over a short period of time). This design will be more problematic when conducting longitudinal experiments that takes place over weeks, months, or years as such studies provide greater opportunities for attrition.

Otherwise, this design controls for all other threats to internal validity. For example, if history or maturation do occur, they should affect both groups equally (and both are less likely to occur when procedures are kept short). Selection (and by extension interactions between selection and the other threats to validity) is controlled by randomly assigning participants to conditions. As Campbell and Stanley (1963) note, randomization is "the most adequate all-purpose assurance of lack of initial bias between groups" (p. 25). The lack of a pretest eliminates the testing threat to internal validity (i.e., there is no pretest to effect posttest scores). Also, given there is no pretest, this design is less likely to require participants selected based on extreme scores. However, even if participants are selected based on extreme scores using some other method besides a pretest, this design still controls for regression by randomly assigning individuals from the same extreme pool to the experimental and control conditions. As a result, if regression is causing changes to the dependent variable, both groups should regress equally. Finally, if the dependent variables are assessed using the same measures (i.e., the same survey) and using the precautions outlined earlier (i.e., proper training, consistent procedures, and regular calibration), the instrumentation threat can be ruled out; or should affect both groups similarly when it does occur.

## Pretest-Posttest Control-Group Design With Random Assignment

This design entails randomly assigning (R) a pool of participants to conditions, followed by a pretest measuring the dependent variables in each group at the start of the study ($O_1$).

Then, the intervention is shown to the experimental group (X present), but not to the control group (X absent). Finally, both groups complete a posttest measuring the dependent variables at the end of the study ($O_2$). This experimental design is diagramed as follows:

**Design E**

Pretest-Posttest Control-Group Design with Random Assignment

$$R \quad O_1 \quad X \quad O_2$$
$$R \quad O_1 \qquad\; O_2$$

The main advantage of Design E is that the included pretest allows you to assess the effects of attrition. Given that attrition will occur in most longitudinal studies, it is important to include a pretest when a study will take place over days, weeks, months, or years. This way you can check for systematic differences between individuals who drop out of the study and those who do not (both overall and in each condition).

The main reason for not including a pretest is that it can increase the likelihood of a testing threat to internal validity. Recall that a testing threat can be reduced by increasing the time between the pretest and the posttest, but this comes at the expense of increasing the likelihood of other threats to internal validity such as attrition, history, and maturation. These are just a few of the many tradeoffs one must consider in practical experimental design (i.e., the steps taken to reduce the likelihood of one threat often increase the likelihood of another threat).

Fortunately, this design controls for all seven threats by including design features that allow you to assess—and hopefully rule out—such plausible alternative explanations (i.e., they should affect the experimental and control groups similarly). However, it is better to take the necessary steps to prevent the most likely threats to internal validity beforehand than to realize there was a problem only after the fact. With this in mind, this design is most appropriate in longer-term studies where attrition is likely and is best avoided in short-term studies where there will be little to no attrition and a likely testing threat is present instead.

### Factorial Design With Random Assignment

One thing all the designs discussed so far have in common is that their goal is to assess the effects of a single independent variable on the dependent variable(s). Sometimes, however, you may want to assess the effects of more than one independent variable on a dependent variable, which brings us to a discussion on factorial designs.

*Factorial designs* are used when you want to study the effects of two or more independent variables on a dependent variable. For example, suppose you want to develop a way to help college students limit or reduce weight gain during their freshman year. One way to do this is to develop an intervention focusing on exercise. Another way to do this is to develop an intervention focusing on diet. You could try to determine the effects of each these interventions separately using any of the experimental designs described above. However, if you wanted to understand the combined effects of both the exercise intervention (your first independent variable) and the diet intervention (the second independent variable) on weight gain (your dependent variable) you would need to use a factorial design.

More specifically, this example represents a $2 \times 2$ factorial design (note that *factor* is just another word for independent variables in this instance). Each number in the design statement, regardless of what it is, represents an independent variable, and the actual number itself represents the number of levels or groups for that independent variable. Since there are two numbers, that means we have two independent variables (in this case, the exercise intervention and the diet intervention), and since both numbers are 2s, that means both independent variables have two levels or groups. In other words, some participants are exposed to the exercise intervention (group one for the first independent variable) and some are not (group two for the first independent variable); and some participants are exposed to the diet intervention (group one for the second independent variable), and some do not (group two for the second independent). Since these groups are crossed, that means we have four groups total (this is easy to remember because $2 \times 2 = 4$).

One way to illustrate this factorial design using our now familiar notation would look like this (where subscript A represents the exercise intervention, subscript B represents the diet intervention, subscript 1 represents that participants are exposed to the intervention, and subscript 0 represents that participants are not exposed to the intervention):

**Design F**

Factorial Design with Random Assignment

$$R \quad X_{A1B1} \quad O_1$$
$$R \quad X_{A1B0} \quad O_1$$
$$R \quad X_{A0B1} \quad O_1$$
$$R \quad X_{A0B0} \quad O_1$$

In other words, participants are first randomly assigned (R) to one of the four groups, making this a true experimental design. Then, each group is or is not exposed to each of the two independent variables as follows:

Group 1 ($X_{A1B1}$) views both the exercise intervention and the diet intervention,

Group 2 ($X_{A1B0}$) views just the exercise intervention and not the diet intervention,

Group 3 ($X_{A0B1}$) views just the diet intervention and not the exercise intervention,

Group 4 ($X_{A0B0}$) views neither the exercise intervention nor the diet intervention.

Finally, the posttest measures are completed ($O_1$). I know that is a lot to keep track of, and fortunately there is another, easier way to diagram this study:

|  | | Diet Intervention | |
|---|---|---|---|
|  | | **Yes** | **No** |
| **Exercise Intervention** | **Yes** | *Group 1:* Views both the exercise and diet interventions | *Group 2:* Views just the exercise intervention |
| | **No** | *Group 3:* Views just the diet intervention | *Group 4:* Views no intervention |

Factorial designs are especially powerful because they allow us to test main effects for each independent variable, as well as the interaction effect when two or more independent variables are combined (i.e., do two or more independent variables work together in a non-additive fashion). For example, a researcher might learn that both the exercise intervention and the diet intervention work well individually (main effects) by comparing Groups 2 and 4 and Groups 3 and 4, respectively. However, when combined (as is the case for Group 1 which received both the exercise and diet intervention) they have an interaction effect that is greater than either of the two main effects combined.

Keep in mind that this is the simplest of the factorial designs. Sometimes a study might have a 2 × 3 design. Since there are still two numbers in the design statement that means we still have two independent variables, and since one of the numbers is a "2" that means there are still two groups for that variable. But, since one of the numbers is now a "3" that means there are three groups for the second independent variable. Finally, since 2 × 3 = 6, we now have a total of six groups in the experiment. Alternatively, you might run into a 2 × 2 × 2 experiment, which simply tells you have three independent variables, each with two groups, which when crossed gives you eight groups total.

## QUASI-EXPERIMENTAL DESIGNS

Dictionary.com defines *quasi-* (2017) as "resembling" or "having some, but not all of the features of." Hence, quasi-experimental designs are similar to, but lack one or two important features of a true experimental design, such as random assignment or a control group. These are important omissions, so quasi-experimental should only be used when a true experimental design is not feasible (as will often be the case when evaluating public health communication interventions). Even then they must be used with caution and clearly reported as such. Despite their limitations, quasi-experimental designs are often used when evaluating public health communication interventions in the field as it is usually impossible or impractical to randomize individuals to conditions in such settings. However, this practical necessity makes quasi-experimental designs more susceptible to internal validity threats discussed earlier in this chapter (which can reduce the strength of the causal claims that can be made when using such designs).

There are three steps you can take to get more accurate results when using quasi-experimental designs (Baldwin & Berkeljon, 2010; Shadish et al., 2002; Shadish et al., 2008). First, you should not let participants self-select into experimental and control groups. Letting participants self-select into groups increases the likelihood of a selection a threat to internal validity; and the likelihood that selection will add to or interact with one or more of the other threats to internal validity (which can be difficult or impossible to detect). Therefore, quasi-experimental designs work best when the assignment of the intervention to one group or the other is random or under the experimenter's control. Second, you should include a pretest to assess the amount of selection bias that exists between the experimental and control groups. Third, you should treat the experimental and control groups the same in all other important ways. As much as possible, the only difference between the two conditions is that the experimental group is exposed to the independent variable while the control group is not. Otherwise, the procedures for the two groups should be identical as possible. This includes collecting data from all conditions at or around the same time and at the same or similar locations. In sum, while it can be more difficult to draw causal inferences when using the following quasi-experimental designs, careful planning and the addition of important design features can lead to designs that allow for stronger causal inference.

### *Pretest-Posttest Control-Group Design Without Random Assignment (a.k.a., Nonequivalent Control-Group Design)*

This design begins with two nonrandomly formed groups (NR); such as two classrooms, schools, organizations, etc. Then, both groups complete a pretest measuring the dependent and other important variables under investigation at the start of the study ($O_1$). Next, the intervention is shown to the treatment group (X present) but not to the control group (X absent). Finally, the same groups of individuals complete a posttest measuring the dependent variables at the end of the study ($O_2$). This quasi-experimental design is diagramed as follows:

**Design G**

Pretest-Posttest Control-Group Design without Random Assignment

$$NR \quad O_1 \quad X \quad O_2$$
$$\text{-------------}$$
$$NR \quad O_1 \quad\quad O_2$$

While this design does have some weaknesses, it is a commonly used and generally accepted option when a true experiment with random assignment is not possible (Cook & Campbell, 1979). This is because when following the three steps presented at the outset of this section (i.e., not letting participants self-select into groups, using a pretest, and treating both groups the same in all other important ways), this design controls for most of basic threats to internal validity introduced earlier in this chapter.

To illustrate, this design controls for history, maturation, testing, instrumentation. That is, if any of these threats were causing changes in the dependent variable, you would also see changes in the control group over time. As a result, if there are changes in the dependent variable between the pretest and posttest in the experimental group but not in the control group, you can generally rule out these threats to internal validity as an alternate explanation for your findings. Nor is regression a plausible threat if individuals are not selected—and especially not self-selected—into different conditions based on extreme scores.

The use of pretest also allows you to assess the amount and nature of attrition in each group. For example, you can track how many participants drop out (both overall and in each condition) and compare those who drop out to those who do not. Attrition represents less of a threat when few participants drop out, when there are no systematic differences between those who drop out and those who do, and when the number or type of individuals that do drop out are similar in each condition.

The main concern with this design is that since the groups are nonrandomly formed, they may not be similar at the start of the experiment (which you should recognize by now as a selection threat to internal validity). Comparing pretest scores allows you to estimate the size and direction of any bias on any measured variables. Unfortunately, since participants were not randomly assigned to groups, the possibility always exists that the two groups are different on some important but unmeasured variable(s). A related limitation of this design is that it does not control for interactions between selection and the other basic threats to internal validity. That is, when pretest differences exist, the possibility increases that selection will combine or interact with one or more other threats to internal validity.

In sum, under the right circumstances, the pretest-posttest control group design without random assignment can be an acceptable quasi-experimental and is the best alternative when a true experimental design is not possible. Below I introduce two additional quasi-experimental designs that might also come in handy from time to time and under certain circumstances.

### Interrupted Time Series Design With a Nonequivalent Control Group

The interrupted time series designs can take on many forms, the most basic of which looks like this (Shadish et al., 2002):

$$O_1 \quad O_2 \quad O_3 \quad O_4 \quad O_5 \quad X \quad O_6 \quad O_7 \quad O_8 \quad O_9 \quad O_{10}$$

As you can see, this design takes many observations from the same or a similar group of individuals both before ($O_{1-5}$) and after ($O_{6-10}$) an intervention (X). For example, you might track the number of fatal traffic crashes each month for 48 months before and 48 months after a new law banning texting while driving takes effect. If the law had an impact, the observations taken after it went into effect should differ from those taken before it went into effect.

Unfortunately, the basic time series design requires more data points than is typically practical when evaluating most public health communication interventions (Shadish et al., 2002). Fortunately, the addition of a control group greatly strengthens shorter time-series designs. Thus, this section focuses on the interrupted time-series design with a nonequivalent control group. This design is diagramed as follows:

**Design H**

Interrupted Time Series Design with a Nonequivalent Control Group

| NR | $O_1$ | $O_2$ | $O_3$ | X | $O_4$ | $O_5$ | $O_6$ |
|----|-------|-------|-------|---|-------|-------|-------|
| NR | $O_1$ | $O_2$ | $O_3$ |   | $O_4$ | $O_5$ | $O_6$ |

The interrupted time-series design with a nonequivalent control group begins with two non-randomly formed groups (NR); such as two classrooms, schools, organizations, cities, etc. Then, the same or similar participants from each group complete the pretest at multiple points in time ($O_{1-3}$). Next, the intervention is shown to the treatment group (X present) but not to the control group (X absent); ideally with X assigned randomly (Campbell

& Stanley, 1963). Finally, the same or similar participants from each group complete the posttest at multiple points in time ($O_{4-6}$).

Design H has much in common with Design G (i.e., the pretest-posttest control-group design without random assignment), but it offers some additional advantages. For example, the extra pretests allow you to assess whether the dependent variable naturally increases, decreases, or remain stable over time (e.g., due to maturation). Also, for example, the extra posttests allow you to assess when the effect occurs (i.e., is it immediate or delayed?) and how long it lasts (i.e., does it persist or decay over time?).

I will conclude this discussion on interrupted time series designs by noting that there are other, even stronger versions of this design. For example, consider the interrupted time series design with a nonequivalent control group and switching replications, which might look like this:

$$
\begin{array}{llllllll}
\text{NR} & O_1 & O_2 & \text{X} & O_3 & O_4 & O_5 & O_6 \\
\hline
\text{NR} & O_1 & O_2 & & O_3 & O_4 & \text{X} & O_5 & O_6
\end{array}
$$

This scenario also begins with two non-randomly formed groups (NR) where the same or similar participants from each group complete the pretest at multiple points in time ($O_{1-6}$). However, in this scenario, each group receives the intervention, and each group serves as the control group, at a different time. Those interested in learning more about the interrupted time series design with a nonequivalent control group and switching replications are referred to Palmgreen (2009), who provides an excellent illustration and discussion of this design in action.

### Separate-Sample Pretest-Posttest Design With Random Assignment

With this design, participants are randomly assigned to conditions (R). The control group completes the survey measuring the dependent variables before viewing to the intervention (indicated by the $O_1$ before the parenthetical X, which comes after and therefore should have no impact on this observation). The experimental group completes the survey measuring the dependent variables after viewing the intervention. This quasi-experimental design, where one group is measured before X and an equivalent group is measured after X, is diagramed as follows:

**Design I**

Separate-Sample Pretest-Posttest Design with Random Assignment

$$
\begin{array}{lll}
\text{R} & O_1 & \text{(X)} \\
\text{R} & & \text{X} & O_2
\end{array}
$$

To illustrate, random assignment to conditions can be accomplished by randomly distributing one of the two versions of the survey to participants in a large envelope (Roberto et al., 2000; Roberto et al., 2017). Participants are then instructed to take out and complete part one of the survey. After completing and placing part one of the survey back in the envelope, participants view the intervention. Then, participants are instructed to take out and complete part two of the survey.

While the procedures and surveys appear identical to participants for all practical purposes, each group is actually asked the questions in a different order. For the control group, the dependent variables are measured on part one, which they completed before viewing the intervention. Part two of the control group survey consists of demographic and filler items unrelated to the dependent variables. For the experimental group, the demographic and filler items are asked on part one of the survey. Part two of the experimental group survey measures the dependent variables under investigation, which they complete after viewing the video.

The major threats to internal validity for this design—history, maturation, and attrition—all have one thing in common; they are directly impacted by the length of the study (i.e., the longer the study, the more plausible history, maturation, and mortality become; and vice versa). With this in mind, this design is most appropriate for short-term studies where participants can be sequestered (i.e., when X and O are administered in single session) and should be avoided when conducting longitudinal studies. This design also controls for selection with random assignment, testing, and regression by not using a pretest (and therefore not selecting participants based on extreme pretest scores), and instrumentation when the appropriate protections are taken (i.e., proper training, consistent procedures, and regular calibration—all of which are less likely with a self-administered survey).

A few final notes about this design: First, there is a variation of this design without random assignment (i.e., the cohort control group design; Shadish et al., 2002). However, as you have probably already guessed, this variation is weaker in terms of selection (i.e., since groups are not randomly assigned to conditions and there is no pretest) and history (i.e., since data is collected from the different groups at different times). There are ways to improve the cohort control group design (e.g., by adding a pretest to both cohorts), but these are beyond the scope of this chapter. Second, I have seen the separate-sample pretest-posttest design with random assignment discussed as an experimental design (Kviz, 2020), likely because it includes random assignment to conditions. However, it was originally introduced as a quasi-experimental design (Campbell & Stanley, 1963), so I decided to treat it as such since it suffers from multiple threats to internal validity under all but the most controlled circumstances (which is not the case for the other experimental designs discussed in that section).

## CONCLUSION

In conclusion, practical experimental design is the key mechanism through which the impacts of public health communication interventions are evaluated. The two main goals of this chapter were to (1) identify the ways intervention evaluators gain control in experiments, and (2) to review a variety of practical experimental and quasi-experimental designs that allow evaluators to more confidently conclude whether an intervention caused the desired changes in the intended audience's beliefs, attitudes, intentions, or behavior. Whenever possible, intervention evaluators should use an experimental design with random assignment to conditions as this represents the best opportunity to rule out initial differences between the groups. Even when random assignment to conditions is possible, it may still be important to also include a pretest under certain circumstances, such as during longitudinal studies where attrition is likely. When random assignment to conditions is not possible, as will often be the case for evaluations taking place in a natural field setting, a pretest becomes necessary to assess, rule out, and potentially control for initial differences between groups.

## REFERENCES

Baldwin, S., & Berkeljon, A. (2010). Quasi-experimental design. N. J. Salkind (Ed.), *Encyclopedia of research design* (pp. 1171–1176). SAGE.

Barnett, A. G., van der Pols, J. C., & Dobson, A. J. (2005). Regression to the mean: What it is and how to deal with it. *International Journal of Epidemiology, 34*, 215–220. https://doi.org/10.1093/ije/dyh299

Campbell, D. T., & Stanley, J. C. (1963). *Experimental and quasi-experimental designs for research.* Houghton Mifflin.

Cook, T. D., & Campbell, D. T. (1979). *Quasi-experimentation: Design & analysis issues for field settings.* Houghton Mifflin.

Craig, S. B., & Hannum, K. M. (2007). Experimental and quasi-experimental evaluations. In K. M. Hannum, J. W. Martineau, & C. Reinelt (Eds.), *The handbook of leadership development evaluation* (pp. 19–47). John Wiley & Sons.

De Vaus, D. A. (2001). *Research design in social science.* SAGE.

Frey, L. R., Botan, C. H., & Kreps, G. L. (2000). *Investigating communication: An introduction to research methods* (2nd ed.). Needham Heights, MA: Allyn & Bacon.

Hornik, R. C. (2002). Epilog: Evaluation design for public health communicating programs. In R. C. Hornik (Ed.), *Public health communication: Evidence for behavior change* (pp. 385–405). Lawrence Erlbaum Associates.

Kviz, F. J. (2020). *Conducting health research: Principles, process, and methods.* SAGE.

Lloyd-Richardson, E. E., Bailey, S., Fava, J. L., & Wing, R. (2009). A prospective study of weight gain during the freshman and sophomore years. *Preventive Medicine, 48*, 256–261. https://doi.org/10.1016/j.ypmed.2008.12.009

Oakley, A. (2010). Randomized control trials. M. S. Lewis-Beck, A. Bryman, & T. F. Liao (Eds.), *The SAGE encyclopedia of social science research methods* (pp. 918–919). SAGE.

Palmgreen, P. (2009). Interrupted time-series designs for evaluating health communication campaigns. *Communication Methods and Measures, 3*, 29–46. https://doi.org/10.1080/19312450902809672

quasi-. (2012). Dictionary.com. http://www.dictionary.com/browse/quasi

Roberto, A. J., Eden, J., Deiss, D. M., Savage, M. W., & Ramos-Salazar, L. (2017). The short-term effects of a cyberbullying prevention intervention for parents of middle school students. *International Journal of Environmental Research and Public Health, 14*(9), 1–8. https://doi.org/10.3390/ijerph14091038

Roberto, A. J., Meyer, G., Johnson, A. J., & Atkin, C. K. (2000). Using the extended parallel process model to prevent firearm injury and death: Field experiment results of a video-based intervention. *Journal of Communication, 50*(4), 157–175. https://doi.org/10.1111/j.1460-2466.2000.tb02867.x

Shadish, W. R., Clark, M. H., & Steiner, P. M. (2008). Can nonrandomized experiments yield accurate answers? A randomized experiment comparing random and nonrandom assignment. *Journal of the American Statistical Association, 103*(484), 1353–1356. https://doi.org/10.1198/016214508000000733

Shadish, W. R., Cook, T. D., & Campbell, D. T. (2002). *Experimental and quasi-experimental designs for generalized causal inference.* Houghton Mifflin Company.

Shadish, W. R., & Ragsdale, K. (1996), Random versus nonrandom assignment in controlled experiments: Do you get the same answer? *Journal of Consulting and Clinical Psychology, 64*(6), 1290–1305. https://doi.org/10.1037/0022-006X.64.6.1290

Snyder, L. B., & Hamilton, M. A. (2002). A meta-analysis of U.S. health campaign effects on behavior: Emphasize enforcement, exposure, and new information, and beware the secular trend. In R. C. Hornik (Ed.), *Public health communication: Evidence for behavior change* (pp. 357–383). Lawrence Erlbaum Associates.

Trochim, W. M. K. (2001). *The research methods knowledge base.* Atomic Dog Publishing.

# INDEX

## A

Accidents, 8
Achievable objective, 40, 41
Activities, as logic model component, 36
Actual product, 69–70
Additive effects threat, 336
Additive hypothesis, 188
Administrative and policy assessment, 96
Administrative and policy assessment and intervention alignment, 90, 91, 92, 96–97
  intervention alignment, 97
  mapping, 97
  matching, 97
  patching, 97
  pooling, 97
Aerobics, 34
Alcohol, 4, 5, 9
Alcoholics Anonymous, 22
All things considered question, 270
Alzheimer's Disease, 8, 9
American Cancer Society, 129
*American Journal of Public Health*, 43
Anonymous data, 297
Applegate, Christina, 134
Area of consequence, 158
Assessment, as public health component, 10, 11
Assurance, as public health component, 10, 11
ATLAS.ti, 280
Attitude, 87, 88, 95, 108, 113, 201, 202, 203, 204, 206, 226. *See also* Experiential attitude, Instrumental attitude
  defined, 112, 176, 199, 203
  measurement of, 183, 211

Attrition threat, 331
Audience research
  outcome or impact evaluation, 63
  primary postproduction formative evaluation, 63
  primary preproduction formative evaluation, 62
  process evaluation monitoring, 63
  secondary formative evaluation, 63
Audience segmentation, 63–68, 265
  generic messages, 64–66
  tailored messages, 67–68
  targeted audience process, 63
  targeted messages, 66
  TARPARE approach, 63–64
Augmented product, 70
Autonomy, 206
  defined, 199
  measurement of, 213
  *vs.* capacity, 208–209

## B

Background variables, 201–204
Bacteria, 7, 14
Barriers, 113, 130. *See also* Cons, Costs, Perceived barriers, Price
  defined, 35, 131
  measurement of, 138
Behavior, 61, 92, 113, 130, 154, 202, 206. *See also* Product
  defined, 112, 131, 152, 155, 176, 199, 201
  defining, 209–210
  measurement of, 138, 162, 183

---

*Italics* signify publications

# T